Surgical Innovations in Bladder Cancer

Surgical Innovations in Bladder Cancer

Edited by **June Stewart**

New Jersey

Published by Foster Academics,
61 Van Reypen Street,
Jersey City, NJ 07306, USA
www.fosteracademics.com

Surgical Innovations in Bladder Cancer
Edited by June Stewart

International Standard Book Number: 978-1-63242-384-9 (Hardback)

Printed in the United States of America.

Contents

Preface

It is often said that books are a boon to humankind. They document every progress and pass on the knowledge from one generation to the other. They play a crucial role in our lives. Thus I was both excited and nervous while editing this book. I was pleased by the thought of being able to make a mark but I was also nervous to do it right because the future of students depends upon it. Hence, I took a few months to research further into the discipline, revise my knowledge and also explore some more aspects. Post this process, I begun with the editing of this book.

The cases of bladder cancer have gone up in the recent years. This book discusses various aspects of bladder cancer disease. It also consists of current knowledge, in a disciplined and simple format, focusing on the treatment of bladder cancer inclusive of surgical procedure, chemotherapy and radiation therapy. The book also looks at future avenues for the treatment of bladder cancer. The aim of this book is to help its readers to gain more knowledge regarding this form of cancer.

I thank my publisher with all my heart for considering me worthy of this unparalleled opportunity and for showing unwavering faith in my skills. I would also like to thank the editorial team who worked closely with me at every step and contributed immensely towards the successful completion of this book. Last but not the least, I wish to thank my friends and colleagues for their support.

                                                                                    Editor

Part 1

Non-Muscle Invasive Disease

Hemocyanins in the Immunotherapy of Superficial Bladder Cancer

Sergio Arancibia[1], Fabián Salazar[1] and María Inés Becker[1,2]
[1]Fundación Ciencia y Tecnología para el Desarrollo (FUCITED)
[2]Biosonda Corporation
[1,2]Chile

1. Introduction

Chemo- and immunotherapeutic approaches have been used to prevent recurrence of transitional cell carcinoma (TCC), the most common type of superficial bladder cancer (SBC). The bacillus Calmette-Guérin (BCG) vaccine for tuberculosis, which consists of an attenuated form of *Mycobacterium bovis*, is the most commonly used immunotherapeutic agent (Morales et al., 1976). Despite the successful results achieved with BCG, its serious side effects have led researchers to investigate other immunostimulatory substances. In the early 1970s, Olsson and collaborators reported that subcutaneous stimulation with keyhole limpet hemocyanin (KLH) from the Californian marine gastropod *Megathura crenulata* significantly reduced SBC recurrence frequency in TCC patients without any toxic side effects, making it ideal for long-term repetitive treatments (Olsson et al., 1974). These results provided promising support for the use of mollusk hemocyanins as alternative agents in SBC immunotherapy.

Hemocyanins, blue respiratory glycoproteins that were discovered in 1878 by Léon Fredericq (Ghiretti-Magaldi & Ghiretti, 1992), are found freely dissolved in the blood of some mollusks and arthropods. These proteins are giant structures with molecular weights between 4 and 8 MDa, and they exhibit some of the most complex and sophisticated quaternary structures known. Hemocyanins are part of the type-3 group of copper proteins that includes phenoloxidases and tyrosinases (Decker & Tuczek, 2000). These proteins contain active copper-containing sites in which the Cu(I,I) state is oxidized to the Cu(II,II) state, thus accounting for their distinctive deep blue color. Because of these properties, the biochemistry of hemocyanins has been intensively studied (van Holde & Miller, 1995). The pioneering work of Weigle in the 1960s on the immunochemical properties of KLH demonstrated its remarkable immunostimulatory properties in an experimental animal model (Weigle, 1964). These results were quickly incorporated into clinical studies to evaluate its immunological effects.

Because the primary amino acid sequences of mollusk hemocyanins are highly divergent from mammalian sequences, they are strongly recognized by the immune system, resulting in potent immunogenicity; these proteins can be used therapeutically as non-specific immunostimulants with beneficial clinical outcomes. Moreover, hemocyanins have been extensively used as carriers to generate antibodies against diverse hapten molecules and peptides and to induce antigen-specific CD8+ and CD4+ T cell responses (Harris & Markl, 1999). Currently, hemocyanins are used as carrier-adjuvants for several tumor-associated antigens (TAAs), such as glycolipid and glycoprotein (mucin-like) antigens, in experimental therapeutic vaccines against certain cancers, including melanomas, sarcomas, breast, prostate, ovary and lung (Musselli et al., 2001; Schumacher, 2001; Zhu et al., 2009; Del Campo et al., 2011). Other therapeutic strategies that use hemocyanins include dendritic cell (DC) vaccines pulsed with tumor lysates to enhance interferon gamma (IFN-γ) production by tumor-reactive T cells (Timmerman & Levy, 2000; Shimizu et al., 2001; Millard et al., 2003; Lopez et al., 2009; Jacobs et al., 2010; Lesterhuis et al., 2011) and anti-idiotype vaccines for some types of B cell malignancies (Leitch & Connors, 2005; Kafi et al., 2009). KLH has been the gold standard for these applications for over 40 years simply because it was used in earlier studies instead of other hemocyanins (Harris & Markl, 1999). The first studies used a research-grade KLH (non-GMP) containing different levels of endotoxin (Vandenbark et al., 1981); since then, several companies have produced clinical-grade KLH.

The versatile properties of KLH in biomedical and biotechnological applications have led to increasing commercial demand and growing interest in finding new, alternative hemocyanins with similar or more potent immunomodulatory properties. Although the KLH gene has been cloned, and its amino acid sequence is known, it has not been possible to express a heterologous protein, mainly because of its complex structure (Lieb et al., 2001; Markl et al., 2001; Altenhein et al., 2002). Therefore, this protein can be obtained only from its natural source. Several hemocyanins from other species of mollusks have been studied biochemically and immunologically, including *Haliotis tuberculata* (HtH, Abalon) (Markl et al., 2001); *Helix vulgarix* (HpH, Vineyard snail), *Rapana venosa* (RvH, Asian rapa whelk), and *Rapana thomasiana* (RtH, Black sea murex) (Dolashka-Angelova et al., 2003; 2008; 2010); and *Concholepas concholepas* (CCH, Loco), which is found on the pacific Chilean coast (De Ioannes et al., 2004). Only CCH has been pre-clinically evaluated in a murine experimental model of SBC and may be considered a safe alternative therapy (Moltedo et al., 2006; Atala, 2006). Although KLH and CCH have different origins and structure they have similar immunostimulatory capacities, suggesting that a conserved pattern common to both hemocyanins induces an ancient immunological mechanism (Moltedo et al., 2006). Interestingly, we have described a new hemocyanin from *Fissuerella latimarginata* (FLH) that exhibits higher immunogenicity than either CCH or KLH, opening a new avenue for research on the use of hemocyanins (Espinoza et al., 2006; Arancibia et al., 2010).

Notwithstanding the biomedical interest in mollusk hemocyanins, the molecular and cellular bases of their adjuvant/immunostimulatory capacity in SBC remain poorly understood. Currently, we know that hemocyanins are able to drive the differentiation of T helper (Th) cells toward a Th1 phenotype, characterized by increased secretion of IFN-γ and the production of IgG2a isotype antibodies (Moltedo et al., 2006).

In this chapter, we will review what is currently known about the experimental and clinical uses of mollusk hemocyanins as non-specific immunostimulants to prevent SBC recurrence, including the details of their intricate structure and the immunologic mechanisms that have been proposed to explain their antitumor activity.

2. Structure of the mollusk hemocyanins

Because of their enormous size, mollusk hemocyanins are easily observed by transmission electron microscopy (TEM) using negative staining. These molecules have a cylindrical form with an external diameter of approximately 350 nm and length of approximately 400 nm. Fig. 1 shows the characteristic appearance of gastropod hemocyanins under TEM.

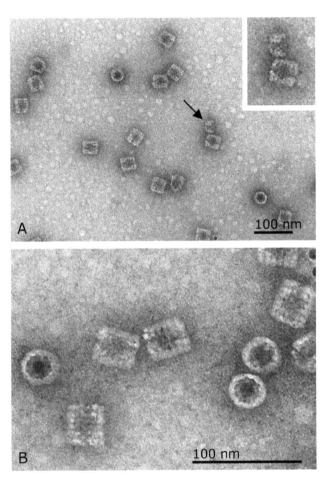

Fig. 1. Electron microscopy of negatively stained *C. concholepas* hemocyanin molecules. **A.** Low magnification micrographs of a preparation of the protein showing their characteristic hollow cylinder form. The images show the top (circles) and lateral (rectangles) views of the molecule. The arrow shows a decamer. **B.** High magnification images of hemocyanin molecules showing their intricate structure. The side views show the proteins' characteristic didecameric form with subunits arranged in layers.

Many experimental studies on hemocyanins, using different dissociation and association conditions and physicochemical and biochemical methods, have helped to elucidate their hierarchically organized structure (van Holde & Miller, 1995; Harris & Markl, 1999). As shown in Fig. 2, the basic structure of hemocyanins is composed of ten subunits that are self-assembled into a hollow cylinder, a structure known as a decamer, with a lumen that is narrowed by a complex collar (Harris et al., 1993; Cuff et al., 1998; Decker et al., 2007). In gastropods, the decamers can self-associate face-to-face to form stable dimers or didecamers, which display an intricate internal arrangement and result in the formation of extremely large structures with approximate D5 symmetry (Orlova et al., 1997). Hemocyanin subunits have a molecular weight ranging from 350 to 450 kDa and are composed of a string of seven or eight globular domains called functional units (FUs), each with a molecular weight between 35 and 50 kDa. These FUs are connected by a short flexible linker peptide strand of 10 to 15 amino acid residues. Each FU has two well-separated copper atoms that reversibly capture O_2 molecules; one is called the A site, which is located towards the N-terminus, and the other is called the B site and is located downstream of the polypeptide (van Holde et al., 2001).

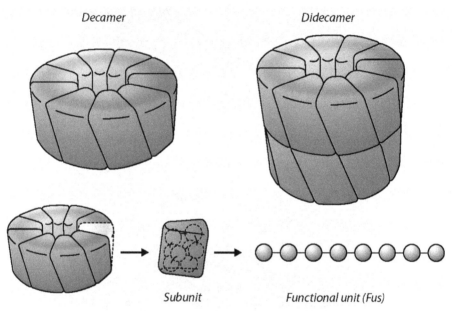

Fig. 2. Model of the structure of mollusk hemocyanin. The basic structure of a mollusk hemocyanin is a decamer, which is formed by the association of 10 polypeptides or subunits. In hemocyanins from some species of mollusk, such as gastropods, including KLH and CCH, the decamers are associated in pairs to form very large molecules called didecamers. The subunit consists of seven or eight globular domains linked by a peptide spacer consisting of 10 to 15 amino acid residues, similar to a pearl necklace. Each of these globular domains has a pair of copper atoms that reversibly bind one oxygen molecule, which is why they are called functional units.

Knowledge of the carbohydrate moieties present in mollusk hemocyanins has been essential for understanding their organization, antigenicity and biomedical properties (Paccagnella et al., 2004; Siddiqui et al., 2007). In fact, several authors have reported that hemocyanin carbohydrates may play a role in their immunostimulatory effects. The high carbohydrate content of hemocyanins, up to 9% (w/w), has been measured by different methods, including the use of lectins and high-pressure liquid chromatography–tandem mass spectrometry (HPLC-MS/MS). The presence of numerous N-glycosylation sites and a reduced number of O-glycosylation sites has been established (Dolashka-Angelova et al., 2003; Gielens et al., 2004; Idakieva et al., 2004; Gatsogiannis & Markl, 2009; Dolashka et al., 2010). Mollusk hemocyanins contain diverse sugar moieties, including mannose, D-galactose, fucose, N-acetyl-D-galactosamine and N-acetyl-glucosamine residues, with mannose being the most abundant (Harris & Markl, 1999). Hemocyanins also contain monosaccharides that are not usually found in animal proteins, such as xylose (Lommerse et al., 1997).

2.1 KLH and CCH

Although KLH and CCH each have two subunits that constitute the basic structure known as a decamer, closer analysis revealed unique differences. Native gel electrophoresis has shown that KLH is made up of two different non-covalently linked subunits called KLH1 (350 KDa) and KLH2 (350 KDa) that do not display shared epitopes (Swerdlow et al., 1996). Using the same approach, it was demonstrated that CCH is also made up of two different subunits, CCHA (405 kDa) and CCHB (350 kDa), that contain common and specific epitopes (Oliva et al., 2002; De Ioannes et al., 2004). In KLH, the subunits form homodidecamers (i.e., the molecules are formed from either KLH1 or KLH2 subunits). However, in CCH the subunits form heterodidecamers (i.e., the molecules are formed by pairing the two different subunits). In addition, purified KLH requires divalent cations in storage buffers to maintain the stability of its quaternary structure, whereas CCH does not (De Ioannes et al., 2004); this is probably a consequence of the higher hydrophobicity of CCH (Leyton et al., 2005). Despite these differences, the immunogenic properties of CCH and KLH are similar. CCH has been successfully used as a carrier protein to generate antibodies against hapten molecules and peptides (Becker et al., 1998; Torres et al., 1999; Mura et al., 2002; Duvillie et al., 2003; Manosalva et al., 2004; Cancino et al., 2007; Gravotta et al., 2007; Matus et al., 2007; Grenegard et al., 2008); as a carrier in vaccines (Miller et al., 2006; Mauldin & Miller, 2007; Pilon et al., 2007) and as an experimental antigen (Becker et al., 2007; Moltedo et al., 2009).

Several studies have demonstrated that KLH contains approximately 3.2% (w/w) carbohydrate residues, displaying specific structural motifs on N-glycans, such as Fuc(alpha1-3)GalNAc, Gal-(beta1-6)Man-, Gal(beta1-4)Fuc-, and Gal(beta1-4)Gal(beta(1-4)Fuc-, which are thought to contribute to its non-specific immunostimulatory capacities in SBC (Wuhrer et al., 2004). Our knowledge of the corresponding oligosaccharide composition of CCH is very limited. However, we have demonstrated using selective glycosidase treatments and electrophoretic analysis that sugar moieties account for 3.1% (w/w) of the mass of CCH. A comparative analysis using lectin staining indicated that mannose is the only exposed carbohydrate common to CCH and KLH (Becker et al., 2009). It is important to note that, despite the differences in carbohydrate composition between KLH and CCH, both proteins have similar immunogenicity and immunotherapeutic capacity in SBC, suggesting that other factors are responsible for this effect. We assume that the primary structure of these proteins contains the determining factor because they share regions of high sequence homology (van Holde et al., 2001; Manubens et al., 2010). These regions were confirmed in antibody cross-reactivity experiments that revealed the presence of common or mimetic epitopes in CCH and KLH (Oliva et al., 2002).

3. Use of hemocyanins in experimental SBC

Rats and various strains of mice have been used as *in vivo* SBC models to evaluate therapeutic agents because bladder tumors in these rodents have similarities with human tumors. In addition, tumor cells can be established subcutaneously (heterotopically) or in the bladder (orthotopically) by either transplantation or chemical induction, allowing the investigation of clinical aspects such as pharmacokinetics and toxicity (Gunther et al., 1999; Linn et al., 2000; Arentsen et al., 2009).

The first controlled study of a hemocyanin as immunotherapy in the treatment of superficial bladder cancer was published in the 1980s by the Lamm group (Lamm et al., 1981). They developed the mouse bladder tumor-2 cell (MBT-2) transplantable murine model of SBC and demonstrated that pre-immunization with 200 µg of KLH three weeks prior to subcutaneous injection with MBT-2, followed by intralesional immunotherapy with 50 µg one and seven days after inoculation, resulted in a significant reduction in tumor growth and a prolongation of animal survival. Later, other studies by the same researchers evaluated non-specific immunotherapeutic regimens (Lamm et al., 1982). Animals received an intradermal MBT-2 inoculation, and the immunotherapy was administered intralesionally one day after tumor transplantation. Tumors were excised at a volume of 400 mm^3, and the animals were re-challenged with tumor cells, treated again, and followed for tumor incidence, growth rate and survival. This study demonstrated that KLH had a weak antitumor effect compared with the response to BCG. In 1986, Lau and collaborators studied the same response, this time comparing intraperitoneal and intralesional administration of the agents. C3H/He mice were injected subcutaneously with 5×10^4 tumor cells. After that, the mice received either intraperitoneal or intralesional treatments (50 µg KLH); these experiments demonstrated that the intralesional route was more effective than intraperitoneal administration for tumor growth inhibition (Lau et al., 1986).

Lamm´s group also evaluated the possible additive and/or synergistic effects of KLH immunotherapy in the MBT-2 model in conjunction with other treatments, such as IFN-α. Tumor cells were transplanted subcutaneously without prior immunization. Treatment was given intraperitoneally twice weekly for three weeks, except for BCG, which was administered once a week. Significant reductions in tumor incidence relative to the controls were observed in groups receiving KLH (42%), IFN-α (42%) and KLH + IFN-α (17%) (Riggs et al., 1992). The following year, the same group compared two alternative immunotherapies in the MBT-2 model: crude KLH and Immucothel, a clinical-grade KLH from Biosyn Arzneimittel GmbH. Mice were sensitized with 50 or 100 µg KLH, and 21 days later, 10^3 tumor cells were injected. Intralesional treatment with 50 or 100 µg KLH was performed on days 1, 7 and 13 or 14. Crude KLH required either immunization before tumor transplant or frequent therapy after transplantation to be effective. In addition, Immucothel required pre-immunization to be effective, even with an increased frequency and dosage of the post-transplant immunizations. In a subsequent study, the endotoxin contamination of KLH was demonstrated to be partly responsible for the antitumor activity because treatment with endotoxin alone resulted in a significant reduction of tumor growth and mortality (50% survival) (Lamm et al., 1993). Moreover, KLH + 100 Endotoxin Units (EU) resulted in complete inhibition of tumor growth and 100% survival. KLH + 1000 EU appeared to reduce the antitumor response (50% survival), suggesting that endotoxin may interfere with the response to purified KLH. Finally, endotoxin-free KLH induced antitumor responses (50% survival). However, pre-immunization was required for KLH to exert a significant (75% survival) antitumor effect (Lamm et al., 1993).

Walsh and collaborators studied KLH immunotherapy in two different models with no promising results. First, they transplanted 2.5×10^6 MBT-2 tumor cells subcutaneously after pre-immunization 20 days prior. Treatment was given on days 1, 8 and 18 in the form of subcutaneous or intralesional injection of 50 µg KLH. The results showed no difference between the control and treated groups in terms of either tumor growth or animal survival. Alternatively, they transplanted 2.1 x 10^6 MBT-2 tumor cells into the bladder of C3H/He mice. The bladder was irrigated with 1.5 mg N-methyl-N-nitrosourea 48 hours prior. The treatment group was injected with 50 µg KLH on day 1, and the bladders were instilled with 200 µg KLH on days 14 and 21. There was no significant difference from the control group (Walsh et al., 1983). Using a similar model, Marsh and collaborators demonstrated that intravesical immunotherapy with *Corynebacterium parvum* and *Allium sativum* was more effective than KLH and slightly more effective than BCG. MBT-2 cells were delivered into the bladder transurethrally using a small catheter, and the immunotherapy was administered directly into the bladder via this catheter on day 1 or day 6, or both. The authors associated the lack of a significant effect with inappropriate dosage or insufficient stimulation of the immune system (Marsh et al., 1987). Later, the antitumor activity and potential toxicity of a clinical grade KLH preparation named KLH-Immune Activator (KLH-IA) was examined. Mice were immunized subcutaneously with KLH-IA two weeks prior to intravesical implantation with 2 x 10^4 MB-49 tumor cells. Treatment consisted of intravesical KLH-IA (10 or 100 µg) 1, 4, 7, 14 and 21 days after implantation. By four weeks after implantation, tumor outgrowth in the treated groups was significantly decreased. Prior subcutaneous immunization was required to elicit the antitumor activity of KLH-IA. Animals treated with a dissociated form of KLH showed decreased tumor outgrowth, but this was not significant. A separate toxicity study in which KLH-IA was given subcutaneously (4 mg/kg), intraperitoneally (40 mg/kg) or intravesically (40 mg/kg) reported no significant gross or histopathological abnormalities, except for mild to moderate papillary hyperplasia in all catheterized animals (Swerdlow et al., 1994).

A third model developed by Recker and collaborators also showed the effectiveness of KLH. Bladder carcinoma was induced in Wistar rats using N-butyl-N-(4-hydroxybutyl) nitrosamine (BBN). Stimulation of the rats with 12.5 mg of KLH administered intravesically and 0.5 mg administered subcutaneously twice weekly after sensitization with 1 mg subcutaneous KLH resulted in a reduction in BBN-induced bladder tumors. These results confirmed that effective induction of an immune response is important for the control of tumor development because immune-suppressed rats treated with cyclosporine A (CsA) showed enhanced bladder tumor expansion compared with rats treated with 0.05% BBN alone (Recker & Rubben, 1989). A subsequent study distinguished between intravesical and subcutaneous application to determine the most effective treatment regime. Five weeks after the completion of tumor induction with 0.05% BBN solution, exophytic bladder tumors appeared in all control animals. In group 2, which was given KLH via intravesical instillation, tumors developed in 73.5% of cases. In group 1, with subcutaneous administration, tumors developed in only 50% of cases. The tumor growth was significantly slower in group 1 than group 2 (Linn et al., 2000).

The results described above demonstrated promising potential for the use of KLH in SBC therapy. More recently, preclinical studies have proven hemocyanin from *Concholepas concholepas* (CCH) to be a reliable alternative to KLH (Moltedo et al., 2006). C3H/He mice were primed with CCH before subcutaneous implantation of MBT-2 cells. Treatment consisted of a subcutaneous dose of CCH (1 mg or 100 µg) at different intervals after implantation. The results demonstrated a significant antitumor effect, as indicated by decreased tumor growth and incidence, prolonged survival and a lack of toxic effects. These results were similar to those achieved with KLH.

Model	Priming[1]	Via Administration	Therapeutic Dosage and Schedule[2]	Results	Reference
Mouse, MBT-2	Yes 200 μg	Intralesional	50 μg Days: 1 and 7.	Significant reduction of tumor growth and survival with KLH.	Lamm et al.1981
	No	Intralesional	Day: 1	KLH presented a minor antitumor effect compared with BCG.	Lamm et al. 1982
	Yes	Subcutaneous or intralesional	50 or 200 μg Days: 1, 8 and 18 or 1, 14 and 21.	KLH do not show difference with controls in tumor growth or animal survival.	Walsh et al. 1983
	No	Intraperitoneal v/s intralesional	50 μg	Intralesional route of inoculation of KLH was more effective.	Lau et al. 1986
	No	Intravesical	50 μg Days: 1 or 6, or both.	Immunotherapy with C. parvum and A. sativum was more effective than KLH.	Marsh et al.1987
	No	Intraperitoneal	50 μg Twice weekly for 3 weeks.	Better response in the animals treated with KLH more INF-α.	Riggs et al. 1992
	Yes 50 or 100 μg	Intralesional	50 or 100 μg Days: 1, 7 and 13 or 14.	Required pre-immunization of KLH and Immucothel to be effective.	Lamm et al. 1993a
	Yes 50 or 100 μg	Intralesional	50 or 100 μg Days: 1, 7 and 13 or 14.	Endotoxin contamination of KLH was responsible in part for the antitumor activity.	Lamm et al. 1993b
	Yes 200 to 400 μg	Subcutaneous	1 mg Days: 1 to 6 or 100 μg Days: 1, 3, 5, 7 and 9.	Significant reduction of tumor growth and survival with CCH.	Moltedo et al. 2006
	Yes 200 μg	Subcutaneous	100 μg Days: 1, 3, 5, 7 and 9.	Better antitumor effect with CCHA subunit than CCHB subunit.	Becker et al. 2009
Mouse, MB-49	Yes 100 μg	Intravesical	10 or 100 μg Days: 1, 4, 7, 14 and 21.	Prior immunization of KLH-IA was required to elicit antitumor activity.	Swerdlow et al. 1994
Rats, tumor induction with BBN[3]	Yes 1 mg	Intravesical and subcutaneous	12.5 mg and 500 μg Twice weekly.	Reduction of bladder tumors with KLH.	Recker et al. 1989
	Yes 1 mg	Intravesical v/s subcutaneous	500 μg Twice weekly for 8 weeks.	Subcutaneous route of KLH was more effective than intravesical route.	Linn et al. 2000

[1] Priming: Usually, around two weeks prior to tumor challenge. [2] Immunotherapy after tumor transplantation. [3] BNN: N-butyl-N-(4-hydroxybutyl) nitrosamine

Table 1. Preclinical studies in different animal models of SBC with KLH or CCH as an immunotherapeutic agent.

Later, the individual contributions of the CCHA and CCHB subunits of CCH as immunotherapeutic agents in the same bladder cancer model were studied. C3He/He mice were subcutaneously primed with CCHA or CCHB; whole CCH and PBS were used as positive and negative controls, respectively. After day 15, mice were challenged with a subcutaneous injection of 2×10^5 MBT-2 cells, and the antitumor treatment was started; treatment consisted of a subcutaneous dose of either subunit or a control on alternate days for 9 days. Surprisingly, either subunit alone showed an antitumor effect in the MBT-2 model. However, the tumor incidence was lower in animals treated with CCHA (44% incidence) than with CCHB (60% incidence) or whole CCH (62.5% incidence). Moreover, the survival probability increased in mice under immunotherapy with CCHA (69.5%) compared with CCHB- (64%), CCH- (60%) and PBS-treated (46.5%) mice. In conclusion, this study indicated that the CCHA subunit accounts for the most important immunogenic effects of CCH (Becker et al., 2009). Together, these preclinical studies (summarized in Table 1) demonstrated that hemocyanins have beneficial effects in animal models of SBC that resemble human disease without the negative side effects of BCG (Schenkman & Lamm, 2004).

4. Use of hemocyanins in clinical studies of SBC

Surgical procedures such as transurethral resection (TUR) are commonly used as the first option to treat SBC. However, there are some tumors that must be treated by other strategies, due to the difficulties of fully removing them and the high risk of recurrence. Thus, intravesical administration of chemotherapeutic and biological agents has been demonstrated to be an effective method in the early stages of the disease, either to treat an existing tumor or to prevent recurrence and tumor progression after TUR (Perabo & Muller, 2004). BCG is one biological therapy that is used as a non-specific immunostimulant to treat several malignant tumors (Edwards & Whitwell, 1974; Milas & Withers, 1976), including SBC (Morales et al., 1976). BCG has become the first-line treatment and the most effective intravesical immunotherapy, lowering the risk of recurrence to an average of 27% of cases (Nseyo & Lamm, 1997). Despite these successful results, BCG therapy causes numerous side effects, such as dysuria, urinary frequency, cystitis (90% of cases), hematuria and, in rare cases, sepsis, indicating the need for new approaches that provide the same or a better response without toxic effects (Lamm, 2003).

In a 1974 delayed-type hypersensitivity (DTH) experiment to measure the immune competence of patients with TCC, Olson and collaborators reported the unexpected result that patients subcutaneously primed with 5 mg of KLH and then subcutaneous immunized with 200 μg of KLH had a significantly diminished tumor recurrence rate over a study period of two years. Those patients that were DTH positive to KLH, and therefore immune competent, had almost no recurrences (Olsson et al., 1974). This outstanding effect was confirmed many years later in a controlled study of patients in stages Ta and T1 who had previously been subject to TUR. In this study, the ability of KLH to prevent tumor recurrence was compared to mitomycin C (MMC). The patients were subcutaneously immunized with 1 mg of KLH and then received monthly intravesical administrations of 10 mg of KLH. Only 14% of the patients treated with KLH had recurrences, in contrast to the MMC patients, 39% of whom reported recurrences, demonstrating that KLH was significantly more effective than MMC (Jurincic et al., 1988).

A prospective randomized trial compared the effects of ethoglucid and KLH in patients who were unresponsive to the chemotherapeutic treatments, doxorubicin or MMC. The recurrence rate and the tumor progression rate for the two therapies showed no statistical differences (Flamm et al., 1990). Wishahi et al., reported that the incidence of recurrence in patients with TCC associated with urinary schistosomiasis was 15% after KLH treatment compared with 77% before therapy (Wishahi et al., 1995). This result was similar to the results obtained by Olson et al., (1974) and Jurincic et al., (1998) confirming the outstanding immunotherapeutic properties of KLH (Olsson et al., 1974; Jurincic et al., 1988). The efficacy of this treatment in patients with carcinoma *in situ* (CIS) grade 3 was studied in a long-term follow-up. The patients received an intravesical instillation of KLH weekly for 6 weeks, monthly for 1 year and bimonthly for the following 2 years. Patients who were unresponsive to KLH were treated with BCG. CIS long-term remission was observed only in a limited number of cases, and most cases progressed over time, indicating the aggressiveness of this disease (Jurincic-Winkler et al., 1995a). In Table 2, we summarize the clinical studies previously described.

Currently, Immucothel, a clinical-grade KLH preparation, is being evaluated in a Phase III clinical trial in Germany for its efficacy in SBC treatment (Biosyn). The Food and Drug Administration (FDA) has also authorized another Phase III trial to evaluate the efficacy and safety of KLH BCI-Immune Activator (Intracell, USA) versus doxorubicin in BCG refractory or intolerant patients with carcinoma *in situ*, with or without resected SBC. However, this study has been suspended.

The mechanism associated with the immunotherapeutic effect of KLH in this disease is still poorly understood. However, there are immunohistological studies on biopsies of TCC patients treated with KLH that show strong cellular activation characterized by the infiltration of large numbers of mononuclear cells and CD4+ lymphocytes, and to a lesser extent, CD8+ T cells and granulocytes, nine months after the beginning of therapy (Jurincic-Winkler et al., 1995b). This result suggests that the effect of KLH might be strongly related to a non-specific immunostimulation of the immune system leading to the development of an antitumor response.

5. Immunologic mechanisms involved in the immunotherapy of SBC with hemocyanins

Although hemocyanins are widely used as thymus-dependent model antigens, the relationship between the structure of hemocyanins and the molecular and cellular basis of their immunostimulatory capacity is still largely unknown. Investigations into the antitumor effect of hemocyanins in human and murine models of SBC have demonstrated a systemic activation of the immune response. In these experiments, priming with hemocyanins is crucial for the induction of antitumor activity (Lamm et al., 2000; Moltedo et al., 2006). This could partially explain why hemocyanins stimulate the immune system. In patients with TCC under intravesical KLH therapy, DTH reactions occur. As mentioned previously, studies on biopsies of TCC patients treated with KLH showed a higher increase in CD4+ cell infiltration than CD8+ T lymphocytes in the submucosa and urothelial cells (Jurincic-Winkler et al., 1995b). Currently, we know that such responses are characteristic of Th1 type responses, which mediate inflammatory functions critical for the development of cell-mediated immune responses (Szabo et al., 2003). Other investigations demonstrated that during immunization with KLH, the T CD4+ lymphocyte response showed a mixed profile of IL-4 and IFN-γ with an increase in T CD8+ cells in the lymphatic nodules (Doyle et al., 1998).

Patients	Control Group	Priming	Therapeutic Dosage and Schedule	Recurrence Rate	Reference
19	10	5 mg subcutaneous	200 μg Subcutaneous	11%	Olsson et al. 1974
44	23	1 mg subcutaneous	10 mg Intravesical, monthly for 21 months, approximately.	14%	Jurincic et al. 1988
84	46	1 mg subcutaneous	30 mg Intravesical, weekly for six weeks and then monthly for one year.	55%	Flamm et al. 1990
13	Own controls	1 mg subcutaneous for five days until DTH	10 mg Intravesical, for seven days.	15%	Wishashi et al. 1995
21	Own controls	No	20 mg Intravesical, weekly for six weeks and then monthly for one year or bimonthly for two years.	43% of patients presented long-term remission 57% had to be cystectomized because of CIS progression	Jurincic-Winkler et al. 1995a

Table 2. Clinical studies using KLH as an immunotherapeutic agent in SBC patients.

The fact that the non-specific immunotherapeutic effects of hemocyanins are not due to any super-antigen-like activity, but rather rely on adequate priming, strongly suggests that their therapeutic properties could be attributable to a bystander effect on the tumor due to either a loss of tolerance toward tumor antigens or an enhancement of the immune response to the tumor. This kind of response would favor a milieu that augments the antigen-specific activity of cytotoxic T lymphocytes (CTLs) and natural killer (NK) cell responses. These hypotheses are supported by the observation that IFN-γ and IL-2 are secreted in the regional lymph nodes in response to hemocyanin treatment (Gilliet et al., 2003; Verdijk et al., 2009). NK cells are strongly stimulated by IL-2 secreted by T lymphocytes, leading to their differentiation into lymphokine-activated killer cells (LAK) and increasing the destructive elements acting on tumor cells. It has been reported that

MBT-2 cells do not grow when they are injected into the bladders of mice treated with a combination of IL-2 and the cytotoxic agent cyclophosphamide (Ikemoto et al., 1997). Moreover, KLH has been shown to enhance NK cell activity and stimulate IFN-γ secretion in SBC patients (Molto et al., 1991). Our later results confirm these observations; mice treated with KLH or CCH increase NK cell activity and serum levels of IFN-γ (Moltedo et al., 2006). This is a very important result because, in primary tumors, IFN-γ is a tumor suppressor cytokine that coordinates T and NK cell activities (Kaplan et al., 1998). Indeed, it has been demonstrated that the depletion of NK cells abolishes the immunotherapeutic effect of BCG on bladder cancer in mice, confirming that these cells play a key role in the destruction of primary tumors (Brandau & Bohle, 2001).

In addition to the antitumor effect provided by the secretion of IFN-γ, NK cells can delay tumor growth by means of antibody-dependent cell-mediated cytotoxicity (ADCC), which induces effector cells to kill bladder tumor target cells. We have observed that, in the MBT-2 model, intralesional CCH or KLH induce an increase in the humoral immune response against cell surface tumor antigens in addition to the CCH or KLH antibody response. Biopsies taken from the surrounding bladder tissues in SBC patients treated with KLH showed an increase in the B lymphocyte population in the lymph follicles, suggesting that humoral mechanism are also involved in the immune response induced by hemocyanins (Jurincic-Winkler et al., 1995b).

Finally, the fact that the immunotherapeutic effects of KLH and CCH on bladder cancer do not require an adjuvant raises intriguing questions regarding the means by which hemocyanins initiate the non-specific anti-tumor immune response and which cells are involved. It is possible that hemocyanins interact with a putative receptor on the cell surface of antigen presenting cells, leading to their internalization and processing. A promising candidate was the mannose receptor because of the high levels of this sugar residue in KLH and CCH and the fact that this receptor is highly expressed in antigen presenting cells. However, experiments on endocytosis inhibition performed in human DCs cultured *in vitro* with an anti-mannose receptor antibody and KLH showed that while KLH incorporation by DCs was partially inhibited, KLH still promoted the activation and maturation of DCs as assessed by the up-regulation of the cell surface expression of Major Histocompatibility Complex (MHC) class II and co-stimulatory molecules (Presicce et al., 2008). In contrast, Teitz-Tennenbaum and collaborators (2008) demonstrated that murine DCs pulsed with KLH for 18 hours *in vitro* did not undergo DC maturation, a result that is consistent with *in vivo* experiments (Teitz-Tennenbaum et al., 2008; Moltedo et al., 2009) and our current results. We observed that DCs internalized (Fig. 3) but did not mature within 72 hours of culture *in vitro* with this protein

It is not known whether hemocyanins might be processed and presented by bladder tumor cells themselves, leading to the stimulation of the cytotoxic killer cell antitumor activity. Murine bladder tumor cells have been shown to be able to present BCG antigens to specific CD4+ T lymphocytes in a classic MHC Class II (Ia)-dependent fashion (Lattime et al., 1992). Experiments performed in our laboratory demonstrated that primary cultures of mouse bladder epithelial cells and MBT-2 cells cultured *in vitro* incorporate hemocyanin; however, we did not observe any changes in the expression pattern of MHC I and MHC II antigens (Del Campo et al., 2007). In addition, *in vitro* anti-cancer effects of KLH against breast, esophageal, prostate and pancreas cancer has been reported (Riggs et al., 2002), also in melanoma (Somasundar et al., 2005), however if this effect have an *in vivo* implication is unknown.

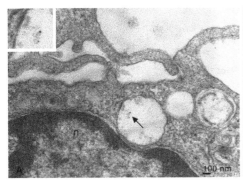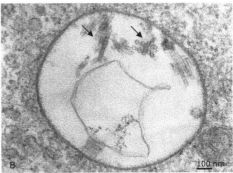

Fig. 3. Incorporation of *Concholepas* hemocyanin by mouse myeloid dendritic cells cultured *in vitro*, analyzed by transmission electron microscopy. Mouse myeloid DCs of 5th day of culture *in vitro* as described (Inaba et al., 1992), previously isolated by positive selection with immunomagnetic beads, and later culture with CCH during different times. **A.** Dendritic cell cultured during 30 minutes with CCH. The photograph shows its characteristic superficial membrane process, the nucleus (n), and hemocyanin molecules inside a clear vacuole (arrow) that resemble a primary lysosome. **B.** Because of the large size of CCH, and because of its peculiar structure as a hollow cylinder, we were able to identify the presence of whole hemocyanin molecules inside secondary lysosome like vesicles (arrows) containing membrane debris (Del Campo et al., 2007).

Macrophages are another potential cell type through which hemocyanins could initiate anti-tumor immune responses. Indeed, IL-1α, a pro-inflammatory cytokine produced by activated macrophages, has been shown to be increased in the urine after intravesical instillation with KLH in patients with SBC (Jurincic-Winkler et al., 1995c). Similarly, this cytokine, in addition to other pro-inflammatory cytokines, has been detected in the urine after BCG instillation along with an influx of mononuclear cells into the bladder (Teppema et al., 1992; Brandau & Bohle, 2001; Brandau et al., 2001).

In summary, considering that BCG is a whole organism, whereas KLH or CCH are single molecules, it is amazing that it induces a similar response. In both cases, however, it is not clear which cytokines and cells contribute directly to the anti-tumor activity and which represent a secondary phenomenon.

6. Conclusions

Hemocyanins have proven to be safe and useful in the immunotherapy and prophylaxis of patients with superficial bladder cancer who have failed or are intolerant to the current BCG therapy. Moreover, KLH has been shown to produce a more predictable reaction than BCG, eliminating the risk of further infections. Despite the fact that biomedical interest in mollusk hemocyanins goes back more than 40 years, the precise molecular and cellular mechanisms underlying the non-specific immunostimulatory capacities of KLH and, more recently, CCH, are poorly understood. The current evidence shows that these huge proteins can induce an inflammatory milieu and activate innate immunity, driving a vigorous antitumor adaptive immune response characterized by long-lasting HLA-DR+ cell infiltration into the bladder and the secretion of a Th1-type cytokine profile.

7. Acknowledgments

We thank Alfredo De Ioannes, Cristóbal Dünner and Augusto Manubens (Biosonda Corporation) and Miguel Del Campo, Pablo De Ioannes and Bruno Moltedo (Fundación Ciencia y Tecnología para el Desarrollo, FUCITED) for their valuable discussions during the course of this work. The authors are grateful to Gabriel De Ioannes for the mollusk hemocyanin structure model.
This study was partially supported by FONDECYT grant 1110651 (to María Inés Becker). Sergio Arancibia is a CONICYT (National Commission for Sciences and Technology of Chile) doctoral fellow.

8. References

Altenhein, B., Markl, J. & Lieb, B. (2002). Gene structure and hemocyanin isoform HtH2 from the mollusc *Haliotis tuberculata* indicate early and late intron hot spots. *Gene*, Vol.301, No.1-2: pp. 53-60, 0378-1119

Arancibia, S., Espinoza, C., Del Campo, M., Salazar, F. & Becker, M.I. (2010). Exceptional immunological and anticancer properties of a new hemocyanin from *Fissurella Latimarginata* (FLH). *Proceedings of International Society for Biological Therapy of Cancer*. Washington, USA. October, 2010

Arentsen, H.C., Hendricksen, K., Oosterwijk, E. & Witjes, J.A. (2009). Experimental rat bladder urothelial cell carcinoma models. *World J Urol*, Vol.27, No.3: pp. 313-317, 1433-8726

Atala, A. (2006). This month in investigative urology. *J Urol* 2006. *J Urol*, Vol.176, No.6 Pt 1: pp. 2335-2336, 0022-5347

Becker, M.I., Carrasco, I., Beltran, C., Torres, M., Jaureguiberry, B. & De Ioannes, A.E. (1998). Development of monoclonal antibodies to gizzerosine, a toxic component present in fish meal. *Hybridoma*, Vol.17, No.4: pp. 373-381, 0272-457X

Becker, M.I., De Ioannes, A.E., Leon, C. & Ebensperger, L.A. (2007). Females of the communally breeding rodent, *Octodon degus*, transfer antibodies to their offspring during pregnancy and lactation. *J Reprod Immunol*, Vol.74, No.1-2: pp. 68-77, 0165-0378

Becker, M.I., Fuentes, A., Del Campo, M., Manubens, A., Nova, E., Oliva, H., Faunes, F., Valenzuela, M.A., Campos-Vallette, M., Aliaga, A., Ferreira, J., De Ioannes, A.E., De Ioannes, P. & Moltedo, B. (2009). Immunodominant role of CCHA subunit of *Concholepas* hemocyanin is associated with unique biochemical properties. *Int Immunopharmacol*, Vol.9, No.3: pp. 330-339, 1878-1705

Biosyn. In: *Vacmune Immucothel*, July 2011, Available from: http://www.biosyncorp.com/bc_downloads/vacmune.pdf.

Brandau, S. & Bohle, A. (2001). Activation of natural killer cells by Bacillus Calmette-Guerin. *Eur Urol*, Vol.39, No.5: pp. 518-524, 0302-2838

Brandau, S., Riemensberger, J., Jacobsen, M., Kemp, D., Zhao, W., Zhao, X., Jocham, D., Ratliff, T.L. & Bohle, A. (2001). NK cells are essential for effective BCG immunotherapy. *Int J Cancer*, Vol.92, No.5: pp. 697-702, 0020-7136

Cancino, J., Torrealba, C., Soza, A., Yuseff, M.I., Gravotta, D., Henklein, P., Rodriguez-Boulan, E. & Gonzalez, A. (2007). Antibody to AP1B adaptor blocks biosynthetic and recycling routes of basolateral proteins at recycling endosomes. *Mol Biol Cell*, Vol.18, No.12: pp. 4872-4884, 1059-1524

Cuff, M.E., Miller, K.I., van Holde, K.E. & Hendrickson, W.A. (1998). Crystal structure of a functional unit from *Octopus* hemocyanin. *J Mol Biol*, Vol.278, No.4: pp. 855-870, 0022-2836

De Ioannes, P., Moltedo, B., Oliva, H., Pacheco, R., Faunes, F., De Ioannes, A.E. & Becker, M.I. (2004). Hemocyanin of the molluscan *Concholepas concholepas* exhibits an unusual heterodecameric array of subunits. *J Biol Chem*, Vol.279, No.25: pp. 26134-26142, 0021-9258

Decker, H. & Tuczek, F. (2000). Tyrosinase/catecholoxidase activity of hemocyanins: structural basis and molecular mechanism. *Trends Biochem Sci*, Vol.25, No.8: pp. 392-397, 0968-0004

Decker, H., Hellmann, N., Jaenicke, E., Lieb, B., Meissner, U. & Markl, J. (2007). Minireview: Recent progress in hemocyanin research. *Integr Comp Biol*, Vol.47, No.4: pp. 631-644, 1540-7063

Del Campo, M., Lagos, L., Manubens, A., Ioannes, A., Moltedo, B. & Becker, M.I. (2007). Efecto de la hemocianina de C. *Concholepas* (CCH) en la maduración de células dendríticas. *Proceedings of XXX Reunión Anual de la Sociedad de Bioquímica y Biología Molecular de Chile*. Chillán, Chile. September, 2007.

Del Campo, M., Arancibia, S., Nova, E., Salazar, F., Gonzalez, A., Moltedo, B., De Ioannes, P., Ferreira, J., Manubens, A. & Becker, M.I. (2011). Hemocyanins as immunostimulants. *Rev. méd. Chile*, Vol.139, No.2: pp. 236-246

Dolashka-Angelova, P., Beck, A., Dolashki, A., Beltramini, M., Stevanovic, S., Salvato, B. & Voelter, W. (2003). Characterization of the carbohydrate moieties of the functional unit RvH1-a of *Rapana venosa* haemocyanin using HPLC/electrospray ionization MS and glycosidase digestion. *Biochem J*, Vol.374, No.Pt 1: pp. 185-192, 0264-6021

Dolashka-Angelova, P., Stefanova, T., Livaniou, E., Velkova, L., Klimentzou, P., Stevanovic, S., Salvato, B., Neychev, H. & Voelter, W. (2008). Immunological potential of *Helix vulgaris* and *Rapana venosa* hemocyanins. *Immunol Invest*, Vol.37, No.8: pp. 822-840, 1532-4311

Dolashka, P., Velkova, L., Shishkov, S., Kostova, K., Dolashki, A., Dimitrov, I., Atanasov, B., Devreese, B., Voelter, W. & Van Beeumen, J. (2010). Glycan structures and antiviral effect of the structural subunit RvH2 of *Rapana* hemocyanin. *Carbohydr Res*, Vol.345, No.16: pp. 2361-2367, 1873-426X

Doyle, A.G., Ramm, L. & Kelso, A. (1998). The CD4+ T-cell response to protein immunization is independent of accompanying IFN-gamma-producing CD8+ T cells. *Immunology*, Vol.93, No.3: pp. 341-349, 0019-2805

Duvillie, B., Attali, M., Aiello, V., Quemeneur, E. & Scharfmann, R. (2003). Label-retaining cells in the rat pancreas: location and differentiation potential in vitro. *Diabetes*, Vol.52, No.8: pp. 2035-2042, 0012-1797

Edwards, F.R. & Whitwell, F. (1974). Use of BCG as an immunostimulant in the surgical treatment of carcinoma of the lung. *Thorax*, Vol.29, No.6: pp. 654-658, 0040-6376

Espinoza, C., De Ioannes, A.E. & Becker, M.I. (2006). Caracterización bioquímica e inmunoquímica de la hemocianina de tres especies de lapas chilenas de la Familia

Fissurellidae. Proceedings of XXIX Reunión Anual de la Sociedad de Bioquímica y Biología Molecular de Chile. Pucón, Chile. November, 2006.

FDA. In: *ClinicalTrials.gov,* July 2011, Available from: http://clinicaltrials.gov/ct2/results?tem=KLH

Flamm, J., Bucher, A., Holtl, W. & Albrecht, W. (1990). Recurrent superficial transitional cell carcinoma of the bladder: adjuvant topical chemotherapy versus immunotherapy. A prospective randomized trial. *J Urol,* Vol.144, No.2 Pt 1: pp. 260-263, 0022-5347

Gatsogiannis, C. & Markl, J. (2009). Keyhole limpet hemocyanin: 9-A CryoEM structure and molecular model of the KLH1 didecamer reveal the interfaces and intricate topology of the 160 functional units. *J Mol Biol,* Vol.385, No.3: pp. 963-983, 1089-8638

Ghiretti-Magaldi, A. & Ghiretti, F. (1992). The pre-history of hemocyanin. The discovery of copper in the blood of molluscs. *Experientia,* Vol.48: pp. 971-972

Gielens, C., De Geest, N., Compernolle, F. & Preaux, G. (2004). Glycosylation sites of hemocyanins of *Helix pomatia* and *Sepia officinalis. Micron,* Vol.35, No.1-2: pp. 99-100, 0968-4328

Gilliet, M., Kleinhans, M., Lantelme, E., Schadendorf, D., Burg, G. & Nestle, F.O. (2003). Intranodal injection of semimature monocyte-derived dendritic cells induces T helper type 1 responses to protein neoantigen. *Blood,* Vol.102, No.1: pp. 36-42, 0006-4971

Gravotta, D., Deora, A., Perret, E., Oyanadel, C., Soza, A., Schreiner, R., Gonzalez, A. & Rodriguez-Boulan, E. (2007). AP1B sorts basolateral proteins in recycling and biosynthetic routes of MDCK cells. *Proc Natl Acad Sci U S A,* Vol.104, No.5: pp. 1564-1569, 0027-8424

Grenegard, M., Vretenbrant-Oberg, K., Nylander, M., Desilets, S., Lindstrom, E.G., Larsson, A., Ramstrom, I., Ramstrom, S. & Lindahl, T.L. (2008). The ATP-gated P2X1 receptor plays a pivotal role in activation of aspirin-treated platelets by thrombin and epinephrine. *J Biol Chem,* Vol.283, No.27: pp. 18493-18504, 0021-9258

Gunther, J.H., Jurczok, A., Wulf, T., Brandau, S., Deinert, I., Jocham, D. & Bohle, A. (1999). Optimizing syngeneic orthotopic murine bladder cancer (MB49). *Cancer Res,* Vol.59, No.12: pp. 2834-2837, 0008-5472

Harris, J.R., Gebauer, W. & Markl, J. (1993). Immunoelectron Microscopy od Hemocyanin from the Keyhole Limpet (*Megathura crenulata*): A Parallel Subunit Model. *J Struct Biol,* Vol.111: pp. 96-104

Harris, J.R. & Markl, J. (1999). Keyhole limpet hemocyanin (KLH): a biomedical review. *Micron,* Vol.30, No.6: pp. 597-623, 0968-4328

Idakieva, K., Stoeva, S., Voelter, W. & Gielens, C. (2004). Glycosylation of *Rapana thomasiana* hemocyanin. Comparison with other prosobranch (gastropod) hemocyanins. *Comp Biochem Physiol B Biochem Mol Biol,* Vol.138, No.3: pp. 221-228, 1096-4959

Ikemoto, S., Kamizuru, M., Wada, S., Asai, Y. & Kishimoto, T. (1997). Changes in lymphocyte subsets following administration of interleukin 2 and cyclophosphamide in mice with transitional cell carcinoma. *Oncol Res,* Vol.9, No.2: pp. 71-75, 0965-0407

Inaba, K., Inaba, M., Romani, N., Aya, H., Deguchi, M., Ikehara, S., Muramatsu, S. & Steinman, R.M. (1992). Generation of large numbers of dendritic cells from mouse bone marrow cultures supplemented with granulocyte/macrophage colony-stimulating factor. *J Exp Med*, Vol.176, No.6: pp. 1693-1702, 0022-1007

Jacobs, J.F., Punt, C.J., Lesterhuis, W.J., Sutmuller, R.P., Brouwer, H.M., Scharenborg, N.M., Klasen, I.S., Hilbrands, L.B., Figdor, C.G., de Vries, I.J. & Adema, G.J. (2010). Dendritic cell vaccination in combination with anti-CD25 monoclonal antibody treatment: a phase I/II study in metastatic melanoma patients. *Clin Cancer Res*, Vol.16, No.20: pp. 5067-5078, 1078-0432

Jurincic-Winkler, C., Metz, K.A., Beuth, J., Sippel, J. & Klippel, K.F. (1995a). Effect of keyhole limpet hemocyanin (KLH) and bacillus Calmette-Guerin (BCG) instillation on carcinoma in situ of the urinary bladder. *Anticancer Res*, Vol.15, No.6B: pp. 2771-2776, 0250-7005

Jurincic-Winkler, C., Metz, K.A., Beuth, J., Engelmann, U. & Klippel, K.F. (1995b). Immunohistological findings in patients with superficial bladder carcinoma after intravesical instillation of keyhole limpet haemocyanin. *Br J Urol*, Vol.76, No.6: pp. 702-707, 0007-1331

Jurincic-Winkler, C.D., Gallati, H., Alvarez-Mon, M., Sippel, J., Carballido, J. & Klippel, K.F. (1995c). Urinary interleukin-1 alpha levels are increased by intravesical instillation with keyhole limpet hemocyanin in patients with superficial transitional cell carcinoma of the bladder. *Eur Urol*, Vol.28, No.4: pp. 334-339, 0302-2838

Jurincic, C.D., Engelmann, U., Gasch, J. & Klippel, K.F. (1988). Immunotherapy in bladder cancer with keyhole-limpet hemocyanin: a randomized study. *J Urol*, Vol.139, No.4: pp. 723-726, 0022-5347

Kafi, K., Betting, D.J., Yamada, R.E., Bacica, M., Steward, K.K. & Timmerman, J.M. (2009). Maleimide conjugation markedly enhances the immunogenicity of both human and murine idiotype-KLH vaccines. *Mol Immunol*, Vol.46, No.3: pp. 448-456, 0161-5890

Kaplan, D.H., Shankaran, V., Dighe, A.S., Stockert, E., Aguet, M., Old, L.J. & Schreiber, R.D. (1998). Demonstration of an interferon gamma-dependent tumor surveillance system in immunocompetent mice. *Proc Natl Acad Sci U S A*, Vol.95, No.13: pp. 7556-7561, 0027-8424

Lamm, D.L., Reyna, J.A. & Reichert, D.F. (1981). Keyhole-limpet haemacyanin and immune ribonucleic acid immunotherapy of murine transitional cell carcinoma. *Urol Res*, Vol.9, No.5: pp. 227-230, 0300-5623

Lamm, D.L., Reichert, D.F., Harris, S.C. & Lucio, R.M. (1982). Immunotherapy of murine transitional cell carcinoma. *J Urol*, Vol.128, No.5: pp. 1104-1108, 0022-5347

Lamm, D.L., DeHaven, J.I., Riggs, D.R. & Ebert, R.F. (1993a). Immunotherapy of murine bladder cancer with keyhole limpet hemocyanin (KLH). *J Urol*, Vol.149, No.3: pp. 648-652, 0022-5347

Lamm, D.L., DeHaven, J.I., Riggs, D.R., Delgra, C. & Burrell, R. (1993b). Keyhole limpet hemocyanin immunotherapy of murine bladder cancer. *Urol Res*, Vol.21, No.1: pp. 33-37, 0300-5623

Lamm, D.L., Dehaven, J.I. & Riggs, D.R. (2000). Keyhole limpet hemocyanin immunotherapy of bladder cancer: laboratory and clinical studies. *Eur Urol*, Vol.37 Suppl 3: pp. 41-44, 0302-2838

Lamm, D.L. (2003). Laboratory and Clinical Experience with Keyhole limpet hemocyanin (Immunocothel) in superficial bladder cancer. *J. Urol.*, Vol.10, No.2: pp. 18-21

Lattime, E.C., Gomella, L.G. & McCue, P.A. (1992). Murine bladder carcinoma cells present antigen to BCG-specific CD4+ T-cells. *Cancer Res*, Vol.52, No.15: pp. 4286-4290, 0008-5472

Lau, B.H., Woolley, J.L., Marsh, C.L., Barker, G.R., Koobs, D.H. & Torrey, R.R. (1986). Superiority of intralesional immunotherapy with *Corynebacterium parvum* and *Allium sativum* in control of murine transitional cell carcinoma. *J Urol*, Vol.136, No.3: pp. 701-705, 0022-5347

Leitch, H.A. & Connors, J.M. (2005). Vaccine therapy for non-Hodgkin's lymphoma and other B-cell malignancies. *Curr Opin Investig Drugs*, Vol.6, No.6: pp. 597-604, 1472-4472

Lesterhuis, W.J., Schreibelt, G., Scharenborg, N.M., Brouwer, H.M., Gerritsen, M.J., Croockewit, S., Coulie, P.G., Torensma, R., Adema, G.J., Figdor, C.G., de Vries, I.J. & Punt, C.J. (2011). Wild-type and modified gp100 peptide-pulsed dendritic cell vaccination of advanced melanoma patients can lead to long-term clinical responses independent of the peptide used. *Cancer Immunol Immunother*, Vol.60, No.2: pp. 249-260, 1432-0851

Leyton, P., Lizama-Vergara, P.A., Campos-Vallete, M.M., Becker, M.I., Clavijo, E., Cordova Reyes, I., Vera, M. & Jerez, C.A. (2005). Surface enhanced Raman spectrum of nanometric molecular systems. *J. Chile. Chem. Soc.*, Vol.50, No.4: pp. 725-730, 0717-9707

Lieb, B., Altenhein, B., Markl, J., Vincent, A., van Olden, E., van Holde, K.E. & Miller, K.I. (2001). Structures of two molluscan hemocyanin genes: significance for gene evolution. *Proc Natl Acad Sci U S A*, Vol.98, No.8: pp. 4546-4551, 0027-8424

Linn, J.F., Black, P., Derksen, K., Rubben, H. & Thuroff, J.W. (2000). Keyhole limpet haemocyanin in experimental bladder cancer: literature review and own results. *Eur Urol*, Vol.37 Suppl 3: pp. 34-40, 0302-2838

Lommerse, J.P., Thomas-Oates, J.E., Gielens, C., Preaux, G., Kamerling, J.P. & Vliegenthart, J.F. (1997). Primary structure of 21 novel monoantennary and diantennary N-linked carbohydrate chains from alphaD-hemocyanin of *Helix pomatia*. *Eur J Biochem*, Vol.249, No.1: pp. 195-222, 0014-2956

Lopez, M.N., Pereda, C., Segal, G., Munoz, L., Aguilera, R., Gonzalez, F.E., Escobar, A., Ginesta, A., Reyes, D., Gonzalez, R., Mendoza-Naranjo, A., Larrondo, M., Compan, A., Ferrada, C. & Salazar-Onfray, F. (2009). Prolonged survival of dendritic cell-vaccinated melanoma patients correlates with tumor-specific delayed type IV hypersensitivity response and reduction of tumor growth factor beta-expressing T cells. *J Clin Oncol*, Vol.27, No.6: pp. 945-952, 1527-7755

Manosalva, H., De Ioannes, A.E. & Becker, M.I. (2004). Development of monoclonal antibodies bearing the internal image of the gizzerosine epitope and application in a competitive ELISA for fish meal. *Hybrid Hybridomics*, Vol.23, No.1: pp. 45-54, 1536-8599

Manubens, A., Salazar, F., Haussmann, D., Figueroa, J., Del Campo, M., Pinto, J.M., Huaquin, L., Venegas, A. & Becker, M.I. (2010). *Concholepas* hemocyanin biosynthesis takes place in the hepatopancreas, with hemocytes being involved in its metabolism. *Cell Tissue Res*, Vol.342, No.3: pp. 423-435, 1432-0878

Markl, J., Lieb, B., Gebauer, W., Altenhein, B., Meissner, U. & Harris, J.R. (2001). Marine tumor vaccine carriers: structure of the molluscan hemocyanins KLH and HtH. *J Cancer Res Clin Oncol*, Vol.127 Suppl 2: pp. R3-9, 0171-5216

Marsh, C.L., Torrey, R.R., Woolley, J.L., Barker, G.R. & Lau, B.H. (1987). Superiority of intravesical immunotherapy with *Corynebacterium parvum* and *Allium sativum* in control of murine bladder cancer. *J Urol*, Vol.137, No.2: pp. 359-362, 0022-5347

Matus, S., Burgos, P.V., Bravo-Zehnder, M., Kraft, R., Porras, O.H., Farias, P., Barros, L.F., Torrealba, F., Massardo, L., Jacobelli, S. & Gonzalez, A. (2007). Antiribosomal-P autoantibodies from psychiatric lupus target a novel neuronal surface protein causing calcium influx and apoptosis. *J Exp Med*, Vol.204, No.13: pp. 3221-3234, 1540-9538

Mauldin, R.E. & Miller, L.A. (2007). Wildlife contraception: targeting the oocyte. Managing Vertebrate Invasive Species: Proceedings of an International Symposium. G.W. Witmer, W.C. Pitt&K.A. Fagerstone. National Wildlife Research Center, Fort Collins, CO.

Milas, L. & Withers, H.R. (1976). Nonspecific immunotherapy of malignant tumors. *Radiology*, Vol.118, No.1: pp. 211-218, 0033-8419

Millard, A.L., Ittelet, D., Schooneman, F. & Bernard, J. (2003). Dendritic cell KLH loading requirements for efficient CD4+ T-cell priming and help to peptide-specific cytotoxic T-cell response, in view of potential use in cancer vaccines. *Vaccine*, Vol.21, No.9-10: pp. 869-876, 0264-410X

Miller, L.A., Talwar, G.P. & Killian, G.J. (2006). Contraceptive effect of a recombinant GnRH vaccine in adult female pigs. Proc. 22nd Vertebr. Pest. Conf. O.B.J. Timm RM, Univ. of Calif: pp. 106-109.

Moltedo, B., Faunes, F., Haussmann, D., De Ioannes, P., De Ioannes, A.E., Puente, J. & Becker, M.I. (2006). Immunotherapeutic effect of *Concholepas* hemocyanin in the murine bladder cancer model: evidence for conserved antitumor properties among hemocyanins. *J Urol*, Vol.176, No.6 Pt 1: pp. 2690-2695, 0022-5347

Moltedo, B., Lopez, C.B., Pazos, M., Becker, M.I., Hermesh, T. & Moran, T.M. (2009). Cutting edge: stealth influenza virus replication precedes the initiation of adaptive immunity. *J Immunol*, Vol.183, No.6: pp. 3569-3573, 1550-6606

Molto, L.M., Carballido, J., Jurincic, C., Lapena, P., Manzano, L., Salmeron, I., Klippel, K.F. & Alvarez-Mon, M. (1991). Keyhole limpet hemocyanine can enhance the natural killer activity of patients with transitional cell carcinoma of the bladder. *Eur Urol*, Vol.19, No.1: pp. 74-78, 0302-2838

Morales, A., Eidinger, D. & Bruce, A.W. (1976). Intracavitary Bacillus Calmette-Guerin in the treatment of superficial bladder tumors. *J Urol*, Vol.116, No.2: pp. 180-183, 0022-5347

Mura, C.V., Becker, M.I., Orellana, A. & Wolff, D. (2002). Immunopurification of Golgi vesicles by magnetic sorting. *J Immunol Methods*, Vol.260, No.1-2: pp. 263-271, 0022-1759

Musselli, C., Livingston, P.O. & Ragupathi, G. (2001). Keyhole limpet hemocyanin conjugate vaccines against cancer: the Memorial Sloan Kettering experience. *J Cancer Res Clin Oncol*, Vol.127 Suppl 2: pp. R20-26, 0171-5216

Nseyo, U.O. & Lamm, D.L. (1997). Immunotherapy of bladder cancer. *Semin Surg Oncol*, Vol.13, No.5: pp. 342-349, 8756-0437

Oliva, H., Moltedo, B., De Ioannes, P., Faunes, F., De Ioannes, A.E. & Becker, M.I. (2002). Monoclonal antibodies to molluskan hemocyanin from *Concholepas concholepas* demonstrate common and specific epitopes among subunits. *Hybrid Hybridomics*, Vol.21, No.5: pp. 365-374, 1536-8599

Olsson, C.A., Chute, R. & Rao, C.N. (1974). Immunologic reduction of bladder cancer recurrence rate. *J Urol*, Vol.111, No.2: pp. 173-176, 0022-5347

Orlova, E.V., Dube, P., Harris, J.R., Beckman, E., Zemlin, F., Markl, J. & van Heel, M. (1997). Structure of keyhole limpet hemocyanin type 1 (KLH1) at 15 A resolution by electron cryomicroscopy and angular reconstitution. *J Mol Biol*, Vol.271, No.3: pp. 417-437, 0022-2836

Paccagnella, M., Bologna, L., Beccaro, M., Micetic, I., Di Muro, P. & Salvato, B. (2004). Structural subunit organization of molluscan hemocyanins. *Micron*, Vol.35, No.1-2: pp. 21-22, 0968-4328

Perabo, F.G. & Muller, S.C. (2004). Current and new strategies in immunotherapy for superficial bladder cancer. *Urology*, Vol.64, No.3: pp. 409-421, 1527-9995

Pilon, J., Loiacono, C., Okeson, D., Lund, S., Vercauteren, K., Rhyan, J. & Miller, L. (2007). Anti-prion activity generated by a novel vaccine formulation. *Neurosci Lett*, Vol.429, No.2-3: pp. 161-164, 0304-3940

Presicce, P., Taddeo, A., Conti, A., Villa, M.L. & Della Bella, S. (2008). Keyhole limpet hemocyanin induces the activation and maturation of human dendritic cells through the involvement of mannose receptor. *Mol Immunol*, Vol.45, No.4: pp. 1136-1145, 0161-5890

Recker, F. & Rubben, H. (1989). Variation of the immunosystem by ciclosporin and keyhole-limpet hemocyanin--are there effects on chemically induced bladder carcinoma? *Urol Int*, Vol.44, No.2: pp. 77-80, 0042-1138

Riggs, D.R., Tarry, W.F., DeHaven, J.I., Sosnowski, J. & Lamm, D.L. (1992). Immunotherapy of murine transitional cell carcinoma of the bladder using alpha and gamma interferon in combination with other forms of immunotherapy. *J Urol*, Vol.147, No.1: pp. 212-214, 0022-5347

Riggs, D.R., Jackson, B., Vona-Davis, L. & McFadden, D. (2002). *In vitro* anticancer effects of a novel immunostimulant: keyhole limpet hemocyanin. *J Surg Res*, Vol.108, No.2: pp. 279-284, 0022-4804

Schenkman, E. & Lamm, D.L. (2004). Superficial bladder cancer therapy. *ScientificWorldJournal*, Vol.4 Suppl 1: pp. 387-399, 1537-744X

Schumacher, K. (2001). Keyhole limpet hemocyanin (KLH) conjugate vaccines as novel therapeutic tools in malignant disorders. *J Cancer Res Clin Oncol*, Vol.127 Suppl 2: pp. R1-2, 0171-5216

Shimizu, K., Thomas, E.K., Giedlin, M. & Mule, J.J. (2001). Enhancement of tumor lysate- and peptide-pulsed dendritic cell-based vaccines by the addition of foreign helper protein. *Cancer Res*, Vol.61, No.6: pp. 2618-2624, 0008-5472

Siddiqui, N.I., Idakieva, K., Demarsin, B., Doumanova, L., Compernolle, F. & Gielens, C. (2007). Involvement of glycan chains in the antigenicity of *Rapana thomasiana* hemocyanin. *Biochem Biophys Res Commun*, Vol.361, No.3: pp. 705-711, 0006-291X

Somasundar, P., Riggs, D.R., Jackson, B.J. & McFadden, D.W. (2005). Inhibition of melanoma growth by hemocyanin occurs via early apoptotic pathways. *Am J Surg*, Vol.190, No.5: pp. 713-716, 0002-9610

Swerdlow, R.D., Ratliff, T.L., La Regina, M., Ritchey, J.K. & Ebert, R.F. (1994). Immunotherapy with keyhole limpet hemocyanin: efficacy and safety in the MB-49 intravesical murine bladder tumor model. *J Urol*, Vol.151, No.6: pp. 1718-1722, 0022-5347

Swerdlow, R.D., Ebert, R.F., Lee, P., Bonaventura, C. & Miller, K.I. (1996). Keyhole limpet hemocyanin: structural and functional characterization of two different subunits and multimers. *Comp Biochem Physiol B Biochem Mol Biol*, Vol.113, No.3: pp. 537-548, 1096-4959

Szabo, S.J., Sullivan, B.M., Peng, S.L. & Glimcher, L.H. (2003). Molecular mechanisms regulating Th1 immune responses. *Annu Rev Immunol*, Vol.21: pp. 713-758, 0732-0582

Teitz-Tennenbaum, S., Li, Q., Davis, M.A. & Chang, A.E. (2008). Dendritic cells pulsed with keyhole limpet hemocyanin and cryopreserved maintain anti-tumor activity in a murine melanoma model. *Clin Immunol*, Vol.129, No.3: pp. 482-491, 1521-7035

Teppema, J.S., de Boer, E.C., Steeremberg, P.A. & van der Meijden, A.P. (1992). Morphological aspects of the interaction of Bacillus Calmette-Guérin with urothelial bladder cells *in vivo* and *in vitro*: relevance for antitumor activity. *Urol. Res.*, Vol.20: pp. 219-228

Timmerman, J.M. & Levy, R. (2000). Linkage of foreign carrier protein to a self-tumor antigen enhances the immunogenicity of a pulsed dendritic cell vaccine. *J Immunol*, Vol.164, No.9: pp. 4797-4803, 0022-1767

Torres, M., Manosalva, H., Carrasco, I., De Ioannes, A.E. & Becker, M.I. (1999). Procedure for radiolabeling gizzerosine and basis for a radioimmunoassay. *J Agric Food Chem*, Vol.47, No.10: pp. 4231-4236, 0021-8561

van Holde, K.E. & Miller, K.I. (1995). Hemocyanins. *Adv Protein Chem*, Vol.47: pp. 1-81, 0065-3233

van Holde, K.E., Miller, K.I. & Decker, H. (2001). Hemocyanins and invertebrate evolution. *J Biol Chem*, Vol.276, No.19: pp. 15563-15566, 0021-9258

Vandenbark, A.A., Yoshihara, P., Carveth, L. & Burger, D.R. (1981). All KLH preparations are not created equal. *Cell Immunol*, Vol.60, No.1: pp. 240-243, 0008-8749

Verdijk, P., Aarntzen, E.H., Lesterhuis, W.J., Boullart, A.C., Kok, E., van Rossum, M.M., Strijk, S., Eijckeler, F., Bonenkamp, J.J., Jacobs, J.F., Blokx, W., Vankrieken, J.H., Joosten, I., Boerman, O.C., Oyen, W.J., Adema, G., Punt, C.J., Figdor, C.G. & de Vries, I.J. (2009). Limited amounts of dendritic cells migrate into the T-cell area of lymph nodes but have high immune activating potential in melanoma patients. *Clin Cancer Res*, Vol.15, No.7: pp. 2531-2540, 1078-0432

Walsh, W.G., Tomashefsky, P., Olsson, C.A. & deVere White, R. (1983). Keyhole-limpet haemocyanin (KLH) immunotherapy of murine transitional cell carcinoma. *Urol Res*, Vol.11, No.6: pp. 263-265, 0300-5623

Weigle, W.O. (1964). Immunochemical Properties of Hemocyanin. *Immunochemistry*, Vol.1: pp. 295-302, 0019-2791

Wishahi, M.M., Ismail, I.M., Ruebben, H. & Otto, T. (1995). Keyhole-limpet hemocyanin immunotherapy in the bilharzial bladder: a new treatment modality? Phase II trial: superficial bladder cancer. *J Urol*, Vol.153, No.3 Pt 2: pp. 926-928, 0022-5347

Wuhrer, M., Robijn, M.L., Koeleman, C.A., Balog, C.I., Geyer, R., Deelder, A.M. & Hokke, C.H. (2004). A novel Gal(beta1-4)Gal(beta1-4)Fuc(alpha1-6)-core modification attached to the proximal N-acetylglucosamine of keyhole limpet haemocyanin (KLH) N-glycans. *Biochem J*, Vol.378, No.Pt 2: pp. 625-632, 1470-8728

Zhu, J., Wan, Q., Lee, D., Yang, G., Spassova, M.K., Ouerfelli, O., Ragupathi, G., Damani, P., Livingston, P.O. & Danishefsky, S.J. (2009). From synthesis to biologics: preclinical data on a chemistry derived anticancer vaccine. *J Am Chem Soc*, Vol.131, No.26: pp. 9298-9303, 1520-5126

The Potential Role of Chemoprevention in the Management of Non-Muscle Invasive Bladder Urothelial Carcinoma

Unyime O. Nseyo[1], Katherine A. Corbyons[2]
and Hari Siva Gurunadha Rao Tunuguntla[3]
[1]North Florida-South Georgia Veterans Health System, Gainesville, Florida,
[2]University of Florida, Gainesville, Florida,
[3]Robert Wood Johnson Medical School, New Brunswick, New Jersey,
USA

1. Introduction

1.1 Epidemiology and bladder carcinogenesis

Cancer represents phenotypic manifestations of abnormal gene expression. Genetic mutations, dysregulation, and gene losses can influence cell proliferation and differentiation, and eventually lead to formation of cancer. Risk factors and etiologic agents involved in the genetic abnormalities influence the distribution of cancer worldwide. This chapter aims at highlighting the epidemiologic significance of urothelial bladder cancer; reviewing its natural history, the roles of industrial and environmental carcinogens and life style factors in urothelial carcinogenesis; and framing possible strategies for chemoprevention in the management of human urothelial cancer of the urinary bladder.

Bladder cancer remains a serious public health problem worldwide, and accounts for 5-10% of all malignancies annually in western countries (*Cancer Treatment of America*). Though the age-adjusted incidence varies in the different parts of the world, the highest rates are found in men from North America (23.3/100,000), North Africa (23.3/100,000) and Southern Europe (22.0/100,000), while the corresponding rates are 5.4, 4.8, and 3.2 per 100000 for women (*Cancer Treatment of America*). These high rates may be influenced by increased industrialization, cigarette smoking, and infection of schistosomiasis (primarily of concern in North Africa). The lowest rates for both sexes have been reported for the Melanesia region of South Pacific and Middle Africa (*Cancer Treatment of America*; Prout, Barton et al. 1992; Grasso 2008; *American Cancer Society* 2010).

Bladder cancer, which is immensely impacted by environmental carcinogens and tobacco smokes, remains a common disease in the United States, and it is estimated that 70, 530 persons (52,760 men and 17,770 women) were diagnosed with cancer of the urinary bladder in 2010, (*Cancer Treatment of America*; *American Cancer Society* 2010) and an estimated 14, 680 died of the disease accounting for 3% and 2% of all cancer deaths in men and women, respectively (*Cancer Treatment of America*; *American Cancer Society* 2010). Estimates of new cancer cases classify *urothelial bladder cancer* (UBC) as the fourth most common in men and the eighth most common in women. The prevalence of UBC in the US is estimated at about one million cases annually, and worldwide, UBC ranks as the ninth most frequent cancer (*Cancer Treatment of America*; Prout, Barton et al. 1992; Grasso 2008; American Cancer Society 2010).

Bladder cancer is a disease of aging; the incidence of UBC rises with age with an average of onset at 69 for men and 67 for women (*Cancer Treatment of America*; Prout, Barton et al. 1992; Dalbagni and Herr 2000; Grasso 2008; *American Cancer Society* 2010). Bladder cancer that occurs at ages 40 or younger tends to be low grade Ta cancer with almost negligible recurrence potential. Given sufficient time, however 50-70% of UBC patients will develop recurrent disease. Recurrences tend to be characterized by multiplicity in time and space, primarily if the initial tumors occurred early in life and were large or multiple in numbers. A majority, 70-75%, of UBC are superficial, that is, non-muscle invasive, and non-lethal, but they are characterized by frequent recurrences. However, the remaining 25-30% of the annual cases of UBC invades into the muscular propria, making them life threatening, because approximately 50% harbor micro-metastases that often manifest within three years out from diagnosis (Droller 2006).

The non-muscle invasive UBC (NMIUBC) that are confined to the mucosa/urothelium Ta, remain non-lethal with a progression rate of less than 5%, and occur often as large or multiple tumors. Ten to twenty percent of the superficially-invasive UBC that is confined to the lamina propria, T1, converts to muscle invasive disease on repeat resection (Dalbagni and Herr 2000).

Variable morphology, natural history, and prognosis demonstrate that transitional cell carcinoma (TCC) or urothelial carcinoma (UC) of the bladder is not a single disease, but occurs in three distinct forms, each possessing characteristic features that include low grade papillary, noninvasive; carcinoma in situ (CIS); and high grade, invasive (Grasso 2008). Seventy to eighty-five percent of new bladder cancer cases, are superficial or *non-muscle invasive* UBC, which include disease confined to the mucosa in CIS: CIS (10%), and Ta (70%), or lamina propria in T1 (20%) (Prout, Barton et al. 1992; Dalbagni and Herr 2000; Droller 2006; Grasso 2008). These types of tumors are considered to have variable invasive potential with a progression rate to invasive cancer of 15% to 50% (Prout, Barton et al. 1992; Dalbagni and Herr 2000; Grasso 2008). However, more than 70% of patients with NMIUBC have one or more recurrences within 5 years of initial diagnosis (Prout, Barton et al. 1992; Dalbagni and Herr 2000; Droller 2006; Grasso 2008). Further analysis shows that approximately 50% of patients diagnosed with solitary bladder cancer will experience recurrences within 4 years, while 70% of multiple bladder tumors reoccur within one year (Prout, Barton et al. 1992; Dalbagni and Herr 2000; Droller 2006; Grasso 2008).

The fact that the bladder serves as a reservoir for urine and its waste product contents predisposes it to the constant cumulative exposure to carcinogens which include industrial toxins and cigarette smoke chemicals. The multiple-step process of carcinogenesis includes induction/activation, promotion and progression, which exists as a continuum in the bladder environment. Consequently, preventive intervention can be difficult to implement under these conditions of cumulative exposures, and the definitive strategy will be to minimize constant cumulative exposure of carcinogenic agents from smoking and industrial sources. Increased carcinogenic exposure by itself cannot explain the 40% increase in bladder cancer incidence in the last 15 years in the US. The explanation certainly includes increased smoking that has added a large population of women, cumulative industrial exposure, and host factors. These host characteristics are likely to influence racial differences in the incidence of bladder cancer. Caucasians have overall bladder cancer risk of 3.9% versus 0.8% overall chance in African Americans: 2.8% in men and 1.5% in women (Droller 2006).

Earliest reported association of industrial carcinogenic exposure and development of bladder cancer was by Rehn (Dietrich and Dietrich 2001). Observations have also documented associations between carcinogen ingestion in animals and development of bladder cancer (Okey, Harper et al. 1998; Sporn and Lippman 2003). Several legislative measures have been implemented in an attempt to decrease the intensity and cumulative nature of the carcinogen exposure. However, cigarette smoking trumps all considerations of environmental and industrial exposure and is the major factor underlying the spread and occurrence of bladder cancer around the globe.

It is estimated that 30% of bladder cancer mortality is attributable to a history of tobacco abuse/dependence (*American Cancer Society*), and studies have tried to characterize the different carcinogenic agents in cigarette smoke that define the causal relationship between smoking and development of urothelial cancer (*American Cancer Society*; Droller 2006). Investigators have tried to correlate bladder cancer risk with the manufacturing processes such as the type of filter used, type of tobacco used, and the curing technique: black versus blonde (Droller 2006). The curing technique determines the concentration of the carcinogens in the cigarette. The smoke of black (air-cured) versus blonde (flue-cured) has been analyzed to show higher concentration of carcinogens in black tobacco. How these commercial practices influence urothelial carcinogenesis remains to be elucidated.

Several specific carcinogens in cigarette smoke have been implicated in the development of urothelial cancer, including polycyclic aromatic hydrocarbons, aromatic and aryl amines (including 4-amino biphenyl), unsaturated aldehydes (e.g. acrolein) and oxygen-free radicals (*American Cancer Society*; Sabichi and Lippman; Droller 2006). Aromatic amines were the first carbon compounds of industrial by-products that were suspected in work- related urothelial cancer, found primarily in those workers who were exposed to the dye, rubber, and plastic manufacturing. These epidemiological data suggest up to 100-fold increased risk that is mediated by cumulative intensity and duration of exposure. Regulatory and legislative efforts to retard the work place risk contributed to the birth of occupational safety and health administration in the industrialized countries around the world.

In spite of extensive efforts since then to curb workplace exposure to industrial carcinogens, textile, dry cleaning, hair dressing, and coal gasification continue to generate the carcinogens in the manufacturing process. The culprit agents are per-chloroethylene (an organic solvent used in dry cleaning), chemical dyes, aromatic amines (used in textile industry), and hair dyes that contain chemical carcinogens. These agents have been associated with bladder cancer development. Other carcinogens, outside of the workplace, that have been associated with the development of urothelial cancer include arsenic in ground water in southeastern Michigan in the US and southwestern Taiwan (Haack, Treccani et al. 2000; Kim, Nriagu et al. 2000; Welch, Westjohn et al. 2000; Droller 2006); ingestion of fang chi (Chinese herb used in weight control); ingestion of ochratoxin A in the Balkan countries resulting indirectly from animals that consumed blackened fern (Droller 2006). Several medications and medical therapies have also been associated with urothelial cancer development including phenacetin used to treat headaches, cyclophosphamide (cytoxan) used to treat pediatric and adult hematologic malignancies (lymphoma and leukemia), and pelvic radiation for cervical and prostate cancer.

In parts of the world with endemicity, there are reports of association between *Schistosoma haematobium* infection and the development of urothelial cancer, primarily squamous cell carcinoma, and some cases of transitional cell cancer (Sabichi and Lippman; Okey, Harper et al. 1998; Sporn and Lippman 2003; Droller 2006). The inciting factors include an inflammatory response to the deposited parasitic ova of *Schistosoma haematobium* in the periurethral areas of the bladder ,as well as conversion of nitrates to nitrites with the nitrosamines mediating the development of urothelial cancer. Other carcinogenic exposures such as fertilizers and cigarette smoke may also play putative roles in the urothelial carcinogenesis in these patients.

In urothelial carcinogenesis, several host factors have been recognized as playing either permissive or protective roles. Acetylation of aromatic amines remains an important mechanism of carcinogenic inactivation in urothelial carcinogenesis. The detoxification of carcinogens is mediated by genes namely NAT1 and NAT2 which are responsible for generating the detoxifying enzymes N-acetyl transferase, and NAT2 remains the predominant gene involved. Individuals who are homozygous for NAT2 are classified as slow acylators and they detoxify carcinogens quite slowly allowing prolonged contact with DNA to induce mutations and carcinogenesis (Sabichi and Lippman; Weber 1987; Droller 2006). These individuals have a two- to four-fold increased risk for the development of urothelial cancer. On the other hand, the heterozygous fast acylators are able to rapidly detoxify these aromatic amines that lower their risk of developing urothelial cancer. Researchers have suggested that the potential differences in racial and ethnic risk of urothelial cancer development are attributable to the difference in the expression of these two genes (Sabichi and Lippman; Weber 1987; Droller 2006; Lattouf 2009).The P450 cytochrome oxidase system is also important in metabolism and detoxification of urothelial carcinogens. The CYP1A2 might be particularly important in metabolizing aromatic amines (Sabichi and Lippman; Okey, Harper et al. 1998; Sporn and Lippman 2003; Droller 2006). Also, individuals deficient in the enzyme glutathione transferase may be at risk for deficient metabolism of polycyclic aromatic amines, which could put them at a 30-50% risk of developing bladder cancer (Okey, Harper et al. 1998; Sporn and Lippman 2003; Droller 2006).

2. Molecular biology of carcinogenesis and chemoprevention

The classic multistep process of carcinogenesis which has been widely accepted includes initiation, promotion, and progression. A clear-cut sequential compartmentalization probably does not always occur, but the multistep structure could be exploited strategically for chemopreventative measures. The first step, initiation, depends upon three cellular functions, namely carcinogen metabolism, DNA repair, and cell proliferation. Cell damage can occur by activation/deactivation mediated by the carcinogen; this cell can cycle through DNA repair or exists as an altered gene (no tumor development) and can be propagated as such, or go through cell proliferation. In the promotion phase, the altered cell continues to undergo repeated bombardment by the promoter agent (initiator or not) leading to additional genomic damage and subsequent clonal expansion into a tumor. In the progression phase, the tumor acquires multicellular defective mutations enhanced by acquired or inherited mutations in the control genes such as p53, Rb, or DNA mismatch repairs (Okey, Harper et al. 1998; Sporn and Lippman 2003; Droller 2006). Consequently a tumor is born that lacks cellular growth controls, and has proliferative autonomy. The challenge in designing a preventive strategy is selecting whether to target genomic or cellular events as well as determining the order of subsequent sequential targeting.

Genotoxic carcinogens can be enzymatically bioactivated and converted into water soluble metabolites to be excreted in urine or bile. These carcinogens can also be inadvertently transformed into electrophiles which react with DNA. Metabolism of carcinogens or broadly biotransformation may depend upon genetic and environmental factors in an individual who is exposed to the carcinogens. The drug metabolizing enzymes are classified into Phase I and Phase II enzymes, with Phase I enzyme being primarily typified by cytochrome P450 mono-oxygenase (CYP) super family. These enzymes function by unmasking the parent substrates (Okey, Harper et al. 1998; Sporn and Lippman 2003; Droller 2006). The Phase II enzymes including sulfotransferase, glutathione transferase (GST), and acetyltransferase primarily detoxify reactive metabolites. They catalyze the conjugation of bulky water insoluble components into hydroxyl groups which can easily be excreted.

As discussed above, carcinogenesis is a multistep process; therefore chemopreventive agents could affect different mechanisms. In practice chemoprevention would require continuous administration of a non-toxic compound over a long period or lifetime of the at-risk individual. However, the chemoprevention strategy would begin with the population approach that advocates a dietary program of increased consumption of fruits and vegetables which have been reported to reduce general cancer risk (Sabichi and Lippman; Sporn and Lippman 2003; Lattouf 2009). At the individual level, the approach would be to reduce the intensity of cumulative exposure through programs that include reduction/elimination of exposure to the carcinogens, dilution and elimination of bladder content by drinking plenty of water and urinating frequently, followed by introduction of the at-risk individual to the chemopreventive agent(s). The potential chemoprevention agents can be broadly classified into two categories: (a) agents that decrease bioactivation or increase detoxification of carcinogens, and (b) agents that alter promotion and progression (Okey, Harper et al. 1998; Sporn and Lippman 2003).

2.1 Agents that decrease bioactivation or increase detoxification of carcinogens

The cytochrome P450 enzyme family, which typifies the Phase I enzymes, acts bidirectionally by bioactivating procarcinogens into reactive metabolites that bind to DNA, but also enhances overall clearance of both the procarcinogens and carcinogens from the body. The first pass clearance of the carcinogen by the high activity of P450 enzymes in the human liver exposes the susceptible peripheral organ/ tissue to reduced concentrations of the carcinogens (Okey, Harper et al. 1998; Sporn and Lippman 2003)..

In bladder cancer, the Phase II enzymes include the detoxifier glutathione transferases which conjugate reactive metabolites with glutathione. These Phase II enzymes can be induced by plant products such as sulforaphane from broccoli. This induction can be highly protective in animals against major carcinogens. However, they can also act bidirectionally to favor Phase I class of enzymes (Okey, Harper et al. 1998; Sporn and Lippman 2003).

Interestingly, oltipraz, an anti-schistosomiasis drug, functions bidirectionally to inhibit the predominant activating enzyme CYP1A2, and also induces a glutathione S-transferase Phase II enzyme that detoxifies carcinogens by conjugation. Another cytochrome P450 modulator is indole-3-carbinole (I3C) which is abundant in broccoli, brussels sprouts, and cruciferous vegetables (Okey, Harper et al. 1998; Sporn and Lippman 2003).

The phytochemicals that reduce adduct formation include vitamin E (α-tocopherol) and vitamin C (ascorbic acid). These act as scavengers of the reactive metabolites, or act as antioxidants (Okey, Harper et al. 1998; Sporn and Lippman 2003). However, they have not been found to decrease the risk of cancer in high-risk populations.

2.2 Agents that alter promotion and progression

Inflammation, increased cell proliferation/decreased differentiation, deficiency of apoptosis, and cumulative genetic instability constitute putative molecular and cellular events that induce promotion and progression during carcinogenesis (Okey, Harper et al. 1998; Sporn and Lippman 2003; Droller 2006). These cellular events are attractive potential targets for chemopreventative intervention.

Synthetic retinoids have been shown to alter gene expression and stimulate apoptosis. However, these have failed as primary chemopreventive agents, but have been shown to delay the appearance of secondary primary cancers of head and neck (Sabichi and Lippman; Okey, Harper et al. 1998; Sporn and Lippman 2003). However, natural retinoids such as β-carotene have shown a paradoxical increase in lung cancer in smokers and asbestos-exposed workers.

Targeting inflammation has become an attractive approach in chemoprevention as scientists gain better understanding of the association between inflammation and increased cancer risk, particularly colon cancer. Both the older-generation non-specific inhibitors of cyclooxygenase including: aspirin and non-steroidal anti-inflammatory agents (NSAIDS) and the newer synthetic selective COX-2 inhibitors such as Celecoxib have shown promising results in preventing colon cancer in rodent models and in humans(Sporn and Lippman 2003).

3. Conventional strategies in preventing recurrence/occurrence and progression

Approaches to bladder cancer prevention include primary prevention which aims at avoiding cancer development in healthy populations, secondary prevention, which aims at preventing premalignant lesions from undergoing promotion and progression into cancer under conducive conditions during carcinogenesis; and tertiary prevention, which aims at aborting cancer progression in patients who have been treated for the cancer. In bladder cancer, primary prevention is widely regarded as impractical. Even if good chemopreventive agents were available the risk-benefit ratio would have to be low in such a large at risk population. The other challenges to primary intervention strategy are discussed in the sections above about the uncertainty of appropriate molecular/cellular targets to prevent tumor initiation. In practice techniques of secondary and tertiary prevention are indistinguishable.

Following the initial diagnosis with transurethral resection of bladder tumor (TURBT), there are several interventions that may be undertaken to retard cancer recurrence and progression: selected patients may undergo repeat TURBT to better delineate the nature of their disease (Prout, Barton et al. 1992; Oosterlinck, Kurth et al. 1993; Lamm, Blumenstein et al. 1995; Dalbagni and Herr 2000), approximately 20% will receive intravesical chemotherapy to potentially eradicate residual disease (Prout, Barton et al. 1992;

Oosterlinck, Kurth et al. 1993; Lamm, Blumenstein et al. 1995; Dalbagni and Herr 2000) and the majority will be placed on some type of endoscopic surveillance schedule. The necessity for early adjuvant treatment, mainly intravesical instillation of immunotherapeutic or chemotherapeutic agents in the management of high-risk CIS, Ta/high grade and T1/any grade is recognized globally (Prout, Barton et al. 1992; Oosterlinck, Kurth et al. 1993; Lamm, Blumenstein et al. 1995; Dalbagni and Herr 2000). The hope is that this treatment, by altering the neoplastic potential of the urothelium, will reduce the risk for recurrence and progression. The subsets of the patients with NMIUBC who fail the conventional intravesical therapies will ultimately be subjected to radical cystectomy with resultant loss of bladder function, body image and sexual function (Prout, Barton et al. 1992; Oosterlinck, Kurth et al. 1993; Lamm, Blumenstein et al. 1995; Dalbagni and Herr 2000). The newest strategy in the management of NMIUBC is Photodynamic Diagnosis (PDD) with Hexvix® (*PhotoCure ASA, Oslo, Norway*) to minimize recurrences/occurrences and progression. PPD uses Hexvix which is an ester derivative of 5-Aminolevulinic Acid (ALA) (Jichlinski, Guillou et al. 2003; Fradet, Grossman et al. 2007) was recently approved by the US Food and Drug Administration (FDA) for management of NMIUBC primarily to improve the diagnostic and staging accuracy of cystoscopy leading to improvement in survival. Photodynamic diagnosis occurs when a photosensitizing agent is first concentrated in malignant or abnormal tissue, and then activated by light (Henderson 1992). The activated photosensitizer either returns to ground state, and releases energy as fluorescence, which can be used in detection (PDD), or the photosensitizer enters into its triplet state, and causes physico-chemical reactions to generate reactive oxygen species (ROS), for therapy as in Photodynamic therapy (PDT). Hexvix-PDD has been reported to improve the diagnostic rate of Ta and T1 papillary bladder cancers by 16.4% and the detection of CIS by 31% (as compared to white light cystoscopy) (Jichlinski, Guillou et al. 2003). Recently, Karl et al., reported that PDD during initial TURBT for T1G3 NMBIC exhibited a significant reduction in recurrence rate; led to detection of additional 35.4% CIS versus 21.8% in the control group (standard white light TURBT).The authors concluded that the initial use of PDD-directed TURBT could provide a superior cancer control and effective treatment of patients with T1G3 NMIBC (Karl 2010).

Bacillus Calmette-Guerin (BCG), an immunotherapy, remains the most effective and widely used intravesical agent to prevent recurrence and progression (Oosterlinck, Kurth et al. 1993; Lamm, Blumenstein et al. 1995; Dalbagni and Herr 2000). Mitomycin, thiotepa and epirubicin are the commonly used intravesical chemotherapeutic agents. while intravesical Valrubicin is FDA-approved as an alternative intravesical therapy to radical cystectomy for BCG refractory CIS patients (Dalbagni and Herr 2000). Administering Mitomycin or epirubicin immediately following TURBT has been reported as effective in preventing tumor implant; however, this approach has failed to ultimately prevent disease progression or mortality (Oosterlinck, Kurth et al. 1993). Of course, each intravesical agent is associated with both local and systemic side effects. Despite current treatment strategies, 30-80% of these patients develop recurrences within 5 years, and this high rate of recurrence of NMIBC invariably leads to a high economic impact (Hedelin, Holmang et al. 2002; Botteman, Pashos et al. 2003; Uchida, Yonou et al. 2007; Hong and Loughlin 2008; Sievert, Amend et al. 2009). The disease progression rate to muscle invasiveness is 42-83% in BCG-treated patients who have concomitant CIS and papillary NMIUBC, and 30-50% in those BCG-treated patients with primary CIS (Oosterlinck, Kurth et al. 1993; Lamm, Blumenstein et al. 1995; Dalbagni and Herr 2000). Frequent follow ups and re-treatment of patients due to the recurrences exert heavy untold burden on the affected patients; eventually leading to morbidity as well as increased expenditure because of continuous treatment (Hedelin, Holmang et al. 2002; Botteman, Pashos et al. 2003; Uchida, Yonou et al. 2007; Hong and Loughlin 2008; Sievert, Amend et al. 2009).

3.1 Chemoprevention in the armamentarium of management of NMIUBC

Early detection and advances in treatments over the last two decades have resulted in an overall reduction in bladder cancer mortality (Cancer Treatment of America; American Cancer Society 2010). The public health and socioeconomic burden of bladder cancer could be reduced through practice of systematic prevention measures including elimination/minimization of exposure to carcinogens, hydration for dilution and frequent urination to expulse potential carcinogens; and practice of active dietary and/or pharmacologic preventative interventions. Unfortunately, in bladder cancer there are still no definite interventions that have been shown to be effective, and research in this area has yielded no evidence-based data to inform on strategies for systematic practice of bladder cancer prevention. Bladder urothelial cancer has biologic and clinical characteristics that favor it as an ideal cancer for chemoprevention. These special features include its susceptibility; carcinogenesis; frequent recurrences, and clinical presentation.

3.2 Cessation of smoking

The most cost-effective measure in bladder cancer prevention strategy would certainly be smoking cessation. This, of course, would be very difficult because of the addictive nature of the current cadre of manufactured cigarettes. In the meantime therapeutic intervention is needed to complement and perhaps even supplant the current socio-cultural as well as the legislative strategies to reduce the economic burden, suffering and death from bladder cancer through tobacco control. In the following section we will review the available evidence for the various chemotherapeutic agents.

4. Bladder cancer chemoprevention strategies: Non-pharmacologic and dietary approach (see also Table 1)

4.1 Fluid intake

The Health Professional Follow Up Study validated the concept that increased fluid intake could substantially lower the risk of UBC due to lowered intensity and cumulative exposure of carcinogens (Michaud, Spiegelman et al. 1999). The study involved mailing questionnaires to 47,903 men; and analysis of their responses regarding daily fluid intake. The data showed inverse association between total daily fluid intake and risk of urothelial cancer (UC) with a relative risk of 0.51 (0.32-0.81, 95% confidence interval: CI) in those who consumed the largest amount of fluid. Daily water consumption offered the best protection when compared with other fluids. However, Geoffrey-Perez and colleagues countered by reporting that there was an absence of association between bladder cancer risk and fluid consumption (Geoffroy-Perez and Cordier 2001). Intuitively it remains logical that dilution of bladder carcinogenic contents with frequent urination would be beneficial and less expensive practice.

4.2 Fat and caloric intake

In the Spanish study, Riboli and associates reported an association between fat consumption and urothelial cancer that showed a 2-fold increase in cancer incidence (Riboli, Gonzalez et al. 1991). Surveillance Epidemiology and End Results (SEER) population-based study data provided further evidence that fat rich diets are associated with an increase in incidence of UC (OR 2.24 for the highest quartile, 95% CI, 1.25-4.03, P=0.006) (Bruemmer, White et al. 1996). A Swedish study suggests a dose dependent effect of fat diet on the incidence of UC (Steineck, Hagman et al. 1990). In a meta-analysis of 36 studies evaluating 6 dietary variables in relation to UC, Steinmaus and group reported a positive association between intake of fat and UC (Relative ratio, RR 1.37, 95% CI, 1.16-1.62), but not with meat consumption (RR 1.08, 95% CI, 0.82-1.42) (Steinmaus, Nunez et al. 2000). However, there was no positive association between total caloric intake and UC over 12 years in the Health Professional Follow-Up Study (Michaud, Spiegelman et al. 2000). The traditional flaws of epidemiologic studies certainly affect the results of these studies including recall bias and lack of prospective randomized data. Other confounding factors include concomitant increased in caloric intake with increased fat intake. Despite these drawbacks of the reports, decreased fat intake should be a recommendation for prevention strategy of UC.

4.3 Green tea

Drinking tea has been reported to confer protective health benefits which include prevention of human cancers including prostate and bladder cancers (Trevisanato and Kim 2000).

The polyphenols found in green tea are potent antioxidants; they also inhibit ornithine decarboxylase which is an enzyme that promotes tumor proliferation via nucleic acid regulation (Steele, Kelloff et al. 2000). The incidence of UC in Asian populations with increased tea consumption is lower than in North America; a weak inverse relationship between tea intake and UC has been reported in one epidemiological study (Kemberling, Hampton et al. 2003). In order to settle the ongoing controversy, NCI-sponsored phase 2 and 3 clinical trials are in progress (National Cancer Institute).

4.4 Soy

Soy products have potential apoptotic and anti-angiogenic actions attributable to their high isoflavone content (Su, Yeh et al. 2000).Their role in UC chemoprevention, unlike in prostate cancer, has yet to be elucidated. Contrary Su and group reported in a Singapore-based population study an increased UC incidence associated with high consumption of soy food (95% CI, 1.1-5.1) (Su, Yeh et al. 2000).This risk was independent of smoking. There is no data yet favoring recommendation of soy for chemoprevention in UC.

5. Bladder cancer chemoprevention strategies: Pharmacologic agents

5.1 Vitamins and supplements

Researchers have long regarded vitamins and the so-called micronutrients as ideal agents for primary chemoprevention for human cancer. For the reasons discussed earlier primary chemoprevention in human bladder cancer lacks an effective agent as well as evidence-based data to encourage wide clinical practice.

5.1.1 Vitamin A and analogues

Epidemiologic data in humans regarding the efficacy of Vitamin A are inconsistent. Many reports have suggested a therapeutic benefit from retinoid supplements. Data includes the SEER database controlled study, which compared 1592 UC participants to a matched neighborhood controls (Castelao, Yuan et al. 2004). Carotenoids were found to be beneficial in previous or current smokers. Authors using fenretinide in a randomized study failed to demonstrate the difference in tumor detection by flow cytometry between treatment and placebo arms in a sample of 99 participants (Decensi, Torrisi et al. 2000). Fenretinide is a synthetic derivative of Vitamin A which is FDA approved for the treatment of macular degeneration, and cystic fibrosis; and it has been investigated for use in cancer chemoprevention. Studer and group treated 90 Ta and T1 patients after transurethral resection with etretinate (Studer, Jenzer et al. 1995). They observed that time to first tumor occurrence was the same in both treatment and placebo groups, however, time to second tumor occurrence was lower for treatment group versus placebo (20.3 v 12.7 months, P>0.006). The data suggests that the agent acts not on established bladder cancer, but acts to prevent new cancer. Vitamin A overdose is known to cause low blood pressure, fever, and pulmonary insufficiency. Synthetic formulations of vitamin A are reported to show less significant adverse events (Sporn and Lippman 2003).

Sabichi and colleagues reported on a negative Phase III chemoprevention trial that showed that Fenretinide was well tolerated but failed to show a significant reduction in high incidence of recurrent non-muscle invasive urothelial bladder cancer (Sabichi, Lerner et al. 2008). The authors speculated that variable of dosing and scheduling could have affected the clinical results. However, data from other randomized clinical studies in contralateral breast cancer, ovarian cancer and oral premalignancy suggested preventative benefit of fenretinide in these malignancies (Sporn and Lippman 2003). In another clinical prevention trial in bladder cancer, this agent was reported as being less toxic and more efficacious than the retinoid etretinate (Sabichi, Lerner et al. 2008).

5.1.2 Vitamin B6 (Pyridoxine)

Vitamin B6 has been evaluated in patients with history of recurrent UC. The Veterans Administration Study by Byar and group showed that Pyridoxine provided the best benefit (P=0.03) in a 3-ARM trial of intravesical thiotepa, Pyridoxine and placebo in 121 patients with history of recurrent NMIUBC (Byar and Blackard 1977). The authors also showed that the efficacy of Pyridoxine was equivalent to that of thiotepa. The theory was that Pyridoxine would correct the abnormalities of Tryptophan metabolism often found in patients with bladder cancer. This data was not supported in a large study of 291 patients in the EORTC trial of Pyridoxine versus placebo with neither treatment showing any benefit in preventing occurrence or recurrence of UC (Newling, Robinson et al. 1995).

5.1.3 Vitamin C

Ascorbic acid (Vitamin C) is a potent antioxidant reported in human epidemiological studies to prevent UC (Shibata, Paganini-Hill et al. 1992; Michaud, Spiegelman et al. 2000). The effect is also thought to be dose dependent, with improved benefit associated with higher consumption (Shibata, Paganini-Hill et al. 1992; Michaud, Spiegelman et al. 2000). Favorable reports are inconsistent in large cohorts.

5.1.4 Vitamin E

Vitamin E is another antioxidant and is capable of reducing the carcinogenic N-nitroso compounds. Vitamin E has been reported in multiple studies to show benefit in reducing incidence of UC (Bruemmer, White et al. 1996; Michaud, Spiegelman et al. 2000). However, a meta-analysis by Miller and associates showed a potential increased in all-cause mortality associated with Vitamin E consumption (Miller, Pastor-Barriuso et al. 2005). This finding has dampened enthusiasm in the use of Vitamin E in chemoprevention for UC.

5.1.5 Selenium

There is no data yet suggesting a chemopreventive role for this oligoelement in UC.

5.1.6 Mega dose vitamins

Vitamins and dietary supplements/modifications have received slightly skewed publicity as alternative protective strategies against bladder cancer (Kamat and Lamm 2002). Individual vitamins including Vitamin A, and its analogues, Vitamin B6 (pyridoxine), Vitamin C, Vitamin E have been studied individually, reported and proposed as dietary supplements to prevent bladder cancer.as discussed above (Byar and Blackard 1977; Shibata, Paganini-Hill et al. 1992; Newling, Robinson et al. 1995; Studer, Jenzer et al. 1995; Decensi, Torrisi et al. 2000; Kamat and Lamm 2002; Castelao, Yuan et al. 2004; Miller, Pastor-Barriuso et al. 2005; Sabichi, Lerner et al. 2008). However, Lamm et al. combined mega doses of Vitamins A(40,000U), B6(100mg), C(2000 mg), E(400U) and Zinc (90mg) in a randomized 2x2 factorial design study in which 65 patients were randomized to receive intraderrmal BCG (Lamm, Riggs et al. 1994). Participants who demonstrated a response to induction intravesical BCG, were randomized to receive either Megadose vitamins or recommended daily allowance (RDA).The use of intradermal BCG did not appear to affect the clinical outcome. The Mega-dose vitamins treatment group showed a 50% reduction in overall NMIUBC recurrence at 4 years, The fact that there was no reduction in tumor recurrence rate in the Megadose vitamins group in the first 10 months, would suggest that these supplements/agents do not affect existing tumors but hinder the formation of new tumors.

5.2 Difluoromethylornithine

Difluoromethylornithine (DFMO) is a competitive inhibitor of ornithine decarboxylase (ODC) which is an enzyme that induces polyamine production necessary for tumor growth. A negative study was reported by Messing and associates who observed that daily oral supplementation of difluoromethylornithine (DFMO) compared with placebo, did not prevent frequent recurrence and progression of low grade NMIBC in patients who had been completely resected at enrollment (Messing, Kim et al. 2006).

5.3 COX Inhibitors

NSAID inhibit the cyclooxygenase (COX) enzyme, which breaks down arachidonic acid into leukotrienes and prostaglandins. Prostaglandin-2 can enhance cell proliferation, angiogenesis, and inhibit apoptosis (Sabichi and Lippman; Okey, Harper et al. 1998; Sporn and Lippman 2003). In vitro evidence suggests that there is an over expression of COX 2 isoform in UC (Okey, Harper et al. 1998; Sporn and Lippman 2003). Theoretically, COX 2 isoform inhibitors could be used in chemoprevention of UC. Castelao and colleagues reported on a population-based, case-control study, in which they evaluated non-steroidal anti-inflammatory drugs (NSAIDs) in NMIUBC (Castelao, Yuan et al. 2000). This study found a 19% decrease in UC risk in those patients treated with oral agents, except those patients treated with phenacetine and pyrazolone derivatives (Castelao, Yuan et al. 2000). Therefore, COX-2 remains a very viable target for future evaluation in bladder cancer chemoprevention.

Preventive Strategy	Methodology	Mechanism	Published studies	Significance	Current status
Fluid intake	Mailing Questionnaires	Increased fluid intake results in lowered cumulative exposure of urothelium to carcinogens with *reduced risk*	The Health Professional Follow up Study (n = 47,903)	High	Recommended (Level 4 evidence; Grade C recommendation)
Fat and calorie intake	Population based study (SEER) and meta-analysis of 36 studies evaluating 6 dietary variables in relation to UC	2-fold increase in cancer with increased fat consumption	Riboli et al & SEER studies: positive correlation; Health Professionals follow up study: no correlation	Intermediate	Recommended (Level 2 evidence; Grade B recommendation)
Green Tea	Epidemiological	Polyphenols contents of green tea are potent antioxidants; also inhibit ornithine decarboxylase which is an enzyme that promotes tumor proliferation via nucleic acid regulation; a *weak inverse relationship between tea intake and UC*	NCI-sponsored phase 2 and 3 clinical trials are in progress	Low	Recommended (Level 4 evidence; Grade C recommendation)

Preventive Strategy	Methodology	Mechanism	Published studies	Significance	Current status
Soy	Population based	potential apoptotic and action attributable to the high isoflavone content; *no data yet favoring recommendation*	Singapore-based population study	Very low	Not recommended
Smoking	Population based	Smoking cessation correlates with decreased incidence	Population based	High - most cost-effective measure in bladder cancer prevention strategy	Highly recommended (Level 3 evidence; Grade B recommendation)
Vitamin A	compared 1592 UC participants to a matched neighborhood controls	Agent does act not on established bladder cancer, but *prevents new cancer*	SEER database controlled study	Low - lacks an effective agent as well as evidence-based data to encourage wide clinical practice	Recommended (Level 3 evidence; Grade B recommendation)
Vitamin B6	3-arm trial; placebo controlled trial	Pyridoxine provided the best benefit (P=0.03) in a 3-Arm trial of intravesical thiotepa, placebo, and Pyridoxine; however, this data was not supported in EORCT trial (n=291) of Pyridoxine versus placebo, *both showing no benefit in preventing occurrence or reoccurrence*	The Veterans Administration Study (Byar et al)	Intermediate	Not recommended
Vitamin C	Human epidemiological studies	potent antioxidant; *effect dose dependent, better with higher consumption*	Large cohort studies	Inconsistent	Not recommended

Preventive Strategy	Methodology	Mechanism	Published studies	Significance	Current status
Vitamin E	meta-analysis	antioxidant capable of reducing carcinogenic N-nitroso compounds in urothelium	Miller et al.	Potential increase in all-cause mortality with Vitamin E consumption	Not recommended
Selenium	No data	no data yet suggesting a chemopreventive role for this oligoelement in UC	No data	N/A	Not recommended
Megadose vitamins	randomized 2x2 design study in which 65 patients were randomized to received intraderrmal BCG or not, and also randomized after response to induction intravesical BCG to receive Megadose vitamins versus daily recommended daily allowance	Possible anti-oxidant role	Small trial from a single institution	Mega-dose vitamins-treated group showed a 50% reduction in overall NMIBC recurrence at 4 years	Not recommended
Difluoromethylornithine (DFMO)	Messing et al	DFMO is a competitive inhibitor of *ornithine decarboxylase* that induces polyamine production necessary for tumor growth	Negative study	daily oral supplementation vs. placebo, did not prevent recurrence and progression of low grade NMIBC following prior TUR-BT	Not recommended

Preventive Strategy	Methodology	Mechanism	Published studies	Significance	Current status
COX inhibitors	Castelao et al.	Prostaglandin-2 can enhance cell proliferation, angiogenesis, and inhibit apoptosis. In vitro evidence suggests over expression of COX 2 isoform in UC	a population-based, case-control study - NSAIDs in NMIUBC showed a19% decrease in UC risk in those treated with oral NSAIDs (except phenacetine and pyrazolone derivatives)	COX-2 remains a very viable target in bladder cancer chemopreventi on	Recommended (non-evidence based)

Table 1. Summary of Reports (discussed above) of various Chemopreventative Strategies (refs:28-51)

6. Future research and experimental cancer chemoprevention

Research continues intensely in the evaluation of pharmaceutical agents for chemoprevention in bladder cancer. However, dietary supplement, multivitamins and phytochemicals/botanical agents are being evaluated in the prevention of many human cancers (Byar and Blackard 1977; Shibata, Paganini-Hill et al. 1992; Lamm, Riggs et al. 1994; Newling, Robinson et al. 1995; Studer, Jenzer et al. 1995; Castelao, Yuan et al. 2000; Decensi, Torrisi et al. 2000; Michaud, Spiegelman et al. 2000; Kamat and Lamm 2002; Castelao, Yuan et al. 2004; Miller, Pastor-Barriuso et al. 2005; Messing, Kim et al. 2006; Sabichi, Lerner et al. 2008). Investigators have reported on results of screening strategies for synthetic pharmaceuticals in an experimental bladder cancer prevention model using the chemically-induced rat bladder tumor model (Sindhwani, Hampton et al. 2001; Lubet, You et al. 2006; Park, Kim et al. 2006; Tian, Wang et al. 2008; Parada, Reis et al. 2011). They reported that low dose aspirin and resveratrol were least effective in preventing large tumor formation, while naproxen and Iressa were most effective (Lubet, You et al. 2006).

In recent years there has been a substantial interest in the application of botanically derived phytochemicals to reduce the incidence of variety of human tumors. Intense research is ongoing to provide evidence-based recommendations to incorporate plant foods or botanical products or dietary modifications into the practice of clinical cancer chemoprevention. There is the salient speculation that Curcumin, a very popular Indian food spice, derived from the rhizome plant called curcuma longa Linn (Zingiberaceae), has been responsible for lower incidence of urothelial malignancies (Sindhwani, Hampton et al. 2001; Tian, Wang et al. 2008)and lower rate of colorectal cancer (Tian, Wang et al. 2008) in the populations that consume Curcumin as a staple part of their diet (Sindhwani, Hampton et al. 2001; Tian, Wang et al. 2008). Investigators have reported on Curcumin induced apoptosis in MBT-2 cells[56] G2/M cell cycle arrest in T-24 cells (Sindhwani, Hampton et al. 2001; Tian, Wang et al. 2008). Curcumin inhibition of intravesical tumor implant in mouse model (Sindhwani, Hampton et al. 2001) and prevention of OH-BBN induced bladder carcinogenesis in rodent, as well as inhibition of tumor development and growth in an intravesical murine bladder model (Sindhwani, Hampton et al. 2001; Tian, Wang et al. 2008).

Seventy-five percent of all pharmaceuticals were discovered by studying the use of plants in traditional medicine. Of the 92 antitumor drugs approved by the FDA between 1983 and 1994, 62 (67%) were either of natural origin or based on a natural compound (Chung, Anscher et al. 2001).

7. Conclusions and clinical practice suggestions

Bladder cancer is a common, but serious health problem globally. It is immensely impacted by environmental carcinogens, tobacco smokes, and infectious etiologies in endemic areas. The bladder urothelial cancer special features which include its susceptibility; carcinogenesis; frequent recurrences, and clinical presentation favor it as an ideal cancer for chemoprevention. Unfortunately, in bladder cancer there are still no definite interventions that have been shown to be effective, and research in this area has yielded no evidence-based data to inform on strategies for systematic practice of bladder cancer prevention. The positive data from the clinical trials with vitamins individually or in combinations suggest that these agents might act not on established bladder cancer, but act to prevent occurring of new cancers, probably by hindering promotion of altered cells to overt cancer. Cessation of smoking will always remain the lofty but impractical goal of prevention strategies in urothelial bladder cancer; however, a plausible paradigm would suggest a chemoprevention strategy that should begin with the population approach that advocates a dietary program of increased consumption of fruits and vegetables which have been reported to reduce general cancer risk. The at-risk individual would embark on additional programs to reduce/eliminate the intensity of cumulative exposure to the carcinogens, dilution and elimination of bladder content by drinking plenty of water and urinating frequently, followed by introduction of the specific chemopreventive agent(s), probably in combination with the vitamins.

8. References

American Cancer Society. "Global Cancer Facts and Figures." Retrieved July 22, 2011, from http://www.acscan.org/tobaccoreports.

American Cancer Society. (2010). "Cancer Facts and Figures 2010." Retrieved July 15, 2010, from http://www.seer.cancer.gov/statfacts/html/urinb.html.

Botteman, M. F., C. L. Pashos, et al. (2003). "The health economics of bladder cancer: a comprehensive review of the published literature." *Pharmacoeconomics* 21(18): 1315-1330.

Bruemmer, B., E. White, et al. (1996). "Nutrient intake in relation to bladder cancer among middle-aged men and women." *Am J Epidemiol* 144(5): 485-495.

Byar, D. and C. Blackard (1977). "Comparisons of placebo, pyridoxine, and topical thiotepa in preventing recurrence of stage I bladder cancer." *Urology* 10(6): 556-561.

Cancer Treatment of America. "World-Class Cancer Center." Retrieved January, 2011, from http://www.cancercenter.com/carethatneverquits.

Castelao, J. E., J. M. Yuan, et al. (2004). "Carotenoids/vitamin C and smoking-related bladder cancer." *Int J Cancer* 110(3): 417-423.

Castelao, J. E., J. M. Yuan, et al. (2000). "Non-steroidal anti-inflammatory drugs and bladder cancer prevention." *Br J Cancer* 82(7): 1364-1369.

Chung, T., M. Anscher, et al. (2001). The role of Hypericum Perforatum in Cancer Research. *Global Science Books.* 5.

Dalbagni, D. and H. Herr (2000). Current clinical questions concerning intravesical bladder cancer. *Urologic Clinic of North America.* Loughlin. 27.

Decensi, A., R. Torrisi, et al. (2000). "Randomized trial of fenretinide in superficial bladder cancer using DNA flow cytometry as an intermediate end point." *Cancer Epidemiol Biomarkers Prev* 9(10): 1071-1078.

Dietrich, H. and B. Dietrich (2001). "Ludwig Rehn (1849-1930)--pioneering findings on the aetiology of bladder tumours." *World J Urol* 19(2): 151-153.

Droller, M. (2006). Introduction. *Textbook of bladder cancer.* S. P. Lerner and M. P. Schoenberg.

Fradet, Y., H. B. Grossman, et al. (2007). "A comparison of hexaminolevulinate fluorescence cystoscopy and white light cystoscopy for the detection of carcinoma in situ in patients with bladder cancer: a phase III, multicenter study." *J Urol* 178(1): 68-73; discussion 73.

Geoffroy-Perez, B. and S. Cordier (2001). "Fluid consumption and the risk of bladder cancer: results of a multicenter case-control study." *Int J Cancer* 93(6): 880-887.

Grasso, M. (2008). "Bladder cancer: a major public health issue." *European Urology Supplements* 7(7): 510-515.

Haack, S., S. Treccani, et al. (2000). *Arsenic concentration and selected geochemical characteristics for ground water and aquifer materials in southeastern Michigan,* US Department of the Interior, US Geological Survey.

Hedelin, H., S. Holmang, et al. (2002). "The cost of bladder tumour treatment and follow-up." *Scand J Urol Nephrol* 36(5): 344-347.

Henderson, B. D., TJ (1992). "How does photodynamic therapy work?" *Photochem Photobiol* 55(1): 145-157.

Hong, Y. M. and K. R. Loughlin (2008). "Economic impact of tumor markers in bladder cancer surveillance." *Urology* 71(1): 131-135.

Jichlinski, P., L. Guillou, et al. (2003). "Hexyl aminolevulinate fluorescence cystoscopy: new diagnostic tool for photodiagnosis of superficial bladder cancer--a multicenter study." *J Urol* 170(1): 226-229.

Kamat, A. and D. L. Lamm (2002). Chemoprevention of bladder cancer. *Urologic Clinics of North America.* Loughlin. 29.

Karl, A. Z., D; Staddler, T. (2010). Influence of photodynamic diagnosis on recurrence rates of T1G3 bladder cancer. *American Urological Association.* San Francisco, CA.

Kemberling, J. K., J. A. Hampton, et al. (2003). "Inhibition of bladder tumor growth by the green tea derivative epigallocatechin-3-gallate." *J Urol* 170(3): 773-776.

Kim, M.-J., J. Nriagu, et al. (2000). "Carbonate ions and arsenic dissolution by groundwater." *Environmental Science and Technology* 34(15): 3094-3100.

Lamm, D. L., B. A. Blumenstein, et al. (1995). "Randomized intergroup comparison of bacillus calmette-guerin immunotherapy and mitomycin C chemotherapy prophylaxis in superficial transitional cell carcinoma of the bladder a southwest oncology group study." *Urol Oncol* 1(3): 119-126.

Lamm, D. L., D. R. Riggs, et al. (1994). "Megadose vitamins in bladder cancer: a double-blind clinical trial." *J Urol* 151(1): 21-26.

Lattouf, J. B. (2009). "Chemoprevention in bladder cancer: What's new?" *Can Urol Assoc J* 3(6 Suppl 4): S184-187.

Lubet, R., M. You, et al. (2006). Chemopreventive effects of Iressa against methylnitrosourea (MNU) induced mammary cancers and 4-hydroxybutyl*butyl)-nitrosamine (OH-BBN) induced urinary bladder cancers. *American Association of Cancer Research*

Messing, E., K. M. Kim, et al. (2006). "Randomized prospective phase III trial of difluoromethylornithine vs placebo in preventing recurrence of completely resected low risk superficial bladder cancer." *J Urol* 176(2): 500-504.

Michaud, D. S., D. Spiegelman, et al. (1999). "Fluid intake and the risk of bladder cancer in men." *N Engl J Med* 340(18): 1390-1397.

Michaud, D. S., D. Spiegelman, et al. (2000). "Prospective study of dietary supplements, macronutrients, micronutrients, and risk of bladder cancer in US men." *Am J Epidemiol* 152(12): 1145-1153.

Miller, E. R., 3rd, R. Pastor-Barriuso, et al. (2005). "Meta-analysis: high-dosage vitamin E supplementation may increase all-cause mortality." *Ann Intern Med* 142(1): 37-46.

National Cancer Institute. "Clinical Trials." Retrieved July 18, 2011, from http://www.cancer.gov/CLINICALTRIALS.

Newling, D. W., M. R. Robinson, et al. (1995). "Tryptophan metabolites, pyridoxine (vitamin B6) and their influence on the recurrence rate of superficial bladder cancer. Results of a prospective, randomised phase III study performed by the EORTC GU Group. EORTC Genito-Urinary Tract Cancer Cooperative Group." *Eur Urol* 27(2): 110-116.

Okey, A., P. Harper, et al. (1998). Chemical and radiation carcinogenesis. *The basic science of oncology*. I. Tannock and R. P. Hill. New York, McGraw-Hill, Health Professions Division: xii, 539 p.

Oosterlinck, W., K. H. Kurth, et al. (1993). "A prospective European Organization for Research and Treatment of Cancer Genitourinary Group randomized trial comparing transurethral resection followed by a single intravesical instillation of epirubicin or water in single stage Ta, T1 papillary carcinoma of the bladder." *J Urol* 149(4): 749-752.

Parada, B., F. Reis, et al. (2011). "Inhibition of bladder tumour growth by sirolimus in an experimental carcinogenesis model." *BJU Int* 107(1): 135-143.

Park, C., G. Y. Kim, et al. (2006). "Induction of G2/M arrest and inhibition of cyclooxygenase-2 activity by curcumin in human bladder cancer T24 cells." *Oncol Rep* 15(5): 1225-1231.

Prout, G. R., Jr., B. A. Barton, et al. (1992). "Treated history of noninvasive grade 1 transitional cell carcinoma. The National Bladder Cancer Group." *J Urol* 148(5): 1413-1419.

Riboli, E., C. A. Gonzalez, et al. (1991). "Diet and bladder cancer in Spain: a multi-centre case-control study." *Int J Cancer* 49(2): 214-219.

Sabichi, A. L., S. P. Lerner, et al. (2008). "Phase III prevention trial of fenretinide in patients with resected non-muscle-invasive bladder cancer." *Clin Cancer Res* 14(1): 224-229.

Sabichi, A. L. and S. M. Lippman Chemoprevention of superficial bladder cancer. *Chemoprevention strategies*.

Shibata, A., A. Paganini-Hill, et al. (1992). "Intake of vegetables, fruits, beta-carotene, vitamin C and vitamin supplements and cancer incidence among the elderly: a prospective study." *Br J Cancer* 66(4): 673-679.

Sievert, K. D., B. Amend, et al. (2009). "Economic aspects of bladder cancer: what are the benefits and costs?" *World J Urol* 27(3): 295-300.

Sindhwani, P., J. A. Hampton, et al. (2001). "Curcumin prevents intravesical tumor implantation of the MBT-2 tumor cell line in C3H mice." *J Urol* 166(4): 1498-1501.

Sporn, M. and S. M. Lippman (2003). Chemoprevention in cancer. *Cancer medicine 6*. D. W. Kufe, J. F. Holland, E. Frei and American Cancer Society. Hamilton, Ont.; Lewiston, NY, BC Decker: 377-388.

Steele, V. E., G. J. Kelloff, et al. (2000). "Comparative chemopreventive mechanisms of green tea, black tea and selected polyphenol extracts measured by in vitro bioassays." *Carcinogenesis* 21(1): 63-67.

Steineck, G., U. Hagman, et al. (1990). "Vitamin A supplements, fried foods, fat and urothelial cancer. A case-referent study in Stockholm in 1985-87." *Int J Cancer* 45(6): 1006-1011.

Steinmaus, C. M., S. Nunez, et al. (2000). "Diet and bladder cancer: a meta-analysis of six dietary variables." *Am J Epidemiol* 151(7): 693-702.

Studer, U. E., S. Jenzer, et al. (1995). "Adjuvant treatment with a vitamin A analogue (etretinate) after transurethral resection of superficial bladder tumors. Final analysis of a prospective, randomized multicenter trial in Switzerland." *Eur Urol* 28(4): 284-290.

Su, S. J., T. M. Yeh, et al. (2000). "The potential of soybean foods as a chemoprevention approach for human urinary tract cancer." *Clin Cancer Res* 6(1): 230-236.

Tian, B., Z. Wang, et al. (2008). "Effects of curcumin on bladder cancer cells and development of urothelial tumors in a rat bladder carcinogenesis model." *Cancer Lett* 264(2): 299-308.

Trevisanato, S. I. and Y. I. Kim (2000). "Tea and health." *Nutr Rev* 58(1): 1-10.

Uchida, A., H. Yonou, et al. (2007). "Intravesical instillation of bacille Calmette-Guerin for superficial bladder cancer: cost-effectiveness analysis." *Urology* 69(2): 275-279.

Weber, W. W. (1987). *The acetylator genes and drug response.* New York, Oxford University Press.

Welch, A., D. Westjohn, et al. (2000). "Arsenic in ground water of the United States-- occurrence and geochemistry." *Ground Water* 38(4): 589-604.

Part 2

Metastatic Disease

3

Chemotherapy for Metastatic Disease

Takehiro Sejima, Shuichi Morizane, Akihisa Yao,
Tadahiro Isoyama and Atsushi Takenaka
Division of Urology, Department of Surgery, Tottori University Faculty of Medicine
Japan

1. Introduction

Bladder cancer occurs with a relatively high incidence in industrial nations. For example, bladder cancer is the fourth most common type of cancer in American men. The estimated U.S. incidence in 2008 was 68,810 cases and the mortality was 14,100 cases (Jemal et al., 2008). Of newly diagnosed bladder cancer cases, approximately 70% - 80% will present with non muscle-invasive disease. Among such cases, 50% - 70% will recur, and 10% - 30% will progress to muscle-invasive disease (Soloway et al., 2002; Saad et al., 2002). Radical cystectomy with or without chemotherapy is the standard therapy for muscle-invasive disease; however, some patients will experience metastatic relapse after radical surgery. A few patients present with metastatic disease upon their initial presentation at the hospital. Such advanced bladder cancer remains an incurable terminal disease, and accounts for 3% of the cancer-related mortality in the United States. Deaths from bladder cancer are mainly related to distant spread; hence, prevention of metastatic disease remains a crucial goal in this disease. Systemic chemotherapy achieves palliation, survival benefit, and occasional long-term remissions. For the last two decades, cisplatin-based combination therapies have evolved as the standard. The MVAC regimen (Sternberg et al., 1988) was reported to demonstrate an impressive complete remission rate of 37% in advanced urothelial carcinoma (UC), and in a subsequent comparative study was found to be superior to the single agent cisplatin (Saxman et al., 1997). In this chapter, we review the recent progress in chemotherapeutic regimens not only for advanced bladder cancer, but also for advanced UC in the upper urinary tract. We also show current data on the efficacy of combination therapy with gemcitabine and platinum anti-cancer drugs, which is mainly used as a second-line treatment in our institution.

2. The first successful chemotherapeutic regimen for advanced Urothelial Carcinoma (UC)

Despite recent developments in anti-cancer drugs, advanced UC remains an incurable disease, with a median survival time of only 12 to 14 months (Jemal et al., 2003). The most reliable treatment option for advanced UC is considered to be combination chemotherapy including a platinum anti-cancer drug. The combination chemotherapy regimen of methotrexate / vinblastine / doxorubicin / cisplatin (MVAC) as reported originally by Sternberg (Sternberg et al., 1988) is currently being used worldwide with superior efficacy. However, MVAC treatment is associated with substantial toxicities and has a toxic death rate of approximately

3 - 4% (Sternberg et al., 1989; Loehrer et al., 1992). Therefore, the need for an alternative less toxic combination chemotherapy that can provide efficacy similar or superior to the MVAC regimen has been identified. Gemcitabine, a nucleoside analogue, has demonstrated activity against a range of solid tumors, including metastatic UC (Gatzemeier et al., Moore, 1996; Stadler et al., 1997). In particular, gemcitabine alone has yielded a response rate of 23 - 29%, with a complete response rate of 4 - 13%, in both previously treated and untreated metastatic UC patients (Sternberg, 2000). The good activity and toxicity profiles of single-agent gemcitabine treatment and its synergism with cisplatin in pre-clinical models (Peters et al., 1995) led to the development of this combination for the treatment of advanced UC. After obtaining results from phase 2 trials of combination therapy comprising gemcitabine plus cisplatin (GC) as first- or second-line treatment for UC, von der Maase et al. published a large multinational phase 3 trial comparing MVAC with GC therapy, with a total of 405 patients accrued (von der Maase et al., 2000). The final results show that the two regimens are similar in terms of response rate, time to progression and survival. However, the GC combination showed a better safety profile and tolerability than MVAC. The representative randomized trials on MVAC and GC are summarized in Table 1. Carboplatin shares a common mechanism of action with cisplatin, but the two have different pharmacokinetic and dose-limiting toxicities (Van Echo et al., 1989). Patients with UC are often elderly, and frequently have clinical or subclinical renal function impairment. Thus, the substitution of carboplatin for cisplatin offers a promising alternative for these patients. There have been several phase 2 reports showing that gemcitabine / carboplatin achieved clinical results equivalent to those of GC (Xu et al., 2007; Dogliotti et al., 2007). It can thus be speculated that the combination of gemcitabine plus a platinum anti-cancer drug (cisplatin or carboplatin) is currently being used worldwide in the treatment of advanced UC.

Therapy	No. of Patients	Response Rate/PFS	Median Survival	Hazard Ratio/P value
MVAC (Sternberg)	263 (MVAC + High dose MVAC)	50 % (CR 9 %) Med PFS 8.1 months	14.9 months (2 year survival 26.2 %) (5 year survival 13.5 %)	HR = 0.76 P = 0.042
High dose MVAC (Sternberg)		64 % (CR 21 %) Med PFS 9.5 months	15.1 months (2 year survival 36.7 %) (5 year survival 21.8 %)	
Cisplatin (Saxman)	122	PR 12 % Med TTP 10 months	8.2 months	P = 0.0002
MVAC (Saxman)	133	PR 39 % Med TTP 4.3 months	12.5 months	
MVAC (Von der Maase)	202	46 % Med PFS 8.3 months	15.2 months	P = 0.75 HR = 0.042
GC (Von der Maase)	203	49 % Med. PFS 7.7 months	14.0 months	

Table 1. Summary of representative randomized trials exploring chemotherapy in metastatic urothelial cancer

3. The efficacy and safety of combination chemotherapy with gemcitabine and a platinum anti-cancer drug. A regimen mainly used as second-line chemotherapy for patients with advanced UC at Tottori university hospital

Our original data regarding the effects of combination therapy with gemcitabine plus platinum anti-cancer drug as second-line chemotherapy for cases of advanced UC are described below. These data were gathered mainly as a result of limitations in the Japanese insurance system, which until recently did not cover the use of gemcitabine for the treatment of UC. That is, before February 2009, the use of gemcitabine was not allowed for general use in Japan, and thus only referral academic institutions such as ours were able to conduct gemcitabine therapy. Because the incurable rate is still high in advanced UC patients to date in spite of the medical progress of many anti-cancer drugs in Japan and other countries, physicians often encounter patients with advanced UC who need to undergo more than one kind of chemotherapy. Therefore sequential data of second-line chemotherapy like ours is considered to be useful for urological oncologists worldwide. In this paragraph, the therapeutic data for cases of upper urinary tract UC are also included. This book is of course about bladder cancer; however, it is often difficult to isolate the therapeutic data for bladder cancer from the data for all cases of UC. Therefore, we regret that we cannot describe the results for bladder cancer data specifically.

3.1 Patients' characteristics

From December 2004 until September 2011, 30 patients received the combination chemotherapy of gemcitabine plus a platinum anti-cancer drug (cisplatin or carboplatin) at

Characteristics	No. of patients (%)	
No. of patients	30	(100%)
Median age, yr (range)	72	(52-83)
Gender		
Male	23	(76.7%)
Female	7	(23.3%)
Previous therapy		
None	4	(13.3%)
Methotrexate/Epirubicin/Cisplatin (MEC)	14	(46.7%)
Methotrexate/Epirubicin/Carboplatin (modified MEC)	9	(30.0%)
Etoposide/ Cisplatin	1	(3.3%)
Radiation + Intraarterial chemotherapy	2	(6.7%)
Primary urothelial tumor site		
Bladder	9	(30.0%)
Renal pelvis ~ ureter	21	(70.0%)
Advanced disease at first visit	7	(23.3%)
Recurrence after surgery for primary tumor	23	(76.7%)
Site of metastasis or recurrence, or invasion from primary tumor		
Lung	6	(20.0%)
Lymph node	18	(60.0%)
Local recurrence	5	(16.7%)
Bone	2	(6.7%)

Table 2. Patient characteristics

our institution. All patients were evaluated for efficacy and for toxicity. The pretreatment characteristics of the patients are listed in Table 2. 23 patients (77%) had previously received combination chemotherapy of methotrexate / epirubicin / cisplatin (MEC).

3.2 Treatment plan

In the first cycle of the therapy, the creatinine clearance (Ccr) (ml / min) of each patient was measured prior to initiation of the therapy. In the patients with Ccr > 60, cisplatin was administered, while in those with Ccr < 60, carboplatin was administered as the platinum anti-cancer drug. Gemcitabine (1,000 mg / m²) was given by intravenous infusion over 30 – 60 min on days 1, 8, and 15. Cisplatin (70 mg / m²) was given by intravenous infusion over 30 – 60 min on day 2 in the cisplatin group, whereas carboplatin dosed to an AUC of 5 was given by intravenous infusion over 30 – 60 minutes on day 2 in the carboplatin group. Basically, each cycle consisted of 21 days. However, an extension of the days in each cycle was permitted based on the judgment of the physician in charge if any severe adverse events were noted. All toxicities were recorded according to the National Cancer Institute Common Toxicity Criteria (NCI-CTC) version 3.0. Dose adjustment during the treatment was based on hematological and non-hematological assessment of toxicities. In the hematological assessment of toxicities, leukocyte and platelet counts were generally measured weekly. For cases where leukocytes < 2,000 / mm³ or platelets < 75,000 / mm³, or where there was evidence of bleeding, gemcitabine was omitted. No new cycle was started unless leukocytes were > 2,000 / mm³ and platelets were > 75,000 / mm³. The platinum anti-cancer drug dose was reduced by 50% for grade 2 neurotoxicity, omitted for grade 3, and stopped for grade 4. For renal toxicity, the dose of platinum anti-cancer drug was reduced by 50% for Ccr 50 – 59, and omitted for Ccr < 50. For other grade 3 non-hematological toxicities (except nausea, vomiting, and alopecia), gemcitabine and platinum anti-cancer drug doses were reduced by 50% or omitted per the physician in charge. For grade 4 toxicities, doses were reduced by 50% or stopped (unless the patient was responding to the therapy).

3.3 Dose administration

The median number of consecutive cycles per patient was 3 (range: 1 – 7). 16 patients (53%) underwent more than 3 cycles of the therapy. Cisplatin was administered in 12 patients (40%), while carboplatin was administered in 18 patients (60%) as the platinum anti-cancer drug (Table 3).

3.4 Efficacy

All 30 patients were assessed with regard to clinical outcome and treatment efficacy according to RECIST criteria at the end of the study. With regard to clinical outcome (Table 3), we observed 2 (7%) cases of complete response (CR) and 7 (23%) cases of partial response (PR), with an overall response rate (ORR) of 30%. The visceral field of metastasis or relapse in patients of CR and PR was the lungs in 3 cases, lymph nodes in 5 cases, and local relapse (post-nephroureterectomy) in 1 case. There were no cases with responses in other visceral fields such as bone. Stable disease (SD) was identified in 10 patients (33%), and progressive disease (PD) in 9 patients (30%). 2 patients (7%) were not evaluated. The median time to follow-up was 11.7 months (range: 0.8 – 65.8 months). The median overall survival (OS) was 11.1 months. Kaplan-Meier curves for OS are shown in Fig. 1.

		No. of patients (%)
No. of chemotherapy cycles	1	6 (20.0)
	2	8 (26.7)
	3	10 (33.3)
	More than 4	6 (20.0)
Platinum drug	Cisplatin	12 (40.0)
	Carboplatin	18 (60.0)
Efficacy according to RECIST	CR	2 (6.7)
	PR	7 (23.3)
	SD	10 (33.3)
	PD	9 (30.0)
	NE	2 (6.7)
Outcome	NED	2 (6.7)
	Alive with cancer	8 (26.7)
	Dead due to cancer	20 (66.6)

Table 3. Treatment profile and efficacy

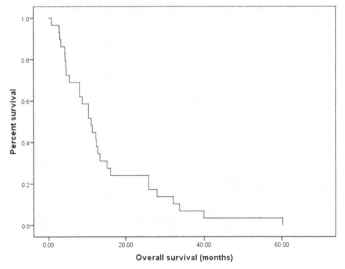

Fig. 1. Overall survival rate of all 30 patients with advance UC treated at Tottori University Hospital

3.5 Toxicity

Only 1 patient discontinued the therapy simply for reasons of toxicity; this patient showed a Grade 2 allergic reaction to gemcitabine, which was administered on day 15. Since this patient eventually received one whole cycle of the therapy, we assessed the efficacy of the treatment as such. Grade 3 / 4 neutropenia was the most frequent toxicity, occurring in 63% of the patients. Grade 3 / 4 thrombocytopenia was also a frequent toxicity, occurring in 57% of the patients. Grade 3 / 4 non-hematologic toxicities included nausea and vomiting in 1 patient (3%). Major toxicities according to NCI-CTC are summarized in Table 4. No other types of major toxicities such as nephrotoxicity or neurotoxicity were observed in any patients. In order to analyze the cumulative damage due to hematologic side effects, the nadir values of blood counts were analyzed. The nadir values of hemoglobin and the nadir counts of leukocytes and platelet cells in the first cycle were practically the same as those in the other progressive cycles. In other words, hematological toxicities were not enhanced by the progressive repetition of cycles (data not shown).

	No. of patients (%)			
	Grade 1	Grade 2	Grade 3	Grade 4
Neutropenia	4 (13.3)	6 (20.0)	16 (53.3)	3 (10.0)
Anemia	3 (10.0)	13 (43.3)	9 (30.0)	4 (13.3)
Thrombocytopenia	6 (20.0)	4 (13.3)	8 (26.7)	9 (30.0)
Vomiting	3 (10.0)	2 (6.7)	1 (3.3)	0 (0)
Allergy	0 (0)	1 (3.3)	0 (0)	0 (0)

Table 4. Mayor toxicities according to NCI-CTC

3.6 Conclusions
The efficacy of gemcitabine plus a platinum anti-cancer drug as a second-line chemotherapy for advanced UC was found to be modest. The toxicity of the therapy was tolerable despite damage from previous chemotherapy and repeated cycles. The present data, obtained as a result of particular limitations in the medical insurance industry in Japan, will be helpful when considering the best course of second-line chemotherapy for cases of advanced UC in the future.

4. Is there any effective combination chemotherapy except MVAC or GC for advanced UC?
— The combination therapy of methotrexate / epirubicin / cisplatin (MEC) —

The combination chemotherapy of methotrexate, epirubicin and cisplatin (MEC) was mainly developed in Japan for the purpose of establishing a regimen less toxic than MVAC but with equal efficacy. Several academic Japanese institutions including the Japanese Urothelial Cancer Research Group promoted a randomized trial comparing MEC and MVAC (Kuroda et al., 1998). Total of 89 patients were assigned to three groups receiving either standard MEC (S-MEC), dose-intensified MEC (I-MEC) or MVAC. The S-MEC regimen consisted of methotrexate (30 mg / m^2), epirubicin (50 mg / m^2) and cisplatin (100 mg / m^2), and that of the I-MEC regimen was methotrexate (36 mg / m^2), epirubicin (60 mg / m^2) and cisplatin (120 mg / m^2). In both groups, methotrexate was administered on day 1 and 15, epirubicin was administered on day 1, and cisplatin was administered on day 2. In the I-MEC group, G-CSF

(2μg / kg) was administered from day 3 until day 12 routinely. The response rates (CR + PR) were 52% with S-MEC, 76% with I-MEC and 47% with MVAC. All of the adverse events were rendered tolerable in the S-MEC and I-MEC groups through the use of G-CSF agents. We had been utilizing MEC as a first choice therapy until 2008 in our institution because it was less toxic than but as effective as MVAC. As a matter of fact, most of the patients in our study of second-line combination chemotherapy with gemcitabine and the platinum anti-cancer drugs described above had been receiving MEC as the first line chemotherapy at other institutions.

5. Prevention of micro metastasis and effort of tumor reduction by neoadjuvant chemotherapy at radical cystectomy

In T2-4 (invasive) bladder cancer, neoadjuvant chemotherapy with MVAC or cisplatin, methotrexate, and vinblastine has demonstrated significant progression-free survival (PFS) and OS benefit in several randomized trials. One representative trial is the Intergroup 8710 trials reported by Grossman et al. in which cystectomy alone was compared with neoadjuvant MVAC followed by radical cystectomy. The group receiving neoadjuvant chemotherapy had an increased likelihood of eliminating residual cancer in the cystectomy specimen (pT0) and had an associated improved survival. Moreover, neoadjuvant chemotherapy did not adversely affect the patient's chance of undergoing a cystectomy and did not increase the risk of postoperative complications (Grossman et al., 2003). In the combined analysis of 2 Nordic studies, neoadjuvant platinum-based combination chemotherapy was associated with an 8% increase in survival at 5 years (Sherif et al., 2004). A meta-analysis of randomized controlled trials demonstrated a survival benefit to receiving neoadjuvant chemotherapy (Winquist et al., 2004). Carboplatin-based regimens have been evaluated in the neoadjuvant setting only in phase 2 trials, and hence their use in the neoadjuvant or adjuvant setting cannot be recommended (Smith et al., 2008; deVele White et al., 2009). The studies of adjuvant chemotherapy have demonstrated conflicting results. They have had design flaws and small sample sizes and are therefore underpowered to give a conclusive answer regarding the benefits.

6. Other recent chemotherapeutic regimens including taxanes

The taxanes are diterpenes produced by the plants of the genus Taxus (yews), and include such compounds as docetaxel and paclitaxel, the latter of which was originally derived from the Pacific yew tree. The principal mechanism of action of the taxane class of drugs is the disruption of microtubule function. Microtubules are essential to cell division, and taxanes stabilize GDP-bound tubulin in the microtubule, thereby inhibiting the process of cell division. Thus, in essence, taxanes are mitotic inhibitors. Both paclitaxel and docetaxel have been studied as chemotherapeutic agents for metastatic bladder cancer. Paclitaxel-based regimens in combination with either cisplatin or carboplatin have been evaluated with response rates between 16% and 36% and median survival ranging from 6 to 10 months depending on the characteristics of the patients enrolled and whether they are ciplatin-sensitive or a refractory population (Vaishampayan et al., 2005; Uhm et al., 2007). A phase 3 study comparing docetaxel and cisplatin (DC) with G-CSF versus MVAC with G-CSF found MVAC to be more effective than DC for metastatic cancer; MVAC demonstrated both a superior median time to progression (9.4 vs 6.1 months; $P = 0.003$) and median survival time (14.2 vs 9.3 months; $P = 0.026$) (Bamias et al., 2004). Other recent representative reports of taxanes with cisplatin therapy are shown in Table 5. Antifolates such as trimetrexate and premetrexed have been better tolerated with promising response rates and should be promising for future evaluation (Witte et al. 1994; Sweeney et al., 2006). Oxaliplatin-based regimens have been evaluated and also shown to be of modest benefit (Carles et al., 2007).

Author	Previous therapy	Dose (mg / m^2)		No. of Cases	Efficacy (%) (CR + PR)	CR rate (%)	Median survival (M)
		Cisplatin	Taxane				
Dreicer	None	75	175 (P)	52	50	8	10.6
Burch	None	70	135 (P)	34	70	32	13
Sengelov	None	75	75 (D)	25	60	26	13.6
Dimopoulos	None	75	75 (D)	66	52	12	8

P, Paclitaxel; D, Docetaxel

Table 5. Recent representative reports of taxanes with cisplatin therapy for advanced urotherial cancer

7. Role of targeted therapies in bladder cancer

The actual clinical advent of targeted therapies has been slower in UC, as compared to other solid tumors due to large variations in histology worldwide, as well as the difficulty in accruing to clinical trials with this malignancy. Vaishampayan et al. evaluated and reported the frequency of overexpression of Her-2 in bladder cancer and correlated with the Her-2 expression in metastatic sites. Interestingly, the overexpression of her-2 by immunohistochemistry (IHC) (2+ or 3+) was 37% in primary bladder tumor tissue, the expression in metastatic sites such as lymph nodes was 63% and the expression in visceral metastases was 86% (Vaishampayan, 2009). 45% of Her-2/neu-negative primaries had Her-2/neu-positive lymph node metastases, while 92% of Her-2-positive primary tumors were associated with Her-2-positive metastasis. This finding suggested that Her-2 over-expression could be a useful therapeutic target for advanced UC. Hence, a phase 2 trial was conducted and reported evaluating the role of trastuzumab with chemotherapy in metastatic UC. An extremely promising 70% response rate and a favorable median survival of 14 months were noted despite 55% of the patients having visceral metastases (Hussain et al., 2007). Another novel approach using molecular targeted therapy for advanced UC patients is the combination therapy of bevacizumab and chemotherapeutic agents. A phase 2 study of bevacizumab in combination with cisplatin and gemcitabine in metastatic or locally advanced bladder cancer involving 36 patients showed a complete response in 6 (17%), and a partial response in 18 (50%); this combination is now being studied in a phase 3 trial (Dovedi & Davies, 2009; Hahn et al., 2011). Another study with anti-angiogenic therapy is the evaluation of sunitinib in a placebo-controlled double-blind trial with the goal of sustaining or prolonging response, after initial chemo-therapy in advanced bladder cancer (Bradley et al., 2007). Epithelial growth factor receptor has also been identified as an exciting target in UC. The over-expression of EGFR by IHC is noted in about 92% (35 of 38) of the bladder cancer cases at Wayne State University; however, its association with survival outcome has not been established (Bellmunt et al., 2003). Given the possibility of EGFR-targeted therapy, a phase 2 randomized trials of cisplatin and gemcitabine with or without cetuximab (a monoclonal antibody to EGFR) is ongoing as a frontline therapy for metastatic UC. Current and future additional trials of targeted therapy are listed in Table 6.

First line for metastatic disease	Therapy	Organization
(not renal insufficiency)		
Phase II	GC + BVZ	CALGB
Phase II	GC + Sorafenib	MSKCC, EORTC
Phase I	GC + Lapatinib	EORTC
First line metastatic disease		
(renal insufficiency)		
Phase II	GEM + CBDCA + BVZ	MSKCC
Phase II	Sunitinib	SOGUG
Second line		
(single agent)		
Phase II	Sunitinib	MSKCC
Phase II	Sunitinib randum	U. Michigan
Phase II	Sorafenib	PMH / SWOG

GC, gemcitabine + cisplatin; BVZ, bevacizumab; GEM, gemcitabine; CBDCA, carboplatin; CALGB, Cancer and Leukemia Group B; MSKCC, Memorial Sloan-Kettering Cancer Center; EORTC, European Organization for Research and Treatment of Cancer; SOGUG, Spanish Oncology Genitourinary Group; U. Michigan, University of Michigan; PMH, Princess Margaret Hospital; SWOG, Southwest Oncology Group

Table 6. Current and future trial with targeted therapy

8. Conclusions

Since the breakthrough progress of development MVAC chemotherapy by Sternberg for advanced UC patients, the survival of such patients has been prolonged compared with those of untreated patients. However, despite the development of anti-cancer drugs, metastatic bladder cancer is still not considered a curable disease. Numerous efforts to achieve improved curability are going, including investigations into molecular targeted therapy, which has just been developed as a breakthrough treatment for patients with advanced renal cell carcinoma in the same field of urologic oncology.

9. References

Bamias A, Aravantinos G, Deliveliotis C, Bafaloukos D, Kalofonos C, Xiros N, Zervas A, Mitropoulos D, Samantas E, Pectasides D, Papakostas P, Gika D, Kourousis C, Koutras A, Papadimitriou C, Bamias C, Kosmidis P, Dimopoulos MA; Hellenic Cooperative Oncology Group (2004): Docetaxel and cisplatin with granulocyte colony-stimulating factor (G-CSF) versus MVAC with G-CSF in advanced urothelial carcinoma: a multicenter, randomized, phase III study from the Hellenic Cooperative Oncology Group. *J Clin Oncol*: Jan 15;22(2):pp. 220-228. Epub 2003 Dec 9. Erratum in: *J Clin Oncol*: May 1;22(9): pp. 1771. PMID: 14665607

Bellmunt J, Hussain M, Dinney CP (2003): Novel approaches with targeted therapies in bladder cancer. Therapy of bladder cancer by blockade of the epidermal growth factor receptor family. *Crit Rev Oncol Hematol*: 46(Suppl): pp. 85-104. PMID: 12850530

Bradley DA, Dunn R, Nanus D, Stadler W, Dreicer R, Rosenberg J, Smith DC, Hussain M (2007): Randomized, double-blind, placebo-controlled phase II trial of maintenance sunitinib versus placebo after chemotherapy for patients with advanced urothelial carcinoma: scientific rationale and study design. *Clin Genitourin*: Dec;5(7): pp. 460-463. PMID: 18272031

Burch PA, Richardson RL, Cha SS, Sargent DJ, Pitot HC 4th, Kaur JS, Camoriano JK (2000): Phase II study of paclitaxel and cisplatin for advanced urothelial cancer. *J Urol*: Nov;164(5): pp. 1538-1542. PMID: 11025699

Carles J, Esteban E, Climent M, Font A, Gonzalez-Larriba JL, Berrocal A, Garcia-Ribas I, Marfa X, Fabregat X, Albanell J, Bellmunt J; Spanish Oncology Genito Urinary Group Study Group (2007): Gemcitabine and oxaliplatin combination: a multicenter phase II trial in unfit patients with locally advanced or metastatic urothelial cancer. *Ann Oncol*: Aug;18(8): pp. 1359-1362. PMID: 17693649

deVere White RW, Lara PN Jr, Goldman B, Tangen CM, Smith DC, Wood DP Jr, Hussain MH, Crawford ED (2009): A sequential treatment approach to myoinvasive urothelial cancer: a phase II Southwest Oncology Group Trial (S0219). *J Urol*: Jun;181(6): pp. 2476-2480; discussion 2480-2481. Epub 2009 Apr 16. PMID: 19371909

Dimopoulos MA, Bakoyannis C, Georgoulias V, Papadimitriou C, Moulopoulos LA, Deliveliotis C, Karayannis A, Varkarakis I, Aravantinos G, Zervas A, Pantazopoulos D, Fountzilas G, Bamias A, Kyriakakis Z, Anagnostopoulos A, Giannopoulos A, Kosmidis P (1999): Docetaxel and cisplatin combination chemotherapy in advanced carcinoma of the urothelium: a multicenter phase II study of the Hellenic Cooperative Oncology Group. *Ann Oncol*: Nov;10(11): pp. 1385-1388. PMID: 10631471

Dogliotti L, Cartenì G, Siena S, Bertetto O, Martoni A, Bono A, Amadori D, Onat H, Marini L (2007): Gemcitabine plus cisplatin versus gemcitabine plus carboplatin as first-line chemotherapy in advanced transitional cell carcinoma of the urothelium: results of a randomized phase 2 trial. *Eur Urol*: Jul;52(1): pp. 134-141. PMID: 17207911

Dovedi SJ, Davies BR (2009): Emerging targeted therapies for bladder cancer: a disease waiting for a drug. *Cancer Metastasis Rev*: Dec;28(3-4): pp. 355-367. PMID: 19997963

Dreicer R, Manola J, Roth BJ, Cohen MB, Hatfield AK, Wilding G (2000): Phase II study of cisplatin and paclitaxel in advanced carcinoma of the urothelium: an Eastern Cooperative Oncology Group Study. *J Clin Oncol*: Mar;18(5): pp. 1058-1561. PMID: 10694557

Gatzemeier U, Shepherd FA, Le Chevalier T, Weynants P, Cottier B, Groen HJ, Rosso R, Mattson K, Cortes-Funes H, Tonato M, Burkes RL, Gottfried M, Voi M (1996): Activity of gemcitabine in patients with non-small cell lung cancer: a multicentre, extended phase II study. *Eur J Cancer*: Feb;32A(2): pp. 243-248. PMID: 8664035

Grossman HB, Natale RB, Tangen CM, Speights VO, Vogelzang NJ, Trump DL, deVere White RW, Sarosdy MF, Wood DP Jr, Raghavan D, Crawford ED (2003): Neoadjuvant chemotherapy plus cystectomy compared with cystectomy alone for locally advanced bladder cancer. *N Engl J*: Aug 28;349(9): pp. 859-866. PMID: 12944571

Hahn NM, Stadler WM, Zon RT, Waterhouse D, Picus J, Nattam S, Johnson CS, Perkins SM, Waddell MJ, Sweeney CJ; Hoosier Oncology Group (2011): Phase II trial of cisplatin, gemcitabine, and bevacizumab as first-line therapy for metastatic urothelial carcinoma: Hoosier Oncology Group GU 04-75. *J Clin Oncol*: Apr 20;29(12): pp. 1525-1530. PMID: 21422406

Hussain MH, MacVicar GR, Petrylak DP, Dunn RL, Vaishampayan U, Lara PN Jr, Chatta GS, Nanus DM, Glode LM, Trump DL, Chen H, Smith DC; National Cancer Institute (2007): Trastuzumab, paclitaxel, carboplatin, and gemcitabine in advanced human epidermal growth factor receptor-2/neu-positive urothelial carcinoma: results of a multicenter phase II National Cancer Institute trial. *J Clin Oncol*: Jun 1;25(16): pp. 2218-2224. Erratum in: *J Clin Oncol*: 2008 Jul 1;26(19): pp. 3295. PMID: 17538166

Jemal A, Murray T, Samuels A, Ghafoor A, Ward E, Thun MJ (2003): Cancer statistics, 2003. *CA Cancer J Clin*: Jan-Feb;53(1):pp. 5-26. PMID: 12568441

Jemal A, Siegel R, Ward E, Hao Y, Xu J, Murray T, Thun MJ (2008): Cancer statistics, 2008. *CA Cancer J Clin*: Mar-Apr;58(2): pp. 71-96. PMID: 18287387

Kuroda M, Kotake T, Akaza H, Hinotsu S, Kakizoe T (1998):Efficacy of dose-intensified MEC (methotrexate, epirubicin and cisplatin) chemotherapy for advanced urothelial carcinoma: a prospective randomized trial comparing MEC and M-VAC (methotrexate, vinblastine, doxorubicin and cisplatin). Japanese Urothelial Cancer Research Group. *Jpn J Clin Oncol*: Aug;28(8): pp. 497-501. PMID: 9769784

Loehrer PJ Sr, Einhorn LH, Elson PJ, Crawford ED, Kuebler P, Tannock I, Raghavan D, Stuart-Harris R, Sarosdy MF, Lowe BA, et al (1992): A randomized comparison of cisplatin alone or in combination with methotrexate, vinblastine, and doxorubicin in patients with metastatic urothelial carcinoma: a cooperative group study. *J Clin Oncol*: Jul;10(7): pp. 1066-1073. Erratum in: *J Clin Oncol* 1993 Feb;11(2): pp. 384. PMID: 1607913

Moore M (1996): Activity of gemcitabine in patients with advanced pancreatic carcinoma. A review. *Cancer*: Aug 1;78(3 Suppl): pp. 633-638. Review. PMID: 8681302

Peters GJ, Bergman AM, Ruiz van Haperen VW, Veerman G, Kuiper CM, Braakhuis BJ (1995): Interaction between cisplatin and gemcitabine in vitro and in vivo. *Semin Oncol*: Aug;22(4 Suppl 11): pp. 72-79. PMID: 7481849

Saad A, Hanbury DC, McNicholas TA, Boustead GB, Morgan S, Woodman AC (2002): A study comparing various noninvasive methods of detecting bladder cancer in urine. *BJU Int*: Mar;89(4): pp. 369-373. PMID: 11872026

Saxman SB, Propert KJ, Einhorn LH, Crawford ED, Tannock I, Raghavan D, Loehrer PJ Sr, Trump D (1997): Long-term follow-up of a phase III intergroup study of cisplatin alone or in combination with methotrexate, vinblastine, and doxorubicin in patients with metastatic urothelial carcinoma: a cooperative group study. *J Clin Oncol*: Jul;15(7): pp. 2564-2569. PMID: 9215826

Sengeløv L, Kamby C, Lund B, Engelholm SA (1998): Docetaxel and cisplatin in metastatic urothelial cancer: a phase II study. *J Clin Oncol*: Oct;16(10): pp. 3392-3397. PMID: 9779718

Sherif A, Holmberg L, Rintala E, Mestad O, Nilsson J, Nilsson S, Malmström PU; Nordic Urothelial Cancer Group. (2004): Neoadjuvant cisplatinum based combination chemotherapy in patients with invasive bladder cancer: a combined analysis of two Nordic studies. *Eur Urol*: Mar;45(3): pp. 297-303. PMID: 15036674

Smith DC, Mackler NJ, Dunn RL, Hussain M, Wood D, Lee CT, Sanda M, Vaishampayan U, Petrylak DP, Quinn DI, Beekman K, Montie JE. (2008): Phase II trial of paclitaxel, carboplatin and gemcitabine in patients with locally advanced carcinoma of the bladder. *J Urol*: Dec;180(6): pp. 2384-2388; discussion pp. 2388. Epub 2008 Oct 18.

Soloway MS, Sofer M, Vaidya A (2002): Contemporary management of stage T1 transitional cell carcinoma of the bladder. *J Urol*: Apr;167(4): pp. 1573-1583. PMID: 18930256

Stadler WM, Kuzel T, Roth B, Raghavan D, Dorr FA (1997): Phase II study of single-agent gemcitabine in previously untreated patients with metastatic urothelial cancer. *J Clin Oncol*: Nov;15(11): pp. 3394-3398. PMID: 9363871

Sternberg CN, Yagoda A, Scher HI, Watson RC, Herr HW, Morse MJ, Sogani PC, Vaughan ED Jr, Bander N, Weiselberg LR, et al (1988): M-VAC (methotrexate, vinblastine, doxorubicin and cisplatin) for advanced transitional cell carcinoma of the urothelium. *J Urol*: Mar;139(3): pp. 461-469. PMID: 3343727

Sternberg CN, Yagoda A, Scher HI, Watson RC, Geller N, Herr HW, Morse MJ, Sogani PC, Vaughan ED, Bander N, et al (1989): Methotrexate, vinblastine, doxorubicin, and cisplatin for advanced transitional cell carcinoma of the urothelium. Efficacy and patterns of response and relapse. *Cancer*: Dec 15;64(12): pp. 2448-2258. PMID: 2819654

Sternberg CN (2000): Gemcitabine in bladder cancer. *Semin Oncol*: Feb;27(1 Suppl 2): pp. 31-39. Review. PMID: 10697034

Sweeney CJ, Roth BJ, Kabbinavar FF, Vaughn DJ, Arning M, Curiel RE, Obasaju CK, Wang Y, Nicol SJ, Kaufman DS (2006): Phase II study of pemetrexed for second-line treatment of transitional cell cancer of the bladder. *J Clin Oncol*: Jul 20;24(21): pp. 3451-3457. PMID: 16849761

Uhm JE, Lim HY, Kim WS (2007): Paclitaxel with cisplatin as salvage treatment for patients with previously treated advanced transitional cell carcinoma of the urothelial tract. *Neoplasia*: Jan;9(1): pp. 18-22. PMID: 17325740

Vaishampayan U (2009): Systemic therapy of advanced urothelial cancer. *Curr Treat Options Oncol*: Aug;10(3-4): pp. 256-266. Epub 2009 Apr 29. Review. PMID: 19408129

Vaishampayan UN, Faulkner JR, Small EJ, Redman BG, Keiser WL, Petrylak DP, Crawford ED (2005): Phase II trial of carboplatin and paclitaxel in cisplatin-pretreated advanced transitional cell carcinoma: a Southwest Oncology Group study. *Cancer*: Oct 15;104(8): pp. 1627-1632. PMID: 16138364

Van Echo DA, Egorin MJ, Aisner J (1989): The pharmacology of carboplatin. *Semin Oncol*: Apr;16(2 Suppl 5): pp. 1-6. Review. PMID: 2655093

von der Maase H, Hansen SW, Roberts JT, Dogliotti L, Oliver T, Moore MJ, Bodrogi I, Albers P, Knuth A, Lippert CM, Kerbrat P, Sanchez Rovira P, Wersall P, Cleall SP, Roychowdhury DF, Tomlin I, Visseren-Grul CM, Conte PF (2000): Gemcitabine and cisplatin versus methotrexate, vinblastine, doxorubicin, and cisplatin in advanced or metastatic bladder cancer: results of a large, randomized, multinational, multicenter, phase III study. *J Clin Oncol*: Sep;18(17): pp. 3068-3077. PMID: 11001674

Winquist E, Kirchner TS, Segal R, Chin J, Lukka H (2004): Neoadjuvant chemotherapy for transitional cell carcinoma of the bladder: a systematic review and meta-analysis. *J Urol*: Feb;171(2 Pt 1): pp. 561-569. PMID: 14713760

Witte RS, Elson P, Khandakar J, Trump DL. (1994): An Eastern Oncology Group phase II trial of trimetrexate in the treatment of advanced urothelial carcinoma. *Cancer*: Feb 1;73(3): pp. 688-691. PMID: 8299090

Xu N, Zhang XC, Xiong JP, Fang WJ, Yu LF, Qian J, Zhang L (2007): A phase II trial of gemcitabine plus carboplatin in advanced transitional cell carcinoma of the urothelium. *BMC Cancer*: Jun 9;7: pp. 98. PMID: 17559681

4

The Molecular Basis of Cisplatin Resistance in Bladder Cancer Cells

Beate Köberle and Andrea Piee-Staffa

Institute of Toxicology, University of Mainz Medical Center, Mainz, Germany

1. Introduction

Bladder cancer is one of the most common cancers among men and women, with men being twice as likely affected from the disease (Jemal et al., 2005). The most common type of bladder cancer is transitional cell carcinoma (TCC), which is derived from the urothelium and constitutes more than 90 % of all bladder cancers (Bischoff & Clark, 2009). Cisplatin-based combination therapy is the standard therapy for the treatment of advanced or metastatic bladder cancers (Cohen et al., 2006, Kaufman, 2006). However, the outcome of patients with metastatic bladder cancer remains poor, as tumors become resistant to cisplatin therapy. It is still not entirely known, which factors influence the response of bladder cancers to the drug and how this cancer acquires cisplatin resistance. Cisplatin is a neutral planar complex (Figure 1A).

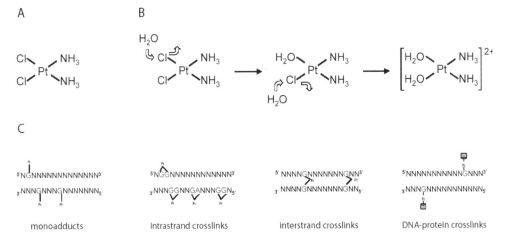

Fig. 1. **A:** The chemical structure of cisplatin. **B:** After entering the cells, cisplatin is transformed to a positively charged molecule that reacts with DNA **C:** Cisplatin induced lesions. Cisplatin preferably binds to the nucleophilic N7 position of the purine bases guanine or adenine, leading to different types of lesions including monoadducts, intrastrand crosslinks, interstrand crosslinks and DNA-protein crosslinks

After entering the cell, it is activated through a series of aquation reactions, in which the chloro ligands are replaced by water molecules (Figure 1B). The resulting positively charged molecule can react with nucleophilic sites on macromolecules, leading to DNA, RNA and protein adducts. It preferably binds to the nucleophilic N7 position of the purine bases guanine or adenine, which leads to different types of lesions (Figure 1C) (Jamieson & Lippard, 1999). In a first reaction, cisplatin binds to DNA, leading to monoadducts, which in a second reaction lead to the formation of DNA crosslinks. The most frequently observed cisplatin DNA lesions are DNA intrastrand crosslinks between adjacent guanines (65 % of all lesions) or intrastrand crosslinks between guanine and adenine (25 %). Interstrand crosslinks between two guanines on the opposite strands of DNA account for less than 5% of all cisplatin-induced lesions. It is still unknown, which of the various DNA lesions ultimately results in cell death (Chu, 1994, Jordan & Carmo-Fonseca, 2000, Kartalou & Essigmann, 2001).

The efficacy of cisplatin in cancer chemotherapy, however, is limited by resistance. While cancers of the bladder, lung and ovary respond initially in 50 % or more of cases, they will almost inevitably relapse with drug-resistant disease. The mechanisms of cisplatin resistance have been studied in numerous cell culture models of cisplatin sensitive and resistant cancer cells lines. It has been shown that a cancer cell can develop cisplatin resistance through different mechanisms (Figure 2). Cisplatin resistance can be due to (i) changes in drug transport, leading to reduced cellular cisplatin accumulation, (ii) increased drug detoxification, also resulting in reduced cellular cisplatin accumulation, (iii) changes in DNA repair mechanisms including nucleotide excision repair, interstrand crosslink repair and mismatch repair, (iv) changes in DNA tolerance mechanisms, and finally (v) alterations in the apoptotic cell death pathways (Köberle et al., 2010, Rabik & Dolan, 2007, Siddik, 2003). In this chapter we describe and discuss the contribution of these mechanisms for the development of cisplatin resistance in bladder cancer cells *in vitro* and compare the preclinical findings to data obtained in clinical studies. A better understanding of the molecular basis of cisplatin resistance may lead to new anticancer strategies that will sensitize unresponsive bladder cancers to cisplatin-based chemotherapy.

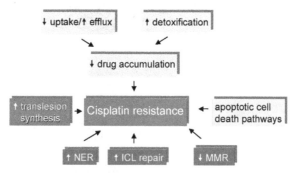

Fig. 2. Mechanisms of resistance towards cisplatin include: Reduced drug accumulation due to changes in drug uptake, efflux or detoxification. Alterations in DNA repair such as increased removal of the damage by nucleotide excision repair (NER) or interstrand crosslink repair (ICL repair) as well as decreased mismatch repair (MMR). Enhanced translesion synthesis (TLS) to tolerate unrepaired cisplatin lesions. Alterations in apoptosis pathways: changes in expression levels of pro- and anti-apoptotic proteins.

2. Intracellular drug accumulation as a determinant of cellular cisplatin sensitivity

2.1 Cellular uptake and efflux of cisplatin

Reduced intracellular cisplatin accumulation has been associated with cisplatin resistance in numerous cancer cell lines (Siddik, 2003). A correlation between intracellular cisplatin accumulation and cisplatin resistance was observed in a series of seven bladder cancer cell lines displaying different sensitivities to cisplatin (Koga et al., 2000). Similarly, using a bladder cancer cell line and its cisplatin-resistant subline, we found reduced accumulation of cisplatin in the resistant subline when compared to its parental cells (Köberle et al., 1996). Reduced accumulation may result from changes in drug transport or increased drug detoxification. Even though the exact mechanism by which cisplatin is taken up by the cells is not fully understood, both passive diffusion and active transport appear to be involved. For active transport the copper transporter 1 (Ctr1), which controls intracellular copper homeostasis, seems to play an important role (Kuo et al., 2007, Safaei, 2006). It has been reported that loss of Ctr1 lead to cisplatin resistance in various cell lines (Holzer et al., 2006, Ishida et al., 2002, Song et al., 2004). However, no data as to Ctr1 expression in bladder cancer cell lines or tumor tissue have been reported to date. Therefore, no conclusion about the importance of uptake for cisplatin response can be drawn for bladder cancer cells (Table 1).

Increased efflux of cisplatin from the cell may also lead to resistance. Efflux pumps such as MRP1/2 (multidrug resistance associated protein) and p-glycoprotein/multidrug resistance 1 (MDR1) are implicated as efflux pumps for cisplatin (Taniguchi et al., 1996, Yeh et al., 2005). Tada and co-workers investigated the relationship between expression of p-glycoprotein expression or MRP1/2 and drug sensitivity in 47 clinical samples of bladder cancer. They showed that expression of p-glycoprotein and MRP1/2 was higher in samples of recurrent tumors than in untreated primary tumors (Tada et al., 2002), indicating that increased efflux can contribute to the development of drug resistance and poor clinical outcome in bladder cancers (Table 1).

2.2 Detoxification of cisplatin by intracellular thiol molecules

Cisplatin resistance can be the result of increased inactivation of the drug by intracellular thiol-containing molecules such as glutathione and metallothionein. Glutathione is a tripeptide that plays an important role for the detoxification of xenobiotic substances by scavenging free radicals. Cisplatin can be conjugated with glutathione, which will inhibit its binding to DNA and other cellular molecules. This reaction is catalyzed by the glutathione-S-transferase (GST) (Mannervik, 1987). Extensive studies about the role of the glutathione system for cisplatin resistance have been carried out in cell lines and in cancer tissue. A correlation between expression of the glutathione system and cisplatin resistance has been reported for ovarian, cervical and lung cancer cell lines (Jansen et al., 2002, Meijer et al., 1992, Mellish et al., 1993). Attempts to correlate expression of the glutathione system with cisplatin resistance in bladder cancer cell lines showed inconsistent findings. Bedford and co-workers investigated the expression of the glutatione system in different bladder cancer cells lines and reported higher levels of glutathione and GST in the less sensitive cells (Bedford et al., 1987). Similarly, using a model system of a bladder cancer cell line and two derived sublines with acquired cisplatin resistance, Kotoh and co-workers observed an increased glutathione content and elevated GST activity in the sublines (Kotoh et al., 1997). Buthionine sulphoximine (BSO), which depletes glutathione, or indomethacin, which blocks

GST, significantly decreased the cisplatin resistance in T24 bladder cancer cells, which is yet another indication that the glutathione-based detoxification system is involved in cisplatin resistance in bladder cancer cells (Byun et al., 2005). However, no correlation between glutathione content and resistance to cisplatin was observed in a study by Koga and co-workers (Koga et al., 2000). In this study, the expression of GST was also not significantly related to cisplatin resistance. In another study with bladder cancer cells, which were either sensitive or progressively resistant to cisplatin, it was observed that expression of GST was increased in the cisplatin resistant cells, however, the increase in glutathione contents did not reach statistical significance (Hour et al., 2000). In conclusion, bladder cancer cells may gain cisplatin resistance through up-regulation of GST, while glutathione contents seems to play a less important role for the development of cisplatin resistance.

Metallothioneins (MT) belong to a family of low molecular weight, thiol-rich proteins that play a role in metal homeostasis and detoxification (Kagi & Schaffer, 1988). MTs can bind to cisplatin, leading to the inactivation of the drug. For numerous cancer cell lines (derived from prostate, lung, ovary and cervical cancer), a correlation between MT expression and cisplatin resistance has been observed (Kasahara et al., 1991, Kondo et al., 1995, Mellish et al., 1993, Surowiak et al., 2007). For bladder cancer cell lines cisplatin resistance, was also correlated with increased levels of MT (Siegsmund et al., 1999, Singh et al., 1995). A role of MT for cisplatin resistance in bladder cancer has been proposed by Satoh and co-workers (Satoh et al., 1994). The authors investigated the effect of modulation of the MT levels for the antitumor activity of cisplatin in nude mice inoculated with human bladder cancer cells. While increasing MT levels reduced the antitumor activity of cisplatin, decreased levels of MT diminished the resistance to the drug (Satoh et al., 1994). Using a different bladder tumor model in mice, it was also suggested that MT might play a role for acquired resistance towards cisplatin (Saga et al., 2004). The clinical relevance of MT levels for cisplatin chemotherapy in bladder cancers has been investigated in a number of studies. In an investigation involving 118 patients with bladder cancer, it was observed that overexpression of MT was associated with a poorer outcome from cisplatin-based chemotherapy (Siu et al., 1998). Similarly, for intrinsic cisplatin resistance of urinary tract TCCs, an involvement of MT has been suggested (Kotoh et al., 1994), and MT overexpression was proposed to be a mechanism for cisplatin resistance in bladder cancer tissue (Wood et al., 1993). In line with this observations are more recent studies, which also reported that high levels of MT expression in bladder cancer tissue were correlated with poor survival after cisplatin chemotherapy (Hinkel et al., 2008, Wülfing et al., 2007). Taken together, the data indicate that high levels of MT in bladder cancers might be a major problem for effective cisplatin-based chemotherapy. In our opinion, expression of MT is one of the main cellular factors for both intrinsic and acquired cisplatin resistance in bladder cancers (Table 1).

3. DNA repair and cisplatin resistance

The contribution of DNA repair for cisplatin resistance has been investigated for many years. In model systems of tumor cell lines and sublines with acquired cisplatin resistance, increased removal of cisplatin induced lesions has been observed in the sublines. For example, ovarian cancer cells with acquired resistance towards cisplatin show an increased removal of cisplatin induced lesions in comparison with their cisplatin sensitive counterparts (Johnson et al., 1994a, Johnson et al., 1994b, Parker et al., 1991). Similarly, colon

Molecular mechanism	Preclinical evidence	Clinical evidence
Intracellular cisplatin accumulation		
Decreased uptake	no data reported	no data reported
Increased efflux	no data reported	observed in resistant tumors
Increased glutathione/ GST levels	conflicting results	Conflicting results
Increased metallothioneine levels	Observed in resistant cancer cell lines	correlated with poor clinical outcome
DNA repair		
Nucleotide excision repair (NER)	High levels of ERCC1 in resistant cancer cells	Conflicting results
ICL repair	Proficiency in resistant bladder cancer cell lines	no data reported
Translesion synthesis (TLS)	no data reported	no data reported
Mismatch repair (MMR)	No association with acquired resistance	Conflicting results
DNA damage response		
p53	Conflicting results	Conflicting results
Bcl-2, Bcl-xL	Overexpression in cisplatin resistant cancer cells	Low levels correlate with better prognosis
Survivin	High levels in bladder cancer cells	Expression as a marker for clinical outcome
XIAP	High expression in bladder cancer cells	High levels correlate with poor prognosis

Table 1. Mechanisms of cisplatin resistance in bladder cancers: preclinical findings and clinical evidence (Table adapted from Köberle et al., 2010)

carcinoma cell lines with acquired cisplatin resistance showed a higher extent of removal of DNA platination compared to the parental cells (Oldenburg et al., 1994), indicating that the acquired resistance to cisplatin might be related to the increased DNA repair capacity. In contrast, when we investigated DNA damage removal in a bladder cancer cell line with acquired cisplatin resistance, we observed no enhanced repair compared to the parental cell line, suggesting that this bladder cancer cell line did not acquire resistance to cisplatin by increasing the DNA repair capacity (Köberle et al., 1996). However, when we compared bladder cancer cell lines with cisplatin sensitive testis tumor cells, we observed that bladder cancer cells are proficient in removing cisplatin damage from the DNA, while testis tumor cells were repair deficient (Köberle et al., 1997), supporting the hypothesis that susceptibility to cisplatin might be related to the repair capacity.

3.1 Nucleotide excision repair

Cisplatin-induced GpG and GpA DNA intrastrand crosslinks are repaired by nucleotide excision repair (NER). NER is a multistep mechanism, which deals with bulky helix-distorting lesions such as UV-induced cyclobutane pyrimidine dimers and 6-4 photoproducts, and DNA lesions induced by many chemotherapeutic drugs (Gillet & Schärer, 2006, Shuck et al., 2008, Wood et al., 2000). The repair of the lesions begins with recognition of the damage and incision on both sides of the lesion, followed by DNA synthesis to replace the excised fragment. The core incision reaction requires the protein factors XPA, RPA, XPC-HR23B, TFIIH, ERCC1-XPF and XPG (Aboussekhra et al., 1995). It is possible to carry out the core NER reaction in a cell free system using cellular protein extracts (Shivji et al., 1999, Shivji et al., 2005). Using this system, it could be confirmed that the increased removal of cisplatin lesions, which has been observed in cisplatin resistant ovarian cancer cells, is in fact due to enhanced NER (Ferry et al., 2000). We found that cellular protein extracts of a bladder cancer cell line were proficient for NER (Köberle et al., 1999). Furthermore, the core NER proteins are expressed to a similar extent in bladder cancer cell lines compared to normal non-cancerous cells (Köberle et al., 1999, Welsh et al., 2004). The removal of cisplatin induced DNA platination, which we previously observed in bladder cancer cell lines (Köberle et al., 1997), is therefore, at least in part, due to NER proficiency in these cells.

Conclusive evidence for functionally increased NER in cisplatin-resistant cancers, however, has not yet been presented. This is due to the lack of methods to easily and reliably measure NER activities in tissue samples. For example, even in protein extracts prepared from cell lines, a significant variability in NER capacity is observed. Even more, in protein extracts prepared from biopsies of human ovarian carcinoma, Jones and co-workers found that the NER capacity varied significantly by as much as ten-fold (Jones et al., 1994). This could be due to either inter-individual variations or to technical problems to obtain active extracts from tissue material. Therefore, as measuring NER capacity in tissue samples is a challenging task, a different approach is to investigate the expression of NER factors on the mRNA or protein level and attempt to correlate these with response to chemotherapy. In these studies, special emphasis was given to ERCC1, the first human DNA repair gene cloned (Westerveld et al., 1984). In preclinical studies, a correlation between ERCC1 expression and cisplatin resistance has been presented (Li et al., 1998, Li et al., 2000, Metzger et al., 1998). By demonstrating that down-regulation of ERCC1 by siRNA sensitized bladder cancer cell lines to cisplatin, we could confirm the importance of ERCC1 for cisplatin resistance in bladder cancer cells (Usanova et al., 2010).

In cancer tissues, ERCC1 mRNA or protein levels show an inverse correlation with the response to platinum therapy or overall survival. High ERCC1 mRNA levels are associated with resistance to cisplatin-based chemotherapy in ovarian, cervical, gastric, colorectal, head and neck, esophageal and lung cancer (Dabholkar et al., 1992, Dabholkar et al., 1994, Gossage & Madhusudan, 2007, Handra-Luca et al., 2007, Jun et al., 2008, Kim et al., 2008, Metzger et al., 1998, Olaussen et al., 2006, Weberpals et al., 2009). Based on these findings, it was suggested that ERCC1 can be used as a predictive and prognostic marker for the outcome of cisplatin-based chemotherapy. For patients with advanced bladder cancer, a significantly higher survival rate was reported when ERCC1 levels in the tumor tissue were low (Bellmunt et al., 2007). However, in another study, no significant difference in overall survival between bladder cancer patients with ERCC1 negative tumors and ERCC1 positive tumors was observed (Kim et al., 2010). On the other hand, the authors reported that progression free survival was longer in patients with ERCC1 negative bladder cancers compared to ERCC1 positive cancers (Kim et al., 2010). Based on these conflicting results, it is difficult to conclude that ERCC1 expression in bladder cancer negatively contributes to the clinical outcome. Furthermore, even though ERCC1 positive tumors would be expected to have a high NER capacity, and ERCC1 negative tumors would be expected to have low NER capacity, these conclusions must be drawn with caution, as functional NER assays for tissue material are still missing. It therefore remains speculative whether altered ERCC1 levels have an impact on NER in tumor tissue. Therefore, the question about the contribution of enhanced NER for cisplatin resistance in cancers, especially in bladder cancers, remains to be solved (Table 1).

3.2 Interstrand crosslink repair
Besides intrastrand adducts, cisplatin induces interstrand crosslinks (ICLs), which are removed by ICL repair, a process less understood than NER (McHugh et al., 2001). Repair of ICLs is a challenging problem for cells. In bacteria and lower eukaryotes, NER and homologous recombination are involved in ICL repair (Cole, 1973, Jachymczyk et al., 1981). In mammalian cells, these both pathways may also operate (De Silva et al., 2000). Besides that, mammalian cells have additional pathways of ICL repair involving DNA polymerases that can bypass the lesion (Sarkar et al., 2006, Shen et al., 2006, Zheng et al., 2005). A contribution of increased ICL repair for acquired resistance to cisplatin has been described for ovarian cancer cells in culture (Zhen et al., 1992). It also seems to play a role for clinical cisplatin resistance, as in paired tumor samples obtained prior to treatment and at relapse following platinum chemotherapy, increased repair of cisplatin ICLs in cells of relapsed ovarian cancer was observed (Wynne et al., 2007). We found that bladder cancer cell lines, which are relatively resistant to cisplatin, are proficient in repairing ICLs (Usanova et al., 2010). Biochemical and cell biological data implicate that ERCC1 is not only involved in NER, but also in ICL repair (Kuraoka et al., 2000, Niedernhofer et al., 2004, Sijbers et al., 1996). Our own experiments revealed that down-regulation of ERCC1 by siRNA affected ICL repair in the bladder cancer cell lines and rendered the cells more sensitive to cisplatin supporting the notion about the importance of ICL repair for cisplatin resistance in cancer cells. However, to date there is no information as to ICL repair in bladder cancer tissue (Table 1).

3.3 Translesion synthesis (TLS)
As described in 3.1 and 3.2, cisplatin damage is removed by NER and ICL repair. However, some lesions may remain. A mechanism, by which cells can tolerate unrepaired DNA

lesions, is translesion synthesis (TLS). TLS is carried out by a group of specialized DNA polymerases, which are capable of bypassing unrepaired DNA lesions. For mammalian cells pol η (POLH), pol ι (POLI), pol κ (POLK), REV1 and pol ζ (REV3 and REV7) are the main TLS polymerases, which have been shown to possess different substrate specificity. Depending on the type of damage, different combinations of TLS polymerases act in concert to bypass the DNA lesions (Shachar et al., 2009). Cisplatin GpG intrastrand crosslinks seem to be bypassed by pol η and pol ζ (Alt et al., 2007, Shachar et al., 2009). For pol κ conflicting results have been reported. While an in vitro assay suggests that pol κ is unable to bypass a GpG intrastrand crosslink, in vivo TLS assays implicated pol κ in combination with pol η for TLS across cisplatin GpG intrastrand crosslinks (Ohashi et al., 2000, Shachar et al., 2009). The importance of TLS in the tolerance towards cisplatin has been shown in cell lines deficient in TLS polymerase activity (Cruet-Hennequart et al., 2008, Cruet-Hennequart et al., 2009, Albertella et al., 2005a, Roos et al., 2009, Wittschieben et al., 2006). Similarly, TLS polymerases may play a role for cisplatin resistance in tumor samples (Albertella et al., 2005b, Ceppi et al., 2009, Wang et al., 2009). However, no data have been reported as to the expression of TLS polymerases in bladder cancer cell lines and tumor specimens. We therefore can neither include nor exclude TLS polymerases as a factor determining efficacy of cisplatin therapy in the clinic (Table 1).

3.4 DNA mismatch repair (MMR)

Mismatch repair (MMR) is the pathway that removes mispaired nucleotides or insertion/deletion loops, which arise during DNA replication or as a result of damage to DNA. MMR consists of following steps: (1) recognition of the mismatch, (2) identification and excision of the mispairs or looped intermediates, and (3) resynthesis of the excised strand (Kunkel & Erie, 2005). In early investigations it has been observed that loss of MMR led to resistance to cisplatin and other platinating agents (Aebi et al., 1996, Fink et al., 1996). A possible explanation for the association of absence of a repair mechanism with increased drug resistance was the observation that MMR proteins can bind to cisplatin damage possibly leading to futile repair and therefore increased drug lethality. The mismatch repair complex MutSα (which is a heterodimer containing MSH2 and MSH6) binds to cisplatin DNA lesions in vitro (Duckett et al., 1996, Mello et al., 1996). Binding of MutSα to cisplatin crosslinks could start the MMR process by recruiting the mismatch repair complex MutLα (consisting of MLH1 and PMS2). It is assumed that lethal intermediates arise by the attempt of the MMR machinery to remove cisplatin lesions, and these lethal intermediates might set off a futile MMR cycle, similar to what has been reported for methylating agents (Dunkern et al., 2001). An alternative model suggests that binding of the MMR complex to cisplatin DNA damage might cause direct activation of the DNA damage response (DDR). A third model is based on the finding that TLS polymerases can bypass of 1,2-intrastrand crosslinks (Alt et al., 2007, Shachar et al., 2009). Since TLS polymerases are error prone causing mis-incorporation of bases, mismatches will be generated that are recognised by the MutSα complex. This in turn causes a futile repair cycle that triggers DDR. New data suggest that mitochondrial pro-death signaling involving cytochrome c and caspases-9 and -3 is required for the execution of MMR protein-mediated induction of cell death by cisplatin (Topping et al., 2009). The importance of MMR for cisplatin resistance has been investigated in a number of cancer cell lines, however, with conflicting results. On the one hand it was observed that

MMR deficient cell lines were more tolerant to cisplatin (Bignami et al., 2003, Fink et al., 1996, Papouli et al., 2004). This was explained by the hypothesis that cisplatin lesions are not processed into lethal intermediates. In other studies, however, it was shown that defective MMR is only a minor contributor for the cisplatin resistance phenotype or is not involved at all (Branch et al., 2000, Claij & te Riele, 2004, Massey et al., 2003). We found that the MMR protein MSH2 was expressed at lower levels in bladder cancer cells compared to cisplatin sensitive testis tumor cells. However, no difference was observed in the expression level of the MMR proteins hMLH1 and PMS2 in this model system of cisplatin resistant and sensitive cell lines. Even more, no difference in the levels of MSH2, MLH1 and PMS2 was observed in parental RT112 bladder cancer cells and the subline with acquired cisplatin resistance (Köberle, unpublished results), suggesting that MMR may not be of importance for cisplatin resistance in our model system.

The clinical relevance of loss of MMR for cisplatin chemotherapy has been investigated in a number of clinical studies, and it was concluded that MMR deficiency is associated with chemotherapy resistance in ovarian and testicular germ cell tumors (Gifford et al., 2004, Helleman et al., 2006, Wei et al., 2002). In 115 patients with bladder cancers, the expression pattern of hMSH2 protein was investigated and a reduced expression of hMSH2 was significantly more frequent in high grade tumors (Jin et al., 1999). Similarly, Catto and co-workers reported that reduced expression of hMLH1 and hMSH2 was seen more commonly in muscle invasive and high grade bladder cancer (Catto et al., 2003). In contrast, in a set of 130 urothelial carcinomas of the bladder, hMSH2 and hMSH6 negative tumors were found to have a favorable impact on overall patient survival (Mylona et al., 2008). In a number of studies, the degree of microsatellite instability (MSI) was investigated in different cancer tissues, such as colorectal-, ovarian- and gastric carcinoma (Dietmaier et al., 1997, Ichikawa et al., 1999, Ottini et al., 1997). MSI is the result from inactivating mutations in MMR genes and suggests MMR deficiency (Parsons et al., 1993, Strand et al., 1993). However, MSI has been observed only infrequently in bladder cancer tissues (Bonnal et al., 2000, Gonzalez-Zulueta et al., 1993, Hartmann et al., 2002). Furthermore, reduced expression of hMLH1 and hMSH2 was not correlated with MSI in bladder cancer (Catto et al., 2003). Based on these conflicting data, a conclusion as to whether MMR impacts the development of cisplatin resistance in bladder cancer in the clinic cannot be drawn to date (Table 1).

4. DNA damage response and apoptosis pathways in cisplatin resistance

It is known that cisplatin treatment induces apoptosis in cells, thereby killing the cells (Chu, 1994). The apoptotic pathways, which are induced following cisplatin treatment, were extensively studied, hence not yet fully understood. Cisplatin-induced apoptosis may be triggered through the extrinsic death receptor pathway, which is mediated through the JNK signaling cascade. Alternatively, the intrinsic mitochondrial pathway may be induced, mediated through p53 and anti- or pro-apoptotic members of the Bcl-2 family proteins (Brozovic et al., 2004, Pabla et al., 2008, Siddik, 2003). Decreased expression or loss of pro-apoptotic proteins may result in cisplatin resistance, similarly may increased expression of anti-apoptotic proteins lead to cisplatin resistance (Brozovic & Osmak, 2007). The contribution of these mechanisms for preclinical and clinical cisplatin resistance of bladder cancer cells will be discussed in the following section.

4.1 p53 and cisplatin resistance of bladder cancer cells

The tumor suppressor protein p53 is activated in cancer cells after treatment with chemotherapeutic drugs and has a central role for the induction of apoptosis. The influence of the p53 status for cisplatin resistance has been studied in numerous cancer cell lines, however, with contradictory results. While no correlation between cisplatin resistance and p53 status was observed in testis and ovarian cancer cell lines (Burger et al., 1997, De Feudis et al., 1997), other studies using breast, lung, colon, kidney, ovarian, leukaemia, melanoma and prostate cancer cell lines showed that p53 mutated cell lines were more resistant to cisplatin compared to p53 wild-type cell lines (Branch et al., 2000, O'Connor et al., 1997).

Contradictory results about the importance of p53 status for cisplatin resistance are also reported for bladder cancer cells. Comparing the cisplatin sensitivity in bladder cancer cell lines with different p53 status revealed that p53 wild type bladder cancer cells were more susceptible to cisplatin, while mutant cell lines were resistant (Kawasaki et al., 1996, Konstantakou et al., 2009). In line with these findings, it was also shown that cisplatin resistance in bladder cancer cells was enhanced by overexpression of mutant p53 protein (Miyake et al., 1999). Our own studies revealed that cisplatin resistant bladder cancer cell lines were mutated for p53, while cisplatin sensitive testis tumor cells showed functional p53 activity after cisplatin treatment (unpublished results). Contrary to these observations, Chang and co-workers investigated the effect of p53 mutations for drug sensitivity and found that bladder cancer cell lines expressing various human mutated p53 proteins displayed enhanced cisplatin sensitivity (Chang & Lai, 2001). Even more, when cisplatin sensitivity was measured in a series using 89 bladder cancer cell lines with different p53 status, it was found that p53 heterozygous cells were most susceptible to cisplatin (Chang & Lai, 2000). Altogether, we therefore conclude that, at least in bladder cancer cell lines, p53 mutations do not always lead to the development of cisplatin resistance.

In a number of studies it has been investigated whether the p53 status can be a predictor for the response to platinum-based chemotherapy in the clinic. Gadducci and co-workers reported that ovarian cancer patients with tumors harbouring p53 mutations experience a lower chance to achieve a complete response following cisplatin therapy, while patients with wild-type p53 tumors have a good chance to respond (Gadducci et al., 2002). In bladder cancers, mutations in the p53 gene are a frequent event (Esrig et al., 1994). However, there are conflicting results whether the p53 status can be used to predict the responsiveness to cisplatin treatment in bladder cancers (Nishiyama et al., 2008). On the one hand, it was shown that in a cohort of patients with TCC only the patients with altered p53 in the tumor would benefit from adjuvant cisplatin chemotherapy (Cote et al., 1997). On the other hand, p53 immunoreactivity could not be used to predict tumor response and patient survival in a cohort of 83 patients (Qureshi et al., 1999). Similarly, no clear conclusion as to whether p53 wild type was related to increased resistance or increased responsiveness could be drawn by Watanabe and co-workers in a study investigating 75 tumor specimens (Watanabe et al., 2004). Therefore, it cannot be concluded to date that the p53 status influences cisplatin responsiveness in bladder cancers (Table 1).

4.2 Anti-apoptotic proteins and cisplatin resistance

Cisplatin resistance has been associated with the expression of a number of anti-apoptotic proteins, both in cell cultures and in clinical samples. Expression of the anti-apoptotic proteins Bcl-2 and Bcl-x$_L$ resulted in cisplatin resistance in ovarian cancer cell lines (Yang et al., 2004). In bladder cancer cell lines, which were resistant to cisplatin and etoposide, Chresta and co-workers also observed high levels of Bcl-2 (Chresta et al., 1996). In addition, levels of the pro-apoptotic protein Bax were very low in the three bladder cancer cell lines under investigation (Chresta et al., 1996). We also observed low endogenous levels of Bax in cisplatin resistant bladder cancer cells compared to cisplatin sensitive testis tumor cell lines (unpublished observations). Furthermore, cisplatin treatment lead to translocation of Bax to the mitochondrial membrane in testis tumor cells, which was not observed in bladder cancer cell lines (unpublished observations). An association between cisplatin resistance, Bcl-2 expression and Bax translocation has also been proposed by Cho and co-workers who observed in cisplatin resistant bladder cancer sublines that Bcl-2 was up-regulated, which resulted in inhibition of Bax translocation to the mitochondrial membrane and reduced cell death (Cho et al., 2006). To elucidate the role of Bcl-2 for cisplatin resistance in bladder cancer cells, Miake and co-workers transfected the human bladder transitional cell carcinoma line KoTTC-1 with an expression plasmid for Bcl-2 and observed that overexpression conferred resistance to cisplatin (Miyake et al., 1998). Stably expressing Bcl-2 cells were then injected subcutaneously into nude mice to determine whether the Bcl-2 status can affect the efficacy of cisplatin treatment. Using this tumor cell implantation model, the authors could show that mice with tumors expressing Bcl-2 have an inferior prognosis compared to mice with tumors with no detectable Bcl-2 protein (Miyake et al., 1998). Altogether, the data suggest that Bcl-2 might be one of the factors influencing cisplatin resistance in bladder cancer cells. In proof of principle experiments, Bcl-2 levels in bladder cancer cells were decreased using Bcl-2 antisense oligonucleotides. These studies revealed that down-regulation of Bcl-2 expression resulted in a significant increase in toxicity of cisplatin in various bladder cancer cell lines (Bolenz et al., 2007, Hong et al., 2002), supporting the notion that expression of Bcl-2 may be associated with cisplatin resistance in bladder cancer cells (Table 1).

Expression levels of the anti-apoptotic factors Bcl-2 and Bcl-xL were determined in tumor samples from a diverse range of tissue to investigate for a possible involvement in clinical resistance, however, with contradictory results. While in ovarian carcinoma patients, expression of Bcl-xL was correlated with a decreased response to platinum chemotherapy (Williams et al., 2005), no association between response and Bcl-2 expression was observed in breast cancer patients (Parton et al., 2002). For bladder cancers, the clinical relevance of Bcl-2 expression for cisplatin resistance has been shown by Cooke and co-workers. The authors observed in a cohort of 51 patients with bladder cell carcinoma who received neo-adjuvant cisplatin chemotherapy that patients with Bcl-2 negative tumors had a significantly better prognosis (Cooke et al., 2000). An improved survival of patients with Bcl-2 negative tumors was also observed in a cohort of 89 patients with invasive bladder cancers who received cisplatin-based chemotherapy (Kong et al., 1998). In conclusion, expression of the anti-apoptotic factor Bcl-2 appears to affect the efficacy of cisplatin therapy for bladder cancers and might be used as a prognostic marker to predict the response to treatment.

The inhibitor of apoptosis (IAP) gene family encodes proteins, which have been reported to play an important role in cellular drug resistance. These proteins have been shown to be endogenous inhibitors of caspases, thus resulting in inhibition of cell death. Survivin, one of the members of the IAP family, is activated by cisplatin, which in part protects cells from cisplatin-induced apoptosis (Belyanskaya et al., 2005). An associated between survivin levels and cisplatin resistance has been reported for a number of cell lines derived from various cancer tissues including thyroid, lung and colon (Tirro et al., 2006) (Belyanskaya et al., 2005,

Hopkins-Donaldson et al., 2006, Pani et al., 2007). Bladder cancer cell lines showed a high expression of survivin compared to non-cancerous uro-epithelial cells (Yang et al., 2010). In clinical studies it has been investigated whether survivin might serve as a prognostic marker to predict clinical outcome. In tumor material of 30 patients with advanced bladder cancer, survivin expression has been identified as a marker for poor clinical outcome (Als et al., 2007). Similarly, Shariat and co-workers identified survivin as an independent predictor for recurrence of the disease in a cohort of 726 patients (Shariat et al., 2009).

The X-linked inhibitor of apoptosis (XIAP) is another member of the family of IAP proteins. Preclinical studies indicate that XIAP expression may be associated with cisplatin resistance. In ovarian carcinoma cell lines, for example, enhanced expression of XIAP was connected to the acquisition of cisplatin resistance (Mansouri et al., 2003). Bilim and co-workers reported considerable levels of XIAP in a panel of 4 bladder cancer cell lines, which are known to be cisplatin resistant (Bilim et al., 2003). The clinical relevance of XIAP for the efficacy of cisplatin treatment has been studied in a number of studies. Parton and co-workers found no association between XIAP expression and response to chemotherapy in ovarian cancer tissue (Parton et al., 2002). An inverse correlation between XIAP expression in the cancer tissue and pathological response was observed for patients with advanced bladder cancer (Pinho et al., 2009). The correlation, however, was not statistically significant. This study also demonstrated that bladder cancer patients with high levels of XIAP-associated factor 1 protein (XAF1) in the cancer tissue had a better prognosis after cisplatin based chemotherapy (Pinho et al., 2009). XAF1 inhibits the anti-caspase activity of XIAP, therefore antagonizing the anti-apoptotic action (Liston et al., 2001). Most likely, this resulted in increased sensitivity towards cisplatin. Another study investigated the expression of XIAP in bladder tumor specimens of 108 patients and found that XIAP was expressed at significantly higher levels in tumors compared to normal urothelium (Bilim et al., 2003). Unfortunately, it was not investigated, whether XIAP positivity was correlated with clinical response to cisplatin. However, it was suggested that XIAP upregulation might play a role in early TCC carcinogenesis (Bilim et al., 2003).

Altogether, information about expression of factors involved in cisplatin-induced apoptotic cell death pathways and its relation to cisplatin resistance is still emerging (Table 1). More information about the clinical relevance of apoptosis-related factors for the clinical outcome is needed, as this may identify new targets for pharmacological intervention.

5. Strategies for overcoming cisplatin resistance

As cisplatin resistance influences the clinical outcome, strategies are needed to circumvent the resistance phenotype. In a number of preclinical studies, modulators of cisplatin resistance were specifically targeted, and it was investigated whether this would influence cisplatin sensitivity. For example, the glutathione system may be modulated by glutathione depletion or GST blocking agents. Using these approaches, Buyn and co-workers could significantly enhance the cisplatin toxicity in bladder cancer cell lines (Byun et al., 2005). Similarly, inhibition of DNA repair has the potential to enhance the cytotoxicity of anticancer agents, as preclinical studies have confirmed that modulation of repair pathways can enhance the sensitivity to DNA damaging agents (Damia & D'Incalci, 2007, Ding et al., 2006). We found that siRNA-mediated down-regulation of the repair factor ERCC1-XFP decreased the repair of cisplatin-induced ICLs in bladder cancer cells and subsequently resulted in reduced cisplatin resistance (Usanova et al., 2010). In a number of studies, the effect of down-regulation of anti-apoptotic proteins for cisplatin resistance was studied. Down-regulation of Bcl-2 and Bcl-xL with antisense oligonucleotides enhanced the cisplatin sensitivity in four human bladder cancer cell lines (Bolenz et al., 2007). Antisense oligonucleotides against Bcl-2 were also used by Schaaf and co-workers who also observed an synergistic effect on cisplatin sensitivity (Schaaf et al., 2004). These findings show that reducing anti-apoptotic proteins positively influences cisplatin efficacy in bladder cancer cell lines and imply that targeting these factors may be a new therapeutic strategy for the treatment of bladder cancer.

6. Novel therapeutic strategies for bladder cancer treatment

Gemcitabine (2´,2´-difluorodeoxycytidine) is a deoxycytidine analogue, which can inhibit the ribonucleotide reductase or may be incorporated into DNA as a false base. Both mechanisms result in inhibition of DNA synthesis thereby leading to induction of apoptosis (Mini et al., 2006). Gemcitabine is used either as a single agent or in combination with other chemotherapeutic drugs for the treatment of cancer. For patients with locally advanced and metastatic bladder cancer, combination treatment of cisplatin or carboplatin and gemcitabine is the current standard chemotherapy regimen (von der Maase et al., 2005). Even though drug resistance is a major clinical problem, the resistance phenotype of bladder cancer cells to gemcitabine has not been investigated in great detail. An increase in expression of the anti-apoptotic protein clusterin has been described as a mechanism for acquired gemcitabine resistance in bladder cancer cells (Muramaki et al., 2009). Knock-down of clusterin sensitized gemcitabine-resistant bladder cancer cells indicating clinical significance (Muramaki et al., 2009). Gemcitabine resistance in bladder cancer cells might differ from cisplatin resistance as gemcitabine has been used for the treatment of cisplatin-refractory metastatic bladder cancer (Soga et al., 2010). The beneficial effect of gemcitabine for the treatment of cisplatin-refractory urothelial carcinoma, however, was not observed in the study of Lin and co-workers who reported that gemcitabine and ifosfamide showed insufficient clinical activity in patients with cisplatin-refractory bladder cancer (Lin et al., 2007). More promising approaches to increase the activity of cisplatin plus gemcitabine for treating metastatic bladder cancer have been reported in a number of recent studies. Addition of vitamin D3 increased the antitumor activity of cisplatin plus gemcitabine in bladder cancer cells and enhanced the antitumor activity in a xenograft model (Ma et al., 2010). The antibody Bevacizumab, which is directed against vascular endothelial growth factor (VEGF), has been shown to have a beneficial effect on cisplatin plus gemcitabine in patients with metastatic bladder cancer (Hahn et al., 2011). More clinical trials combining novel agents with cisplatin and gemcitabine, however, are needed to improve the treatment of bladder cancers.

7. Conclusion

Cisplatin-based combination therapy is the standard therapy for the treatment of advanced or metastatic cancer of the bladder. However, the efficacy of cisplatin is limited by intrinsic or acquired resistance to the drug. Mechanisms determining cisplatin resistance include drug transport, detoxification, DNA repair and expression of pro- and anti-apoptotic proteins. The clinical significance of these mechanisms for bladder cancers is not yet fully understood and still evolving. A better understanding about resistance mechanisms in bladder cancers is essential for developing therapeutic strategies aimed at circumventing cisplatin resistance for improving cancer therapy.

8. References

Aboussekhra, A.; Biggerstaff, M.; Shivji, M. K. K.; Vilpo, J. A.; Moncollin, V.; Podust, V. N.; Protic', M.;Hübscher, U.; Egly, J.-M. & Wood, R. D. (1995). Mammalian DNA nucleotide excision repair reconstituted with purified protein components. *Cell,* Vol. 80, pp. 859-868.

Aebi, S.; Kurdihaidar, B.; Gordon, R.; Cenni, B.; Zheng, H.; Fink, D.; Christen, R. D.; Boland, C. R.; Koi, M.; Fishel, R. & Howell, S. B. (1996). Loss of DNA mismatch repair in acquired-resistance to cisplatin. *Cancer Res,* Vol. 56, pp. 3087-3090.

Albertella, M. R.; Green, C. M.; Lehmann, A. R. & O'Connor, M. J. (2005a). A role for polymerase eta in the cellular tolerance to cisplatin-induced damage. *Cancer Res,* Vol. 65, pp. 9799-9806.

Albertella, M. R.; Lau, A. & O'Connor, M. J. (2005b). The overexpression of specialized DNA polymerases in cancer. *DNA Repair (Amst),* Vol. 4, pp. 583-593.

Als, A. B.; Dyrskjot, L.; von der Maase, H.; Koed, K.; Mansilla, F.; Toldbod, H. E.; Jensen, J. L.; Ulhoi, B. P.; Sengelov, L.; Jensen, K. M. & Orntoft, T. F. (2007). Emmprin and survivin predict response and survival following cisplatin-containing chemotherapy in patients with advanced bladder cancer. *Clin Cancer Res,* Vol. 13, pp. 4407-4414.

Alt, A.; Lammens, K.; Chiocchini, C.; Lammens, A.; Pieck, J. C.; Kuch, D.; Hopfner, K. P. & Carell, T. (2007). Bypass of DNA lesions generated during anticancer treatment with cisplatin by DNA polymerase eta. *Science,* Vol. 318, pp. 967-970.

Bedford, P.; Walker, M. C.; Sharma, H. L.; Perera, A.; McAuliffe, C. A.; Masters, J. R. W. & Hill, B. T. (1987). Factors influencing the sensitivity of two human bladder carcinoma cell lines to cis-diamminedichloro-platinum(II). *Chem-Biol Interactions,* Vol. 61, pp. 1-15.

Bellmunt, J.; Paz-Ares, L.; Cuello, M.; Cecere, F. L.; Albiol, S.; Guillem, V.; Gallardo, E.; Charles, J.; Mendez, P.; de la Cruz, J. J.; et al. (2007). Gene expression of ERCC1 as a novel prognostic marker in advanced bladder cancer patients receiving cisplatin-based chemotherapy. *Annals of Oncology,* Vol. 18, pp. 522-528.

Belyanskaya, L. L.; Hopkins-Donaldson, S.; Kurtz, S.; Simoes-Wust, A. P.; Yousefi, S.; Simon, H. U.; Stahel, R. & Zangemeister-Wittke, U. (2005). Cisplatin activates Akt in small cell lung cancer cells and attenuates apoptosis by survivin upregulation. *Int J Cancer,* Vol. 117, pp. 755-763.

Bignami, M.; Casorelli, I. & Karran, P. (2003). Mismatch repair and response to DNA-damaging antitumour therapies. *Eur J Cancer,* Vol. 39, pp. 2142-2149.

Bilim, V.; Kasahara, T.; Hara, N.; Takahashi, K. & Tomita, Y. (2003). Role of XIAP in the malignant phenotype of transitional cell cancer (TCC) and therapeutic activity of XIAP antisense oligonucleotides against multidrug-resistant TCC in vitro. *Int J Cancer, Vol. 103,* pp. 29-37.

Bischoff, C. J. & Clark, P. E. (2009). Bladder cancer. *Curr Opin Oncol,* Vol. 21, pp. 272-277.

Bolenz, C.; Becker, A.; Trojan, L.; Schaaf, A.; Cao, Y.; Weiss, C.; Alken, P. & Michel, M. S. (2007). Optimizing chemotherapy for transitional cell carcinoma by application of bcl-2 and bcl-xL antisense oligodeoxynucleotides. *Urol Oncol,* Vol. 25, pp. 476-482.

Bonnal, C.; Ravery, V.; Toublanc, M.; Bertrand, G.; Boccon-Gibod, L.; Henin, D. & Grandchamp, B. (2000). Absence of microsatellite instability in transitional cell carcinoma of the bladder. *Urology*, Vol. 55, pp. 287-291.

Branch, P.; Masson, M.; Aquilina, G.; Bignami, M. & Karran, P. (2000). Spontaneous development of drug resistance: mismatch repair and p53 defects in resistance to cisplatin in human tumor cells. *Oncogene*, Vol. 19, pp. 3138-3145.

Brozovic, A.; Fritz, G.; Christmann, M.; Zisowsky, J.; Jaehde, U.; Osmak, M. & Kaina, B. (2004). Long-term activation of SAPK/JNK, p38 kinase and fas-L expression by cisplatin is attenuated in human carcinoma cells that acquired drug resistance. *Int J Cancer*, Vol. 112, pp. 974-985.

Brozovic, A. & Osmak, M. (2007). Activation of mitogen-activated protein kinases by cisplatin and their role in cisplatin-resistance. *Cancer Letters*, Vol. 251, pp. 1-16.

Burger, H.; Nooter, K.; Boersma, A. W.; Kortland, C. J. & Stoter, G. (1997). Lack of correlation between cisplatin-induced apoptosis, p53 status and expression of Bcl-2 family proteins in testicular germ cell tumour cell lines. *Int J Cancer*, Vol. 73, pp. 592-599.

Byun, S.-S.; Kim, S. W.; Choi, H.; Lee, C. & Lee, E. (2005). Augmentation of cisplatin sensitivity in cisplatin-resistant human bladder cancer cells by modulating glutathione concentrations and glutathione- related enzyme activities. *Brit J Urol*, Vol. 95, pp. 1086-1090.

Catto, J. W.; Xinarianos, G.; Burton, J. L.; Meuth, M. & Hamdy, F. C. (2003). Differential expression of hMLH1 and hMSH2 is related to bladder cancer grade, stage and prognosis but not microsatellite instability. *Int J Cancer*, Vol. 105, pp. 484-490.

Ceppi, P.; Novello, S.; Cambieri, A.; Longo, M.; Monica, V.; Lo Iacono, M.; Giaj-Levra, M.; Saviozzi, S.; Volante, M.; Papotti, M. & Scagliotti, G. (2009). Polymerase eta mRNA expression predicts survival of non-small cell lung cancer patients treated with platinum-based chemotherapy. *Clin Cancer Res*, Vol. 15, pp. 1039-1045.

Chang, F. L. & Lai, M. D. (2000). The relationship between p53 status and anticancer drugs-induced apoptosis in nine human bladder cancer cell lines. *Anticancer Res*, Vol. 20, pp. 351-355.

Chang, F. L. & Lai, M. D. (2001). Various forms of mutant p53 confer sensitivity to cisplatin and doxorubicin in bladder cancer cells. *J Urol*, Vol. 166, pp. 304-310.

Cho, H. J.; Kim, J. K.; Kim, K. D.; Yoon, H. K.; Cho, M. Y.; Park, Y. P.; Jeon, J. H.; Lee, E. S.; Byun, S. S.; Lim, H. M. *et al.* (2006). Upregulation of Bcl-2 is associated with cisplatin-resistance via inhibition of Bax translocation in human bladder cancer cells. *Cancer Lett*, Vol. 237, pp. 56-66.

Chresta, C. M.; Masters, J. R. & Hickman, J. A. (1996). Hypersensitivity of human testicular tumors to etoposide-induced apoptosis is associated with functional p53 and a high Bax:Bcl-2 ratio. *Cancer Res*, Vol. 56, pp. 1834- 1841.

Chu, G. (1994). Cellular-responses to cisplatin - the roles of DNA-binding proteins and DNA-repair. *J Biol Chem*, Vol. 269, pp. 787-790.

Claij, N. & te Riele, H. (2004). Msh2 deficiency does not contribute to cisplatin resistance in mouse embryonic stem cells. *Oncogene*, Vol. 23, pp. 260-266.

Cohen, S. M.; Goel, A.; Phillips, J.; Ennis, R. D. & Grossbard, M. L. (2006). The role of perioperative chemotherapy in the treatment of urothelial cancer. *Oncologist*, Vol. 11, pp. 630-640.

Cole, R. S. (1973). Repair of DNA containing interstrand crosslinks in *Escherichia coli*: sequential excision and recombination. *Proc Natl Acad Sci USA*, Vol. 70, pp. 1064-1068.

Cooke, P. W.; James, N. D.; Ganesan, R.; Burton, A.; Young, L. S. & Wallace, D. M. (2000). Bcl-2 expression identifies patients with advanced bladder cancer treated by radiotherapy who benefit from neoadjuvant chemotherapy. *BJU Int*, Vol. 85, pp. 829-835.

Cote, R. J.; Esrig, D.; Groshen, S.; Jones, P. A. & Skinner, D. G. (1997). p53 and treatment of bladder cancer. *Nature*, Vol. 385, pp. 123-125.

Cruet-Hennequart, S.; Glynn, M. T.; Murillo, L. S.; Coyne, S. & Carty, M. P. (2008). Enhanced DNA-PK-mediated RPA2 hyperphosphorylation in DNA polymerase eta-deficient human cells treated with cisplatin and oxaliplatin. *DNA Repair (Amst)*, Vol. 7, pp-582-596.

Cruet-Hennequart, S.; Villalan, S.; Kaczmarczyk, A.; O'Meara, E.; Sokol, A. M. & Carty, M. P. (2009). Characterization of the effects of cisplatin and carboplatin on cell cycle progression and DNA damage response activation in DNA polymerase eta-deficient human cells. *Cell Cycle*, Vol. 8, pp. 3039-3050.

Dabholkar, M.; Bostick-Bruton, F.; Weber, C.; Bohr, V. A.; Egwuagu, C. & Reed, E. (1992). ERCC1 and ERCC2 expression in malignant tissues from ovarian cancer patients. *J Natl Cancer Inst*, Vol. 84, pp. 1512-1517.

Dabholkar, M.; Vionnet, J.; Bostick-Bruton, F.; Yu, J. J. & Reed, E. (1994). Messenger RNA levels of XPAC and ERCC1 in ovarian cancer tissue correlate with response to platinum-based chemotherapy. *J Clin Invest*, Vol. 94, pp. 703-708.

Damia, G. & D'Incalci, M. (2007). Targeting DNA repair as a promising approach in cancer therapy. *Eur J Cancer*, Vol. 43, pp. 1791-1801.

De Feudis, P.; Debernardis, D.; Beccaglia, P.; Valenti, M.; Graniela, S. E.; Arzani, D.; Stanzione, S.; D'Incalci, M.; Russo, P. & Broggini, M. (1997). DDP-induced cytotoxicity is not influenced by p53 in nine human ovarian cancer cell lines with different p53 status. *Br J Cancer*, Vol. 76, pp. 474-479.

De Silva, I. U.; McHugh, P. J.; Clingen, P. H. & Hartley, J. A. (2000). Defining the roles of nucleotide excision repair and recombination in the repair of DNA interstrand cross-links in mammalian cells. *Mol Cell Biol*, Vol. 20, pp. 7980-7990.

Dietmaier, W.; Wallinger, S.; Bocker, T.; Kullmann, F.; Fishel, R. & Ruschoff, J. (1997). Diagnostic microsatellite instability: definition and correlation with mismatch repair protein expression. *Cancer Res*, Vol. 57, pp. 4749-4756.

Ding, J.; Miao, Z.-H.; Meng, L.-H. & Geng, M.-Y. (2006). Emerging cancer therapeutic opportunities target DNA repair systems. *Trends Pharmacol Sci*, Vol. 27, pp. 338-344.

Duckett, D. R.; Drummond, J. T.; Murchie, A. I. H.; Reardon, J. T.; Sancar, A.; Lilley, D. M. & Modrich, P. (1996). Human MutS-alpha recognizes damaged DNA-base pairs containing O-6-methylguanine, O-4-methylthymine, or the cisplatin-d(GpG) adduct. *Proc Natl Acad Sci U S A*, Vol. 93, pp. 6443-6447.

Dunkern, T. R.; Fritz, G. & Kaina, B. (2001). Cisplatin-induced apoptosis in 43-3B and 27-1 cells defective in nucleotide excision repair. *Mutat Res*, Vol. 486, pp. 249-258.

Esrig, D.; Elmajian, D.; Groshen, S.; Freeman, J. A.; Stein, J. P.; Chen, S. C.; Nichols, P. W.; Skinner, D. G.; Jones, P. A. & Cote, R. J. (1994). Accumulation of nuclear p53 and tumor progression in bladder cancer. *N Engl J Med,* Vol. 331, pp. 1259-1264.

Ferry, K. V.; Hamilton, T. C. & Johnson, S. W. (2000). Increased nucleotide excision repair in cisplatin-resistant ovarian cancer cells: role of ERCC1-XPF. *Biochem Pharmacol,* Vol. 60, pp. 1305-1313.

Fink, D.; Nebel, S.; Aebi, S.; Zheng, H.; Cenni, B.; Nehme, A.; Christen, R. D. & Howell, S. B. (1996). The role of DNA mismatch repair in platinum drug-resistance. *Cancer Res,* Vol. 56, pp. 4881-4886.

Gadducci, A.; Cosio, S.; Muraca, S. & Genazzani, A. R. (2002). Molecular mechanisms of apoptosis and chemosensitivity to platinum and paclitaxel in ovarian cancer: biological data and clinical implications. *Eur J Gynaecol Oncol,* Vol. 23, pp. 390-396.

Gifford, G.; Paul, J.; Vasey, P. A.; Kaye, S. B. & Brown, R. (2004). The acquisition of hMLH1 methylation in plasma DNA after chemotherapy predicts poor survival for ovarian cancer patients. *Clin Cancer Res,* Vol. 10, pp. 4420-4426.

Gillet, L. C. & Schärer, O. D. (2006). Molecular mechanisms of mammalian global genome nucleotide excision repair. *Chem Rev,* Vol. 106, pp. 253-276.

Gonzalez-Zulueta, M.; Ruppert, J. M.; Tokino, K.; Tsai, Y. C.; Spruck, C. H.; 3rd, Miyao, N.; Nichols, P. W.; Hermann, G. G.; Horn, T.; Steven, K. & et al. (1993). Microsatellite instability in bladder cancer. *Cancer Res,* Vol. 53, pp. 5620-5623.

Gossage, L. & Madhusudan, S. (2007). Current status of excision repair cross complementation-group 1 (ERCC1) in cancer. *Cancer Treatment Reviews,* Vol. 33, pp. 565-577.

Hahn, N. M.; Stadler, W. M.; Zon, R. T.; Waterhouse, D.; Picus, J.; Nattam, S.; Johnson, C. S.; Perkins, S. M.; Waddell, M. J. & Sweeney, C. J. (2011). Phase II trial of cisplatin, gemcitabine, and bevacizumab as first-line therapy for metastatic urothelial carcinoma: Hoosier Oncology Group GU 04-75. *J Clin Oncol,* Vol. 29, pp. 1525-1530.

Handra-Luca, A.; Hernandez, J.; Mountzios, G.; Taranchon, E.; Lacau-St-Guily, J.; Soria, J.-C. & Fouret, P. (2007). Excision repair cross complementation group 1 immunohistochemical expression predicts objective response and cancer-specific survival in patients treated by cisplatin-based induction chemotherapy for locally advanced head and neck squamous cell carcinoma. *Clin Cancer Res,* Vol. 13, pp. 38553859.

Hartmann, A.; Zanardo, L.; Bocker-Edmonston, T.; Blaszyk, H.; Dietmaier, W.; Stoehr, R.; Cheville, J. C.; Junker, K.; Wieland, W.; Knuechel, R.; *et al.* (2002). Frequent microsatellite instability in sporadic tumors of the upper urinary tract. *Cancer Res,* Vol. 62, pp. 6796-6802.

Helleman, J.; van Staveren, I. L.; Dinjens, W. N. M.; van Kuijk, P. F.; Ritstier, K.; Ewing, P. C.; van cer Burg, M. E. L.; Stoter, G. & Berns, E. M. J. J. (2006). Mismatch repair and treatment resistance in ovarian cancer. *BMC Cancer,* Vol. 6, pp. 201.

Hinkel, A.; Schmidtchen, S.; Palisaar, R. J.; Noldus, J. & Pannek, J. (2008). Identification of bladder cancer patients at risk for recurrence or progression: an immunohistochemical study based on the expression of metallothionein. *J Toxicol Environ Health A,* Vol. 71, pp. 954-959.

Holzer, A. K.; Manorek, G. H. & Howell, S. B. (2006). Contribution of the major copper influx transporter CTR1 to the cellular accumulation of cisplatin, carboplatin, and oxaliplatin. *Mol Pharmacol*, Vol. 70, pp. 1390-1394.

Hong, J. H.; Lee, E.; Hong, J.; Shin, Y. J. & Ahn, H. (2002). Antisense Bcl2 oligonucleotide in cisplatin-resistant bladder cancer cell lines. *BJU Int*, Vol. 90, pp. 113-117.

Hopkins-Donaldson, S.; Belyanskaya, L. L.; Simoes-Wust, A. P.; Sigrist, B.; Kurtz, S.; Zangemeister-Wittke, U. & Stahel, R. (2006). p53-induced apoptosis occurs in the absence of p14(ARF) in malignant pleural mesothelioma. *Neoplasia*, Vol. 8, pp. 551-559.

Hour, T. C.; Chen, J.; Huang, C. Y.; Guan, J. Y.; Lu, S. H.; Hsieh, C. Y. & Pu, Y. S. (2000). Characterization of chemoresistance mechanisms in a series of cisplatin-resistant transitional carcinoma cell lines. *Anticancer Res*, Vol. 20, pp. 3221-3225.

Ichikawa, Y.; Lemon, S. J.; Wang, S.; Franklin, B.; Watson, P.; Knezetic, J. A.; Bewtra, C. & Lynch, H. T. (1999). Microsatellite instability and expression of MLH1 and MSH2 in normal and malignant endometrial and ovarian epithelium in hereditary nonpolyposis colorectal cancer family members. *Cancer Genet Cytogenet*, Vol. 112, pp. 2-8.

Ishida, S.; Lee, J.; Thiele, D. J. & Herskowitz, I. (2002). Uptake of the anticancer drug cisplatin mediated by the copper transporter Ctr1 in yeast and mammals. *Proc Natl Acad Sci*, Vol. 99, pp. 14298-14302.

Jachymczyk, W. J.; von Borstel, R. C.; Mowat, M. R. & Hastings, P. J. (1981). Repair of interstrand cross-links in DNA of Saccharomyces cerevisiae requires two systems for DNA repair: the RAD3 system and the RAD51 system. *Mol Gen Genet*, Vol. 182, pp. 196-205.

Jamieson, E. R. & Lippard, S. J. (1999). Structure, recognition and processing of cisplatin-DNA adducts. *Chem Rev*, Vol. 99, pp. 2467-2498.

Jansen, B. A. J.; Brouwer, J. & Reedijk, J. (2002). Glutathione induces cellular resistance against cationic dinuclear platinum anticancer drugs. *J Inorg Biochem*, Vol. 89, pp. 197-202.

Jemal, A.; Murray, T.; Ward, E.; Samuels, A.; Tiwari, R. C.; Ghafoor, A.; Feuer, E. J. & Thun, M. J. (2005). Cancer statistics, 2005. *CA Cancer J Clin*, Vol. 55, pp. 10-30.

Jin, T. X.; Furihata, M.; Yamasaki, I.; Kamada, M.; Liang, S. B.; Ohtsuki, Y. & Shuin, T. (1999). Human mismatch repair gene (hMSH2) product expression in relation to recurrence of transitional cell carcinoma of the urinary bladder. *Cancer*, Vol. 85, pp. 478-484.

Johnson, S. W.; Perez, R. P.; Godwin, A. K.; Yeung, A. T.; Handel, L. M.; Ozols, R. F. & Hamilton, T. C. (1994a). Role of platinum-DNA adduct formation and removal in cisplatin resistance in human ovarian cancer cell lines. *Biochem Pharmacol*, Vol. 47, pp. 689-697.

Johnson, S. W.; Swiggard, P. A.; Handel, L. M.; Brennan, J. M.; Godwin, A. K.; Ozols, R. F. & Hamilton, T. C. (1994b). Relationship between platinum-DNA adduct formation and removal and cisplatin cytotoxicity in cisplatin-sensitive and cisplatin-resistant human ovarian-cancer cells. *Cancer Res*, Vol. 54, pp. 5911-5916.

Jones, S. L.; Hickson, I. D.; Harris, A. L. & Harnett, P. R. (1994). Repair of cisplatin-DNA adducts by protein extracts from human ovarian-carcinoma. *Int J Cancer*, Vol. 59, pp. 388-393.

Jordan, P. & Carmo-Fonseca, M. (2000). Molecular mechanisms involved in cisplatin cytotoxicity. *Cell Mol Life Sci,* Vol. 57, pp. 1229-1235.

Jun, H. J.; Ahn, M. J.; Kim, H. S.; Sy, S. Y.; Han, J.; Lee, S. K.; Ahn, Y. C.; Jeong, H.-S.; Son, Y.-I.; Baek, J. H. & Park, K. (2008). ERCC1 expression as a predictive marker of squamous cell carcinoma of the head and neck treated with cisplatin-based concurrent chemotherapy. *Br J Cancer,* Vol. 99, pp. 167-172.

Kagi, J. H. & Schaffer, A. (1988). Biochemistry of metallothionein. *Biochemistry,* Vol. 27, pp. 8509-8515.

Kartalou, M. & Essigmann, J. M. (2001). Recognition of cisplatin adducts by cellular proteins. *Mutat Res,* Vol. 478, pp. 1-21.

Kasahara, K.; Fujiwara, Y.; Nishio, K.; Ohmori, T.; Sugimoto, Y.; Komiya, K.; Matsuda, T. & Saijo, N. (1991). Metallothionein content correlates with the sensitivity of human small cell lung cancer cell lines to cisplatin. *Cancer Res,* Vol. 51, pp. 3237-3242.

Kaufman, D. S. (2006). Challenges in the treatment of bladder cancer. *Ann Oncol,* Vol. 17 Suppl 5, pp. 106-112.

Kawasaki, T.; Tomita, Y.; Bilim, V.; Takeda, M.; Takahashi, K. & Kumanishi, T. (1996). Abrogation of apoptosis induced by DNA-damaging agents in human bladder-cancer cell lines with p21/WAF1/CIP1 and/or p53 gene alterations. *Int J Cancer,* Vol. 68, pp. 501-505.

Kim, K. H.; Do, I. G.; Kim, H. S.; Chang, M. H.; Kim, H. S.; Jun, H. J.; Uhm, J.; Yi, S. Y.; Lim do, H.; Ji, S. H.; *et al.* (2010). Excision repair cross-complementation group 1 (ERCC1) expression in advanced urothelial carcinoma patients receiving cisplatin-based chemotherapy. *Apmis,* Vol. 118, pp. 941-948.

Kim, M. K.; Cho, K.-J.; Kwon, G. Y.; Park, S.-I.; Kim, Y. H.; Kim, J. H.; Song, H.-Y.; Shin, J. H.; Jung, H. Y.; Lee, G. H.; *et al.* (2008). Patients with ERCC1-negative locally advanced esophageal cancers may benefit from preoperative chemotherapy. *Clin Cancer Res,* Vol. 14, pp. 4225-4231.

Köberle, B.; Grimaldi, K. A.; Sunters, A.; Hartley, J. A.; Kelland, L. R. & Masters, J. R. (1997). DNA repair capacity and cisplatin sensitivity of human testis tumour cells. *Int J Cancer,* Vol. 70, pp. 551-555.

Köberle, B.; Masters, J. R.; Hartley, J. A. & Wood, R. D. (1999). Defective repair of cisplatin-induced DNA damage caused by reduced XPA protein in testicular germ cell tumours. *Curr Biol,* Vol. 9, pp. 273-276.

Köberle, B.; Payne, J.; Grimaldi, K. A.; Hartley, J. A. & Masters, J. R. W. (1996). DNA-repair in cisplatin-sensitive and resistant human cell-lines measured in specific genes by quantitative polymerase chain- reaction. *Biochem Pharmacol,* Vol. 52, pp. 1729-1734.

Köberle, B.; Tomicic, M.; Usanova, S. & Kaina, B. (2010). Cisplatin resistance: preclinical findings and clinical implications BBA *Reviews on Cancer,* Vol. 1806, pp. 172-182.

Koga, H.; Kotoh, S.; Nakashima, M.; Yokomizo, A.; Tanaka, M. & Naito, S. (2000). Accumulation of intracellular platinum is correlated with intrinsic cisplatin resistance in human bladder cancer cell lines. *Int J Oncol,* Vol. 16, pp. 1003-1007.

Kondo, Y.; Kuo, S.-M.; Watkins, S. C. & Lazo, J. S. (1995). Metallothionein localization and cisplatin resistance in human hormone-independent prostatic tumor cell lines. *Cancer Res,* Vol. 1995, pp. 474-477.

Kong, G.; Shin, K. Y.; Oh, Y. H.; Lee, J. J.; Park, H. Y.; Woo, Y. N. & Lee, J. D. (1998). Bcl-2 and p53 expressions in invasive bladder cancers. *Acta Oncol,* Vol. 37, pp. 715-720.

Konstantakou, E. G.; Voutsinas, G. E.; Karkoulis, P. K.; Aravantinos, G.; Margaritis, L. H. and Stravopodis, D. J. (2009). Human bladder cancer cells undergo cisplatin-induced apoptosis that is associated with p53- dependent and p53-independent responses. *Int J Oncol*, Vol. 35, pp. 401-416.

Kotoh, S.; Naito, S.; Sakamoto, N.; Goto, K. & Kumazawa, J. (1994). Metallothionein expression is correlated with cisplatin resistance in transitional cell carcinoma of the urinary tract. *J Urology*, Vol. 152, pp. 1267- 1270.

Kotoh, S.; Naito, S.; Yokomizo, A.; Kohno, K.; Kuwano, M. & Kumazawa, J. (1997). Enhanced expression of gamma-glutamylcysteine synthetase and glutathione S-transferase genes in cisplatin-resistant bladder cancer cells with multidrug resistance phenotype. *J Urol*, Vol. 157, pp. 1054-1058.

Kunkel, T. A. & Erie, D. A. (2005). DNA mismatch repair. *Annu Rev Biochem*, Vol. 74, pp. 681-710.

Kuo, M. T.; Chen, H. H. W.; Song, I.-S.; Savaraj, N. & Ishikawa, T. (2007). The roles of copper transporters in cisplatin resistance. *Cancer Metastasis Rev*, Vol. 26, pp. 71-83.

Kuraoka, I.; Kobertz, W. R.; Ariza, R. R.; Biggerstaff, M.; Essigmann, J. M. & Wood, R. D. (2000). Repair of an interstrand DNA crosslink initiated by ERCC1-XPF repair/recombination nuclease. *J Biol Chem*, Vol. 275, pp. 26632-26636.

Li, Q.; Gardner, K.; Zhang, L.; Tsang, B.; Bostick-Bruton, F. & Reed, E. (1998). Cisplatin induction of ERCC-1 mRNA expression in A2780/CP70 human ovarian cancer cells. *J Biol Chem*, Vol. 273, pp. 23419-23425.

Li, Q.; Yu, J. J.; Mu, C.; Yunmbam, M. K.; Slavsky, D.; Cross, C. L.; Bostick-Bruton, F. & Reed, E. (2000). Association between the level of ERCC-1 expression and the repair of cisplatin-induced DNA damage in human ovarian cancer cells. *Anticancer Res*, Vol. 20, pp. 645-652.

Lin, C. C.; Hsu, C. H.; Huang, C. Y.; Keng, H. Y.; Tsai, Y. C.; Huang, K. H.; Cheng, A. L. & Pu, Y. S. (2007). Gemcitabine and ifosfamide as a second-line treatment for cisplatin-refractory metastatic urothelial carcinoma: a phase II study. *Anticancer Drugs*, Vol. 18, pp. 487-491.

Liston, P.; Fong, W. G.; Kelly, N. L.; Toji, S.; Miyazaki, T.; Conte, D.; Tamai, K.; Craig, C. G.; McBurney, M. W. & Korneluk, R. G. (2001). Identification of XAF1 as an antagonist of XIAP anti-Caspase activity. *Nat Cell Biol*, Vol. 3, pp. 128-133.

Ma, Y.; Yu, W. D.; Trump, D. L. & Johnson, C. S. (2010). 1,25D3 enhances antitumor activity of gemcitabine and cisplatin in human bladder cancer models. *Cancer*, Vol. 116, pp. 3294-3303.

Mannervik, B. (1987). The enzymes of glutathione metabolism: an overview. *Biochem Soc Trans*, Vol. 15, pp. 717- 718.

Mansouri, A.; Zhang, Q.; Ridgway, L. D.; Tian, L. & Claret, F. X. (2003). Cisplatin resistance in an ovarian carcinoma is associated with a defect in programmed cell death control through XIAP regulation. *Oncol Res*, Vol. 13, pp. 399-404.

Massey, A.; Offman, J.; Macpherson, P. & Karran, P. (2003). DNA mismatch repair and acquired cisplatin resistance in *E. coli* and human ovarian carcinoma cells. *DNA Repair (Amst)*, Vol. 2, pp. 73-89.

McHugh, P. J.; Spanswick, V. J. & Hartley, J. A. (2001). Repair of DNA interstrand crosslinks: molecular mechanisms and clinical relevance. *The Lancet Oncology*, Vol. 2, pp. 483-490.

Meijer, C.; Mulder, N. H.; Timmer-Bosscha, H.; Sluiter, W. J.; Meersma, G. J. & de Vries, E. G. E. (1992). Relationship of cellular glutathione to the cytotoxicity and resistance of seven platinum compounds. *Cancer Res, Vol. 52*, pp. 6885-6889.

Mellish, K. J.; Kelland, L. R. & Harrap, K. R. (1993). In vitro drug chemosensitivity of human cervical squamous cell carcinoma cell lines with intrinsic and acquired resistance to cisplatin. *Br J Cancer, Vol. 68*, pp. 240- 250.

Mello, J. A.; Acharya, S.; Fishel, R. & Essigmann, J. M. (1996). The mismatch-repair protein hMSH2 binds selectively to DNA-adducts of the anticancer drug cisplatin. *Chem Biol, Vol. 3*, pp. 579-589.

Metzger, R.; Leichman, C. G.; Danenberg, K. D.; Danenberg, P. V.; Lenz, H. J.; Hayashi, K.; Groshen, S.; Salonga, D.; Cohen, H.; Laine, L.; *et al.* (1998). ERCC1 mRNA levels complement thymidylate synthase mRNA levels in predicting response and survival for gastric cancer patients receiving combination cisplatin and fluorouracil chemotherapy. *J Clin Oncol, Vol. 16*, pp. 309-316.

Mini, E.; Nobili, S.; Caciagli, B.; Landini, I. & Mazzei, T. (2006). Cellular pharmacology of gemcitabine. *Ann Oncol, Vol. 17* Suppl 5, v7-12.

Miyake, H.; Hanada, N.; Nakamura, H.; Kagawa, S.; Fujiwara, T.; Hara, I.; Eto, H.; Gohji, K.; Arakawa, S.; Kamidono, S. & Saya, H. (1998). Overexpression of Bcl-2 in bladder cancer cells inhibits apoptosis induced by cisplatin and adenoviral-mediated p53 gene transfer. *Oncogene, Vol. 16*, pp. 933-943.

Miyake, H.; Hara, I.; Yamanaka, K.; Arakawa, S. & Kamidono, S. (1999). Synergistic enhancement of resistance to cisplatin in human bladder cancer cells by overexpression of mutant-type p53 and Bcl-2. *J Urol, Vol. 162*, pp. 2176-2181.

Muramaki, M.; So, A.; Hayashi, N.; Sowery, R.; Miyake, H.; Fujisawa, M. & Gleave, M. E. (2009). Chemosensitization of gemcitabine-resistant human bladder cancer cell line both in vitro and in vivo using antisense oligonucleotide targeting the anti-apoptotic gene, clusterin. *BJU Int, Vol. 103*, pp. 384- 390.

Mylona, E.; Zarogiannos, A.; Nomikos, A.; Giannopoulou, I.; Nikolaou, I.; Zervas, A. & Nakopoulou, L. (2008). Prognostic value of microsatellite instability determined by immunohistochemical staining of hMSH2 and hMSH6 in urothelial carcinoma of the bladder. *Apmis, Vol. 116*, 59-65.

Niedernhofer, L. J.; Odijk, H.; Budzowska, M.; van Drunen, E.; Maas, A.; Theil, A. F.; de Wit, J.; Jaspers, N. G.; Beverloo, H. B.; Hoeijmakers, J. H. & Kanaar, R. (2004). The structure-specific endonuclease Ercc1-Xpf is required to resolve DNA interstrand cross-link-induced double-strand breaks. *Mol Cell Biol, Vol. 24*, pp. 5776- 5787.

Nishiyama, H.; Watanabe, J. & Ogawa, O. (2008). p53 and chemosensitivity in bladder cancer. *Int J Clin Oncol, Vol. 13*, pp. 282-286.

O'Connor, P. M.; Jackman, J.; Bae, I.; Myers, T. G.; Fan, S.; Mutoh, M.; Scudiero, D. A.; Monks, A.; Sausville, E. A.; Weinstein, J. N.; *et al.* (1997). Characterization of the p53 tumor suppressor pathway in cell lines of the National Cancer Institute anticancer drug screen and correlations with the growth-inhibitory potency of 123 anticancer agents. *Cancer Res, Vol. 57*, pp. 4285-4300.

Ohashi, E.; Ogi, T.; Kusumoto, R.; Iwai, S.; Masutani, C.; Hanaoka, F. & Ohmori, H. (2000). Error-prone bypass of certain DNA lesions by the human DNA polymerase kappa. *Genes Dev, Vol. 14*, pp. 1589-1594.

Olaussen, K. A.; Dunant, A.; Fouret, P.; Brambilla, E.; Andre, F.; Haddad, V.; Taranchon, E.; Filipits, M.; Pirker, R.; Popper, H. H.; et al. (2006). DNA repair by ERCC1 in non-small-cell lung cancer and cisplatin- based adjuvant chemotherapy. N Engl J Med, Vol. 355, pp. 983-991.

Oldenburg, J.; Begg, A. C.; van Vugt, M. J.; Ruevekamp, M.; Schornagel, J. H.; Pinedo, H. M. & Los, G. (1994). Characterization of resistance mechanisms to cis-diamminedichloroplatinum(II) in three sublines of the CC531 colon adenocarcinoma cell line in vitro. Cancer Res, Vol. 54, pp. 487-493.

Ottini, L.; Palli, D.; Falchetti, M.; D'Amico, C.; Amorosi, A.; Saieva, C.; Calzolari, A.; Cimoli, F.; Tatarelli, C.; De Marchis, L.; et al. (1997). Microsatellite instability in gastric cancer is associated with tumor location and family history in a high-risk population from Tuscany. Cancer Res, Vol. 57, pp. 4523-4529.

Pabla, N.; Huang, S.; Mi, Q.-S.; Daniel, R. & Dong, Z. (2008). ATR-Chk2 signaling in p53 activation and DNA damage response during cisplatin-induced apoptosis. J Biol Chem, Vol. 283, pp. 6572-6583.

Pani, E.; Stojic, L.; El-Shemerly, M.; Jiricny, J. & Ferrari, S. (2007). Mismatch repair status and the response of human cells to cisplatin. Cell Cycle, Vol. 6, pp. 1796-1802.

Papouli, E.; Cejka, P. & Jiricny, J. (2004). Dependence of the cytotoxicity of DNA-damaging agents on the micmatch repair status of human cells. Cancer Res, Vol. 64, pp. 3391-3394.

Parker, R. J.; Eastman, A.; Bostick-Bruton, F. & Reed, E. (1991). Acquired cisplatin resistance in human ovarian cancer cells is associated with enhanced repair of cisplatin-DNA lesions and reduced drug accumulation. J Clin Invest, Vol. 87, pp. 772-777.

Parsons, R.; Li, G. M.; Longley, M. J.; Fang, W. H.; Papadopoulos, N.; Jen, J.; Delachapelle, A.; Kinzler, K. W.; Vogelstein, B. & Modrich, P. (1993). Hypermutability and mismatch repair deficiency in rer+ tumor- cells. Cell, Vol. 75, pp. 1227-1236.

Parton, M.; Krajewski, S.; Smith, I.; Krajewska, M.; Archer, C.; Naito, M.; Ahern, R.; Reed, J. & Dowsett, M. (2002). Coordinate expression of apoptosis-associated proteins in human breast cancer before and during chemotherapy. Clin Cancer Res, Vol 8, pp. 2100-2108.

Pinho, M. B.; Costas, F.; Sellos, J.; Dienstmann, R.; Andrade, P. B.; Herchenhorn, D.; Peixoto, F. A.; Santos, V. O.; Small, I. A.; Guimaraes, D. P. & Ferreira, C. G. (2009). XAF1 mRNA expression improves progression- free and overall survival for patients with advanced bladder cancer treated with neoadjuvant chemotherapy. Urol Oncol. Vol. 27, pp. 382-390.

Qureshi, K. N.; Griffiths, T. R.; Robinson, M. C.; Marsh, C.; Roberts, J. T.; Hall, R. R.; Lunec, J. & Neal, D. E. (1999). TP53 accumulation predicts improved survival in patients resistant to systemic cisplatin-based chemotherapy for muscle-invasive bladder cancer. Clin Cancer Res, Vol. 5, pp. 3500-3507.

Rabik, C. A. & Dolan, M. E. (2007). Molecular mechanisms of resistance and toxicity associated with platinating agents. Cancer Treat Rev, Vol. 33, pp. 9-23.

Roos, W. P.; Tsaalbi-Shtylik, A.; Tsaryk, R.; Guvercin, F.; de Wind, N. & Kaina, B. (2009). The translesion polymerase Rev3L in the tolerance of alkylating anticancer drugs. Mol Pharmacol, Vol. 76, pp. 927-934.

Safaei, R. (2006). Role of copper transporters in the uptake and efflux of platinum containing drugs. Cancer Letters, Vol. 234, pp. 34-39.

Saga, Y.; Hashimoto, H.; Yachiku, S.; Iwata, T. & Tokumitsu, M. (2004). Reversal of acquired cisplatin resistance by modulation of metallothionein in transplanted murine tumors. *Int J Urol,* Vol. 11, pp. 407-415.

Sarkar, S.; A.A.; D.; H.D.; U. & McHugh, P. J. (2006). DNA interstrand crosslink repair during G1 involves nucleotide excision repair and DNA polymerase ζ. *The EMBO J,* Vol. 25, pp. 1285-1294.

Satoh, M.; Cherian, M. G.; Imura, N. & Shimizu, H. (1994). Modulation of resistance to anticancer drugs by inhibition of metallothionein synthesis. *Cancer Res,* Vol. 54, pp. 5255-5257.

Schaaf, A.; Sagi, S.; Langbein, S.; Trojan, L.; Alken, P. & Michel, M. S. (2004). Cytotoxicity of cisplatin in bladder cancer is significantly enhanced by application of bcl-2 antisense oligonucleotides. *Urol Oncol,* Vol. 22, pp. 188-192.

Shachar, S.; Ziv, O.; Avkin, S.; Adar, S.; Wittschieben, J.; Reissner, T.; Chaney, S.; Friedberg, E. C.; Wang, Z.; Carell, T.; *et al.* (2009). Two-polymerase mechanisms dictate error-free and error-prone translesion DNA synthesis in mammals. *Embo J,* Vol. 28, pp. 383-393.

Shariat, S. F.; Karakiewicz, P. I.; Godoy, G.; Karam, J. A.; Ashfaq, R.; Fradet, Y.; Isbarn, H.; Montorsi, F.; Jeldres, C.; Bastian, P. J.; *et al.* (2009). Survivin as a prognostic marker for urothelial carcinoma of the bladder: a multicenter external validation study. *Clin Cancer Res,* Vol. 15, pp. 7012-7019.

Shen, X.; Jun, S.; O"Neal, L. E.; Sonoda, E.; Bemark, M.; Sale, J. E. & Li, L. (2006). REV3 and REV1 play major roles in recombination-independent repair of DNA interstrand cross-links mediated by monoubiquitinated proliferating cell nuclear antigen (PCNA). *J Biol Chem,* Vol. 281, pp. 13869-13872.

Shivji, M. K.; Moggs, J. G.; Kuraoka, I.; & Wood, R. D. (1999). Dual-incision assays for nucleotide excision repair using DNA with a lesion at a specific site. In *DNA Repair Protocols: Eukaryotic Systems, D. S. Henderson, ed. (Totowa, NJ, Humana Press),* pp. 373-392.

Shivji, M. K.; Moggs, J. G.; Kuraoka, I. & Wood, R. D. (2005). Assaying for the dual incisions of nucleotide excision repair using DNA with a lesion at a specific site. In *DNA Repair Protocols: Eukaryotic Systems, Second Edition, D. S. Henderson, ed. (Totowa, NJ, Humana Press),* pp. 435-456.

Shuck, S. C.; Short, E. A. & Turchi, J. J. (2008). Eukaryotic nucleotide excision repair: from understanding mechanisms to influencing biology. *Cell Research,* Vol. 18, pp. 64-72.

Siddik, Z. H. (2003). Cisplatin: mode of action and molecular basis of resistance. *Oncogene,* Vol. 22, pp. 7265- 7279.

Siegsmund, M. J.; Marx, C.; Seemann, O.; Schummer, B.; Steidler, A.; Toktomambetova, L.; Kohrmann, K. U.; Rassweiler, J. & Alken, P. (1999). Cisplatin-resistant bladder carcinoma cells: enhanced expression of metallothioneins. *Urol Res,* Vol. 27, pp. 157-163.

Sijbers, A. M.; de Laat, W. L.; Ariza, R. R.; Biggerstaff, M.; Wei, Y.-F.; Moggs, J. G.; Carter, K. C.; Shell, B. K.; Evans, E.; de Jong, M. C.; *et al.* (1996). Xeroderma pigmentosum group F caused by a defect in a structure- specific DNA repair endonuclease. *Cell,* Vol. 86, pp. 811-822.

Singh, S. V.; Xu, B. H.; Jani, J. P.; Emerson, E. O.; Backes, M. G.; Rihn, C.; Scalamogna, D.; Stemmler, N.; Specht, S.; Blanock, K. & et al. (1995). Mechanism of cross-resistance to cisplatin in a mitomycin C-resistant human bladder cancer cell line. *Int J Cancer*, Vol. 61, pp. 431-436.

Siu, L. L.; Banerjee, D.; Khurana, R. J.; Pan, X.; Pflueger, R.; Tannock, I. F. & Moore, M. J. (1998). The prognostic role of p53, metallothionein, P-glycoprotein, and MIB-1 in muscle-invasive urothelial transitional cell carcinoma. *Clin Cancer Res*, Vol. 4, pp. 559-565.

Soga, N.; Kise, H.; Arima, K. & Sugimura, Y. (2010). Third-line gemcitabine monotherapy for platinum-resistant advanced urothelial cancer. *Int J Clin Oncol*, Vol. 15, pp. 376-381.

Song, I.-S.; Savaraj, N.; Siddik, Z. H.; Liu, P.; Wei, Y.; Wu, C. J. & Kuo, M. T. (2004). Role of human copper transporter Ctr1 in the transport of platinum-based antitumor agents in cisplatin-sensitive and cisplatin-resistant cells. *Molec Cancer Therapeutics*, Vol. 3, pp. 1543-1549.

Strand, M.; Prolla, T. A.; Liskay, R. M. & Petes, T. D. (1993). Destabilization of tracts of simple repetitive DNA in yeast by mutations affecting DNA mismatch repair. *Nature*, Vol. 365, pp. 274-276.

Surowiak, P.; Materna, V.; Maciejczyk, A.; Pudelko, M.; Markwitz, E.; Spaczynski, M.; Dietel, M.; Zabel, M. & Lage, H. (2007). Nuclear metallothionein expression correlates with cisplatin resistance of ovarian cancer cells and poor clinical outcome. *Virchows Arch*, Vol. 450, pp. 279-285.

Tada, Y.; Wada, M.; Migita, T.; Nagayama, J.; Hinoshita, E.; Mochida, Y.; Maehara, Y.; Tsuneyoshi, M.; Kuwano, M. & Naito, S. (2002). Increased expression of multidrug resistance-associated proteins in bladder cancer during clinical course and drug resistance to doxorubicin. *Int J Cancer*, Vol. 98, pp. 630- 635.

Taniguchi, K.; Wada, M.; Kohno, K.; Nakamura, T.; Kawabe, T.; Kawakami, M.; Kagotani, K.; Okumura, K.; Akiyama, S. & Kuwano, M. (1996). A human canalicular multispecific organic anion transporter (cMOAT) gene is overexpressed in cisplatin-resistant human cancer cell lines with decreased drug accumulation. *Cancer Res*, Vol. 56, pp. 4124-4129.

Tirro, E.; Consoli, M. L.; Massimino, M.; Manzella, L.; Frasca, F.; Sciacca, L.; Vicari, L.; Stassi, G.; Messina, L.; Messina, A. & Vigneri, P. (2006). Altered expression of c-IAP1, survivin, and Smac contributes to chemotherapy resistance in thyroid cancer cells. *Cancer Res*, Vol. 66, pp. 4263-4272.

Topping, R. P.; Wilkinson, J. C. & Drotschmann Scarpinato, K. (2009). Mismatch repair protein deficiency compromises cisplatin-induced apoptotic signaling. *J Biol Chem*, Vol. 284, pp. 14029-14039.

Usanova, S.; Piee-Staffa, A.; Sied, U.; Thomale, J.; Schneider, A.; Kaina, B. & Köberle, B. (2010). Cisplatin sensitivity of testis tumour cells is due to deficiency in interstrand-crosslink repair and low ERCC1- XPF expression. *Mol Cancer*, Vol. 9, pp. 248.

von der Maase, H.; Sengelov, L.; Roberts, J. T.; Ricci, S.; Dogliotti, L.; Oliver, T.; Moore, M. J.; Zimmermann, A. & Arning, M. (2005). Long-term survival results of a randomized trial comparing gemcitabine plus cisplatin, with methotrexate, vinblastine, doxorubicin, plus cisplatin in patients with bladder cancer. *J Clin Oncol*, Vol. 23, pp. 4602-4608.

Wang, H.; Zhang, S. Y.; Wang, S.; Lu, J.; Wu, W.; Weng, L.; Chen, D.; Zhang, Y.; Lu, Z.; Yang, J.; *et al.* (2009). REV3L confers chemoresistance to cisplatin in human gliomas: the potential of its RNAi for synergistic therapy. *Neuro Oncol,* Vol. 11, pp. 790-802.

Watanabe, J.; Nishiyama, H.; Okubo, K.; Takahashi, T.; Toda, Y.; Habuchi, T.; Kakehi, Y.; Tada, M. & Ogawa, O. (2004). Clinical evaluation of p53 mutations in urothelial carcinoma by IHC and FASAY. *Urology,* Vol. 63, pp. 989-993.

Weberpals, J.; Garbuio, K.; O'Brien, A.; Clark-Knowles, K.; Doucette, S.; Antoniouk, O.; Goss, G. & Dimitroulakos, J. (2009). The DNA repair proteins BRCA1 and ERCC1 as predictive markers in sporadic ovarian cancer. *Int J Cancer,* Vol. 124, pp. 806-815.

Wei, S. H.; Chen, C. M.; Strathdee, G.; Harnsomburana, J.; Shyu, C. R.; Rahmatpanah, F.; Shi, H.; Ng, S. W.; Yan, P. S.; Nephew, K. P.; *et al.* (2002). Methylation microarray analysis of late-stage ovarian carcinomas distinguishes progression-free survival in patients and identifies candidate epigenetic markers. *Clin Cancer Res,* Vol. 8, pp. 2246-2252.

Welsh, C.; Day, R.; McGurk, C.; Masters, J. R.; Wood, R. D. & Köberle, B. (2004). Reduced levels of XPA, ERCC1 and XPF DNA repair proteins in testis tumor cell lines. *Int J Cancer,* Vol. 110, pp. 352-361.

Westerveld, A.; Hoeijmakers, J. H. J.; van Duin, M.; de Wit, J.; Odijk, H.; Pastink, A.; Wood, R. & Bootsma, D. (1984). Molecular cloning of a human DNA repair gene. *Nature,* Vol. 310, pp. 425-429.

Williams, J.; Lucas, P. C.; Griffith, K. A.; Choi, M.; Fogoros, S.; Hu, Y. Y. & Liu, J. R. (2005). Expression of Bcl-xL in ovarian carcinoma is associated with chemoresistance and recurrent disease. *Gynecol Oncol,* Vol. 96, pp. 287-295.

Wittschieben, J. P.; Reshmi, S. C.; Gollin, S. M. & Wood, R. D. (2006). Loss of DNA polymerase zeta causes chromosomal instability in mammalian cells. *Cancer Res,* Vol. 66, pp. 134-142.

Wood, D. P. J.; Klein, E.; Fair, W. R. & Chaganti, R. S. (1993). Metallothionein gene expression in bladder cancer exposed to cisplatin. *Modern Pathology,* Vol. 6, pp. 33-35.

Wood, R. D.; Araújo, S. J.; Ariza, R. R.; Batty, D. P.; Biggerstaff, M.; Evans, E.; Gaillard, P.-H.; Gunz, D.; Köberle, B.; Kuraoka, I.; *et al.* (2000). DNA damage recognition and nucleotide excision repair in mammalian cells. *Cold Spring Harbor Sym Quant Biol,* Vol. 65, pp. 173-182.

Wülfing, C.; van Ahlen, H.; Eltze, E.; Piechota, H.; Hertle, L. & Schmid, K. W. (2007). Metallothionein in bladder cancer: correlation of overexpression with poor outcome after chemotherapy. *World J Urol,* Vol. 25, pp. 199-205.

Wynne, P.; Newton, C.; Ledermann, J. A.; Olaitan, A.; Mould, T. A. & Hartley, J. A. (2007). Enhanced repair of DNA interstrand crosslinking in ovarian cancer cells from patients following treatment with platinum-based chemotherapy. *Br J Cancer,* Vol. 97, pp. 927-933.

Yang, D.; Song, X.; Zhang, J.; Ye, L.; Wang, S.; Che, X.; Wang, J.; Zhang, Z.; Wang, L. & Shi, W. (2010). Therapeutic potential of siRNA-mediated combined knockdown of the IAP genes (Livin, XIAP, and Survivin) on human bladder cancer T24 cells. *Acta Biochim Biophys Sin (Shanghai),* Vol. 42, pp. 137-144.

Yang, X.; Zheng, F.; Xing, H.; Gao, Q.; Wei, W.; Lu, Y.; Wang, S.; Zhou, J.; Hu, W. & Ma, D. (2004). Resistance to chemotherapy-induced apoptosis via decreased caspase-3 activity and overexpression of antiapoptotic proteins in ovarian cancer. J *Cancer Res Clin Oncol*, Vol. 130, pp. 423-428.

Yeh, J. J.; Hsu, N. Y.; Hsu, W. H.; Tsai, C. H.; Lin, C. C. & Liang, J. A. (2005). Comparison of chemotherapy response with P-glycoprotein, multidrug resistance-related protein-1, and lung resistance-related protein expression in untreated small cell lung cancer. *Lung*, Vol. 183, pp. 177-183.

Zhen, W.; Link, C. J.; Jr.; O'Connor, P. M.; Reed, E.; Parker, R.; Howell, S. B. & Bohr, V. A. (1992). Increased gene-specific repair of cisplatin interstrand cross-links in cisplatin-resistant human ovarian cancer cell lines. *Mol Cell Biol*, Vol. 12, pp. 3689-3698.

Zheng, H.; Tomschik, M.; Zlatanova, J. & Leuba, S. H. (2005). Evanescent field fluorescence microscopy (EFFM) for analysis of protein/DNA interactions at the single-molecule level. In *Protein-protein interactions, a molecular cloning manual, 2nd edition,* E. Golemis, & P. Adams, eds. (Cold Spring Harbor, NY, Cold Spring Harbor Laboratory Press), pp. 1-19 Chapter 20.

Part 3

Invasive Disease, Surgical Treatment and Robotic Approach

5

Robotic-Assisted Laparoscopic Radical Cystoprostatectomy and Intracorporeal Urinary Diversion (Studer Pouch or Ileal Conduit) for Bladder Cancer

Abdullah Erdem Canda, Ali Fuat Atmaca and Mevlana Derya Balbay
Ankara Atatürk Training and Research Hospital, 1st Urology Clinic, Ankara
Turkey

1. Introduction

Bladder cancer is the fourth most common malignancy in American men and almost 25% is muscle invasive at the time of diagnosis (Cancer Facts and Figures, 2009; Nieder et al., 2008).

Currently, most effective local treatment of muscle invasive bladder cancer and non-invasive, high-grade bladder tumors that recur or progress despite intravesical therapies is open radical cystoprostatectomy with urinary diversion (Clinical Practice Guidelines in Oncology, 2010; Huang et al., 2007).

With the advancement of technology, minimally invasive surgical approaches including laparoscopic (Huang et al., 2010; Guazzoni et al., 2003) or robotic-assisted laparoscopic (Akbulut et al., 2011; Rehman et al., 2011; Kauffman et al., 2011; Hellenthal et al., 2010; Kasraeian et al., 2010; Pruthi et al., 2010; Schumacher et al., 2009) cystectomies are increasingly being performed.

This chapter summarizes the current state of the use of the surgical robot in performing radical cystoprostatectomy with urinary diversion in patients with bladder cancer.

2. Why to use a surgical robot?

Radical cystoprostatectomy with bilateral extended lymph node dissection and urinary diversion (Studer pouch reconstruction or ileal conduit formation) are complex and time consuming surgical procedures. Performing these complex procedures in an open surgical approach is well established. To perform these complex procedures pure laparoscopically is extremely difficult. However, the use of a surgical robot enables the operating surgeon to perform these procedures much more easily because it has the advantages of the 3-dimensional and magnified image capability, higher grades of wristed hand movements, decreased hand tremor leading to a shorter learning curve. Besides, having the 4th-robotic arm gives the advantage of additional assistance and tissue retraction and letting the console surgeon to operate in a comfortable sitting position rather than standing position for long hours. Menon et al suggested that robotic approach combines the oncological principles of open surgery with technical advantages of the surgical robot which allows a precise, gentle, quick and safe surgery during performing radical cystectomy for bladder cancer (Menon et al., 2003).

Therefore, following the introduction of da Vinci-S 4-arm surgical robot (Intuitive Surgical, Sunnyvale, California) many centers have started to publish their experiences with the use of a surgical robot in performing these complex surgical procedures (Akbulut et al., 2011; Rehman et al., 2011; Kauffman et al., 2011; Hellenthal et al., 2010; Kasraeian et al., 2010; Pruthi et al., 2010; Schumacher et al., 2009).

3. Open versus robotic approach

3.1 Comparison of complications

A prospective study from Weill Cornell Medical College, Department of Urology, New York, NY, USA has recently evaluated prospective complications of open (n=104) versus robotic (n=83) cystectomy procedures (Ng et al., 2010). Complications were classified due to modified Clavien system. Significantly lower major complications were detected in the robotic group compared to the open surgical approach (17% versus 31%, p=0.03). Robotic cystectomy was found to be an independent predictor of fewer overall and major complications at 0-30 day (perioperative) and 31-90 day periods. Another well known study from The University of North Carolina at Chapel Hill, Division of Urologic Surgery, Chapel Hill, North Carolina, USA randomized 21 patients to robotic approach and 20 to the open technique. No significant difference in regard to overall complication rate or hospital stay was detected between the two groups of patients (Nix et al., 2010). In our initial experience of 12 cases whom we performed robot assisted laparoscopic nerve sparing radical cystoprostatectomy with bilateral extended lymph node dissection and intracorporeal Studer pouch construction, we had 6 minor complications (Grade 1 and 2) 2 major complications (Grade 3-5) in the perioperative period (0-30 day) and 3 minor and 2 major complications in the 31-90 day period due to modified Clavien system (Akbulut et al., 2011). Although the number of prospective and randomized studies comparing these two approaches is limited currently in the literature, robotic approach does not seem to add an additional complication risk when compared to open surgery.

3.2 Comparison of oncologic parameters

Lymph node yield, surgical margins, recurrence-free survival and overall survival are important parameters in evaluating surgical oncologic efficacy. The University of North Carolina study which randomized 21 patients to robotic approach and 20 to the open technique did not find any significant difference in the number of lymph nodes removed between two groups (19 versus 18, p>0.05). Likewise, surgical margins were negative in all patients in both approaches (Nix et al., 2010). The Weill Cornell Medical College study, having larger numbers of patients similarly did not find significant differences concerning these two parameters between the two approaches (Ng et al., 2010). Mean lymph node yield was 15.7 in the open surgical approach and was 17.9 in the robotic approach (p>0.05). Positive surgical margins were detected 8.7% of the patients in open approach and 7.2% of the patients in robotic approach (p>0.05). In our initial series of 12 patients, mean lymph node yield was 21.3±.8.8 (Akbulut et al., 2011).

A recent review from the Memorial Sloan-Kettering Cancer Center has recently evaluated the oncological outcomes after radical cystectomy for bladder cancer comparing open versus minimally invasive approaches (Chade et al., 2010). Although the follow-up is limited in robotic series compared to open surgical approach, robotic assisted studies reported recurrence-free survival rates of 86% to 91% at 1 to 2 years and 90% to 96% overall survival in 1 to 2 years of follow-up. On the other hand, large open surgery studies showed 62% to 68% recurrence-free survival at 5 years and 50% to 60% at 10 years, with overall survival of 59% to 66% at 5 years and 37% to 43% at 10 years.

With these limited current data, robotic approach seems to provide sufficient short-term surgical oncologic efficacy in patients with bladder cancer.

3.3 Comparison of cost

Controversial reports exist regarding the cost analysis of open versus robotic approaches. One study revealed that robotic assisted laparoscopic radical cystectomy is associated with a higher financial cost than the open approach in the perioperative setting (Smith et al., 2010). Whereas, another study suggested that although robotic approach is more expensive in terms of operative costs and robotic supplies, due to decreased hospital stay in robotic approach and higher complication rates with open surgical approach make total actual costs much higher than robotic approach (Martin et al., 2011).

4. Surgical oncologic safety of robotic approach (lymph node yield and surgical margins)

Regarding open radical cystectomy, lymph node yield and positive surgical margin rates are considered as the significant factors related to surgical quality (Herr et al., 2004; Skinner et al., 2007; Stein et al., 2003). Herr et al and Skinner et al suggested a lymph node yield of greater than 10 and a positive surgical margin rate of less than 10% in surgical oncologic adequacy (Herr et al., 2004; Skinner et al., 2007). Stein et al suggested a lymph node yield of greater than 15 obtained during open radical cystectomy in order to be oncologically acceptable and sufficient (Stein et al., 2003).

Guru et al evaluated whether robot assistance allows adequate pelvic lymph node dissection particularly during the initial experience (Guru et al., 2008). In a series of 67 patients, mean number of lymph nodes retrieved was 18 (6-43) (Guru et al., 2008). Mean lymph node yield was 41.8 (18-67) in another series of 15 consecutive patients who underwent robotic radical cystectomy for bladder cancer (Lavery et al., 2010). Recently, International Robotic Cystectomy Consortium (IRCC) evaluated 527 patients who underwent robotic cystectomy for bladder cancer and mean lymph node yield was 17.8 (range 0-68) (Hellenthal et al., 2011). Mean lymph node yield was 21.3 (range, 8-38) and 24.8±.9.2 in our initial series of 12 (Akbulut et al., 2011) and 27 cases (unpublihsed data), respectively.

Positive surgical margin rates were reported as 6.8%, 0%, 7.2% and 2% in 513, 83, 100 and 50 robotic cystectomy patients (Hellenthal et al., 2010; Pruthi et al., 2010; Ng et al., 2010; Shamim Khan et al., 2010). In our initial series of 12 patients, positive surgical margin rate was 0% (Akbulut et al., 2011). We had only one patient with positive surgical margin (3.7%) who had pT4b disease in the total of 27 patients underwent totally intracorporeal robotic cystectomy (unpublihsed data).

5. Learning curve of robotic approach

Robotic-assisted laparoscopic radical cystectomy with bilateral extended lymph node dissection and particularly intracorporeal urinary diversion (Studer or ileal conduit) are complex procedures. Therefore, a learning curve is required in order to perform these procedures successfully.

Regarding the completion of the learning curve of robotic cystectomy, some authors have suggested to perform a certain number of cases in the literature. International Robotic Cystectomy Consortium (IRCC) suggested that 21 cases were needed to be performed for operative time to reach 6.5 hours and 8, 20 and 30 patients were required to reach a lymph node yield of 12, 16 and 20, respectively (Hayn et al., 2010). On the other hand, others reported that after the first 20 cases of robotic cystectomy, no further significant improvement was detected in terms of intraoperative parameters, pathologic outcomes and complication rates (Pruthi et al., 2008). Following evaluation of 100 cases of robotic cystectomy, Guru et al stated that operative results and oncologic outcomes for robotic-assisted radical cystectomy constantly improve as the technique evolves (Guru et al., 2009).

We have started performing robotic urological procedures at our institution in February 2009, following initially performing more than 50 cases of robot assisted laparoscopic radical prostatectomy cases some of which also included pelvic lymph node dissection. We recommend to start performing robotic cystectomy cases after a certain experience gained particularly on robotic radical prostatectomy. Additionally, a good knowledge of the pelvic anatomy and adequate open surgical experience are essential.

6. Surgical technique

6.1 Patient position

Patient is placed in deep (30°) Trendelenburg position at the beginning of the procedure until the completion of robotic cystectomy, bilateral extended lymph node dissection and transposition of the left ureter under the mobilized sigmoid colon. During performing intracorporeal Studer pouch reconstruction or ileal conduit formation, patient position is adjusted to mild (5°) Trendelenburg position.

A Veress needle is introduced into the abdominal cavity about 2 cm above the umbilicus. Intra-abdominal pressure is set to 10-12 mmHg during performing bilateral extended lymph node dissection. Regarding rest of the surgery, intra-abdominal pressure is set to 16-18 mmHg.

6.2 Abdominal port locations

Overall, we use 6 trocars with the 4th-arm of the surgical robot placed on the patient's right which provides easy control to the right-handed console surgeon (Figure 1).

Camera port (12-mm) is placed 2 cm above the umbilicus. Two robotic trocars (8-mm) are placed 8 cm apart from the camera port at the level of the umblicus. An 8-mm sized robotic trocar is placed 3 cm vertically above from the right iliac crest for the 4th-arm. We use 2 assistant trocars on the left abdomen for the assistant surgeon: A 15-mm trocar for introducing for tissue staplers for bowels and endobags for specimens is placed 3 cm vertically above from the left iliac crest and a 12-mm trocar is placed between the camera port and the 2nd-robotic arm.

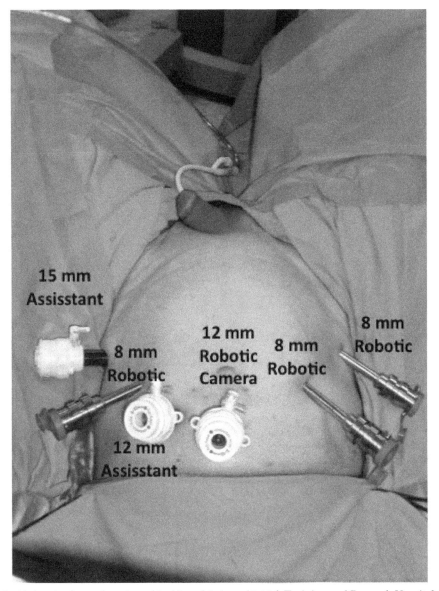

Fig. 1. Abdominal port locations (*Archive of Ankara Atatürk Training and Research Hospital, 1st Urology Clinic, Ankara, Turkey*)

6.3 Robotic-assisted laparoscopic bilateral neurovascular bundle sparing radical cystoprostatectomy in male patients (Akbulut et al., 2011; Canda et al., 2011; Canda et al., 2011; Akbulut et al., 2010)

Surgery starts with dissection of the ureters. They are double clipped and cut where they enter the bladder. Most distal parts are sent for frozen section analysis (Figure 2).

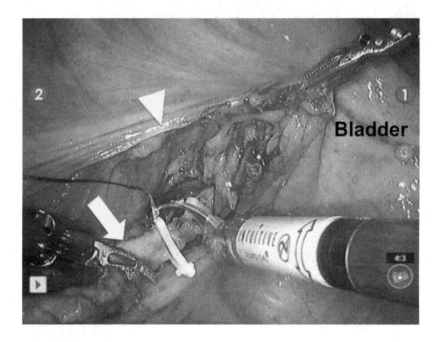

Fig. 2. Ureters are dissected, double clipped and cut where they enter the bladder (left side). Arrow: left ureter, arrowhead: incised and opened peritoneum on the left side. *(Archive of Ankara Atatürk Training and Research Hospital, 1st Urology Clinic, Ankara, Turkey)*

Peritoneum on the anterior wall of the Douglas' pouch is incised and posterior dissection of the prostate is carried out (Figure 3).

Following the identification of seminal vesicles, Denonvilliers' fascia is opened (Figure 4). Tissue lateral to the tip of the seminal vesicles corresponding to the mid point of the pararectal plexus is marked with Hem-o-lok® clips on both sides (Figure 5). Prostate is dissected off of the rectum. Lateral bladder pedicles are severed with vessel sealing system (Ligasure®) until the Hem-o-lok® clips placed at the tips of the seminal vesicles to mark pararectal plexus of which the neurovascular bundles originate (Figure 6). Then, endopelvic fascia is opened on both sides. Dorsal venous complex is ligated by 0/0 vicryl (40 mm ½ RB needle). High anterior release (intra-fascial) neurovascular bundle preservation is performed on both sides by dissecting the periprostatic fascia over the prostatic capsule alongside the prostate down until the dorsal venous complex suture and bilateral neurovascular bundle dissections are completed (Figure 7).

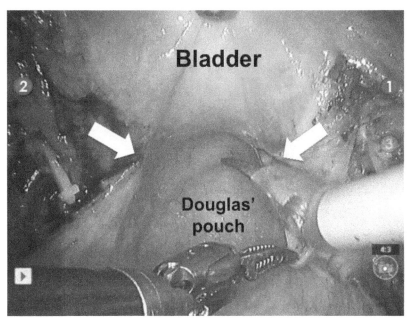

Fig. 3. Incision of the peritoneum on the anterior Douglas' pouch wall (arrows). (*Archive of Ankara Atatürk Training and Research Hospital, 1st Urology Clinic, Ankara, Turkey*)

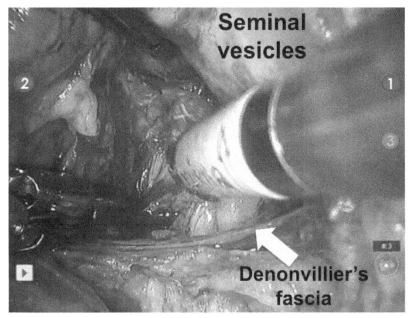

Fig. 4. Opening Denonvilliers' fascia (arrow). (*Archive of Ankara Atatürk Training and Research Hospital, 1st Urology Clinic, Ankara, Turkey*)

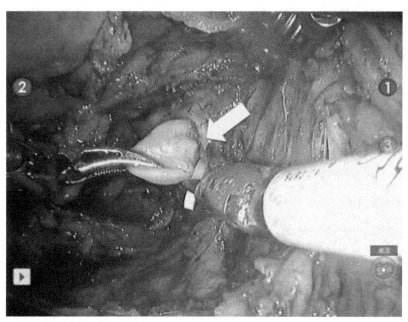

Fig. 5. Tip of the seminal vesicle is marked with a Hem-o-lok® clip and cut (arrow). (*Archive of Ankara Atatürk Training and Research Hospital, 1st Urology Clinic, Ankara, Turkey*)

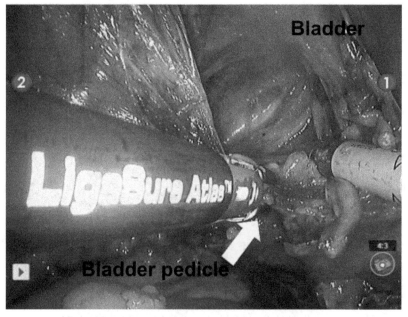

Fig. 6. Severence of lateral bladder pedicles with vessel sealing system (arrow). (*Archive of Ankara Atatürk Training and Research Hospital, 1st Urology Clinic, Ankara, Turkey*)

Robotic-Assisted Laparoscopic Radical Cystoprostatectomy and Intracorporeal Urinary Diversion (Studer Pouch or Ileal Conduit) for Bladder Cancer

95

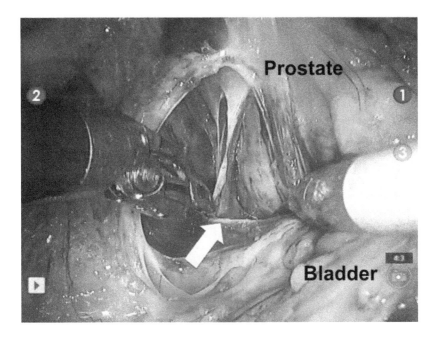

Fig. 7. High anterior release of the periprostatic fascia (arrow) over the prostatic capsule alongside the prostate in preserving neurovascular bundles on the left side. *(Archive of Ankara Atatürk Training and Research Hospital, 1st Urology Clinic, Ankara, Turkey)*

Starting from the umblical level, urachus is dissected by incising lateral to the medial umblical ligaments on the anterior abdominal wall. Puboprostatic ligaments are cut. Ligated dorsal venous complex (Figure 8) and ligated membraneous urethra (Figure 9) with 0/0 vicryl (40 mm ½ RB needle) to prevent tumor spillage are cut. Cystoprostatectomy is completed (Figure 10) and specimen is put into the endobag. Urethral stump is sampled for frozen section analysis.

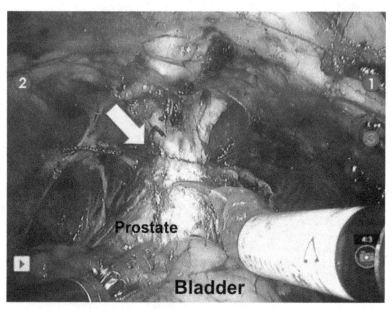

Fig. 8. Dorsal venous complex is ligated and cut (arrow). (Archive of Ankara Atatürk Training and Research Hospital, 1st Urology Clinic, Ankara, Turkey)

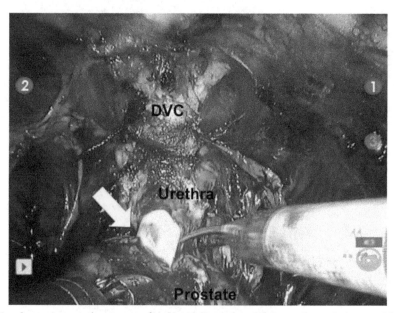

Fig. 9. Membraneous urethra is cut after being ligated and foley catheter is inserted back in until its tip reaches the specimen to show the anatomic details apparently. Arrow: appearance of the urethral catheter. DVC: dorsal venous complex (ligated and cut) *(Archive of Ankara Atatürk Training and Research Hospital, 1st Urology Clinic, Ankara, Turkey)*

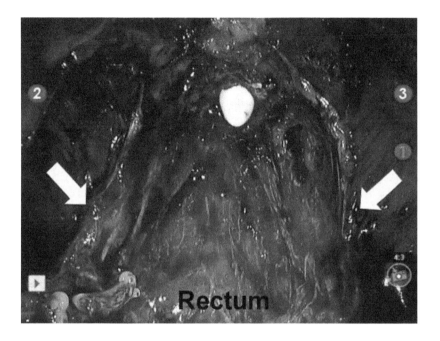

Fig. 10. Bilaterally preserved neurovascular bundles following the removal of the cystoprostatectomy specimen into the endobag (arrows). *(Archive of Ankara Atatürk Training and Research Hospital, 1st Urology Clinic, Ankara, Turkey)*

6.4 Robot assisted laparoscopic bilateral extended lymph node dissection (Canda et al., 2011; Akbulut et al., 2010; Akbulut et al., 2011)

We use the landmarks below during performing robot assisted laparoscopic bilateral extended lymph node dissection:

Superior border: inferior mesenteric artery and accompanying vena cava superior

Inferior border: node of Cloquet and circumflex iliac vein

Medial border: cut edge of the endopelvic fascia over the neurovascular bundles and internal iliac vessels

Lateral border: genitofemoral nerves, psoas muscles and ureters

Initially, starting from the genitofemoral nerve lymphatic tissue around external iliac artery & vein are removed until the obturator nerve is seen (Figure 11).

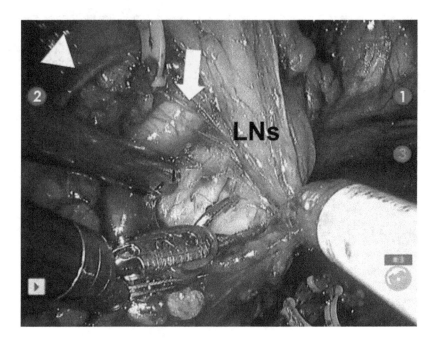

Fig. 11. Arrowhead: Genitofemoral nerve (left). Arrow: External iliac artery (left). LNs: Lymph node tissue. *(Archive of Ankara Atatürk Training and Research Hospital, 1st Urology Clinic, Ankara, Turkey)*

Then, bifurcation of common iliac artery are identified and lymphatic tissues located below the obturator nerve and surrounding the internal iliac artery are removed. Later, lymphatic tissues medial to the genitofemoral nerve and around the common iliac artery are dissected until the aortic bifurcation. Same lymphatic dissection is performed on the other side. Then, lymphatic tissues which are located distal to the aortic bifurcation, overlying and distally located to the vena caval bifurcation and common iliac arteries and veins are removed followed by presacral lymph nodes anterior to the sacrum. Lastly, preaortic and paracaval lymphatic dissections are performed. Inferior mesenteric artery on the aorta makes the most proximal end of the extended lymphatic dissection (Figure 12). Hem-o-lok® clips are used in order to tie off the most distal parts of the lymphatic vessels draining the limbs to prevent or reduce lymphatic leakage and lymphocele formation.

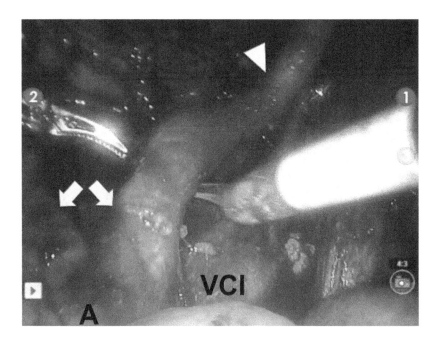

Fig. 12. Completed bilateral extended lymph node dissection and appearance of the major abdominal vasculature that are skeletonized. A: abdominal aorta, VCI: vena cava inferior, Arrows: right and left common iliac arteries, Arrowhead: right external iliac artery. *(Archive of Ankara Atatürk Training and Research Hospital, 1st Urology Clinic, Ankara, Turkey)*

Having completed the extended lymph node dissection, sigmoid colon is mobilized and left ureter is transposed to the right gutter underneath the sigmoid colon above the vasculature.

6.5 Robot assisted laparoscopic intracorporeal Studer pouch reconstruction (Canda et al., 2011; Akbulut et al., 2010; Akbulut et al., 2011)

Using a double armed 3/0 monocryl (17 mm ½c RB needle) urethral remnant is anostomosed to the assigned 1 cm opening on the antimesenteric wall of the most dependent part of the segregated ileum, initially (Figures 13,14). A 10 cm ileal segment on the right and a 40 cm ileal segment on the left side of urethroileal anastomosis are assigned for the pouch sparing the distal 20 cm ileal segment adjacent to the ceacum. Laparoscopic intestinal staplers are introduced through the 15 mm assistant port on the left side and placed perpendicular across the ileum and adjacent mesointestinum of approximately 2 cm (Figure 15). Side-to-side ileoileostomy is performed using two additional laparoscopic intestinal staplers between proximal and distal ends of the ileum (Figure 16).

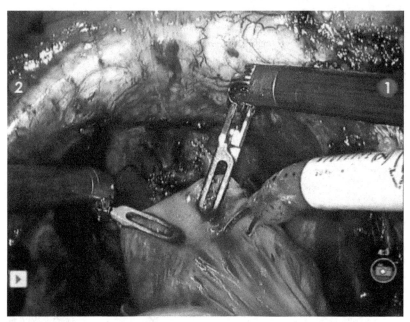

Fig. 13. Segregated antimesenteric ileal wall. (*Archive of Ankara Atatürk Training and Research Hospital, 1st Urology Clinic, Ankara, Turkey*)

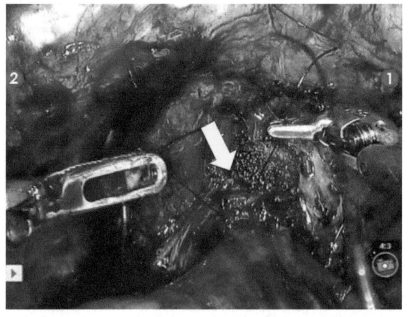

Fig. 14. Urethral remnant is sutured to the assigned antimesenteric ileal wall which is segregated. (*Archive of Ankara Atatürk Training and Research Hospital, 1st Urology Clinic, Ankara, Turkey*)

Robotic-Assisted Laparoscopic Radical Cystoprostatectomy and Intracorporeal Urinary Diversion (Studer Pouch or Ileal Conduit) for Bladder Cancer

101

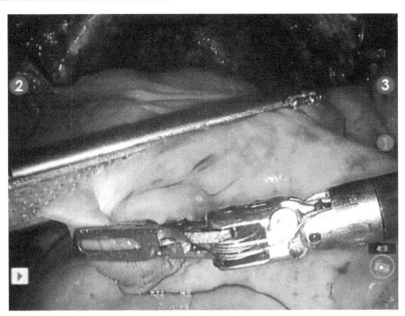

Fig. 15. Laparoscopic intestinal stapler introduced through the 15 mm assistant port on the left side and placed perpendicular across the ileum with adjacent 2 cm of mesointestinum included. *(Archive of Ankara Atatürk Training and Research Hospital, 1st Urology Clinic, Ankara, Turkey)*

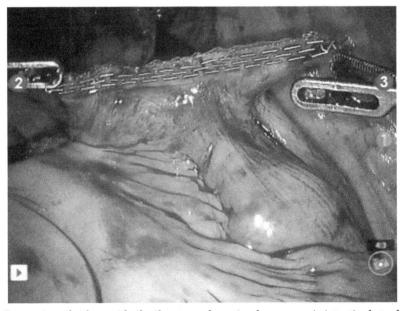

Fig. 16. Formation of side-to-side ileoileostomy by using laparoscopic intestinal staplers between proximal and distal ends of the ileum. *(Archive of Ankara Atatürk Training and Research Hospital, 1st Urology Clinic, Ankara, Turkey)*

Proximal 10 cm segment of the segregated ileum is spared as afferent loop. Then, a 60 cm feeding tube is inserted through the urethra and advanced within the lumen of the ileal segment until the proximal end of the afferent loop. Next, sparing the afferent loop, anti-mesenteric border of the remaining ileal segment is incised. Asymmetric closure of the posterior wall is accomplished with interrupted 2/0 vicryl (30 mm ½c RB needle) sutures followed by a running suture of 3/0 monocryl (26 mm ½c RB needle). Anterior wall anastomosis is accomplished using a running 3/0 monocryl (26 mm ½c RB needle) (Figure 17).

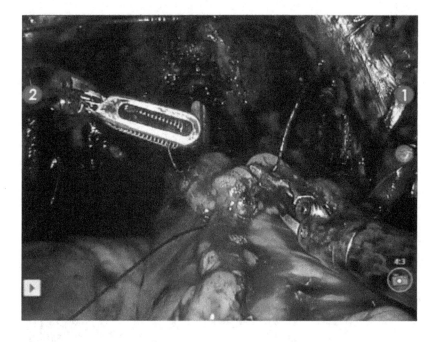

Fig. 17. Anterior wall closure. (*Archive of Ankara Atatürk Training and Research Hospital, 1st Urology Clinic, Ankara, Turkey*)

Distal ureteric ends are spatulated and anastomosed to each other at their medial edges in order to develop a common ureteral duct (Figure 18).

Robotic-Assisted Laparoscopic Radical Cystoprostatectomy and Intracorporeal Urinary Diversion (Studer Pouch or Ileal Conduit) for Bladder Cancer

103

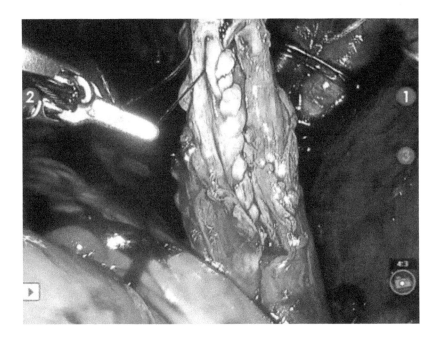

Fig. 18. Distal ureteric ends are spatulated and anastomosed to each other at their medial edges in order to develop a common ureteral duct before reconstruciton of a Wallace type uretero-ureteral and intestinal anastomosis. *(Archive of Ankara Atatürk Training and Research Hospital, 1st Urology Clinic, Ankara, Turkey)*

Double J stents with long strings at their distal ends are passed through inside the feeding tube over a guide wire to the uretero-intestinal anostomosis site and fed up to the ureters and renal pelves (Figure 19). Distal tips of the stents are tied to the tip of a 22F urethral catheter outside the body, which will then be passed through the urethra into the completed Studer pouch over a guide-wire.

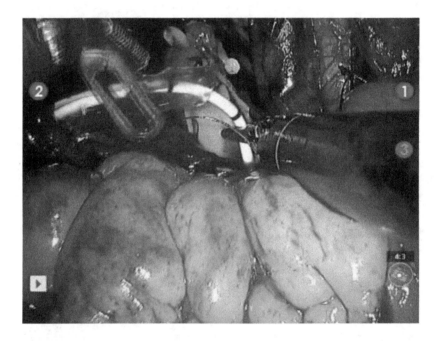

Fig. 19. Use of a feeding tube for inserting the double J catheters through the urethra, within the lumen of the ileum and into the ureters up to the renal pelves. *(Archive of Ankara Atatürk Training and Research Hospital, 1st Urology Clinic, Ankara, Turkey)*

A Wallace type uretero-intestinal anostomosis is performed between common ureteral duct and proximal end of the afferent loop. To do this anostomosis, medial edge of the ureteral duct is sutured to the medial edge of the ileal wall with a double armed 4/0 monocryl (22 mm ½c RB needle) running suture. After internalization of the double-J stents, rest of the ureteroileal anastomosis is completed (Figure 20). Ureteroileal anastomosis is retroperitonealized by using several interrupted sutures in the right gutter laterally.

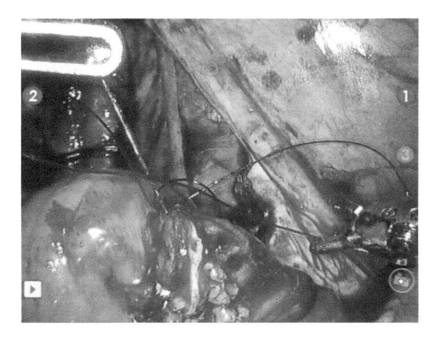

Fig. 20. Stapler line is excised at the proximal end of the afferent loop and posterior wall is anastomosed halfway between the ileal wall and medial edge of the uretero-ureteric anastomosis with a double armed 4/0 monocryl (22 mm ½c RB needle) running suture. *(Archive of Ankara Atatürk Training and Research Hospital, 1st Urology Clinic, Ankara, Turkey)*

Watertightness of the created Studer pouch is tested filling it with 150 cc of saline (Figure 21).

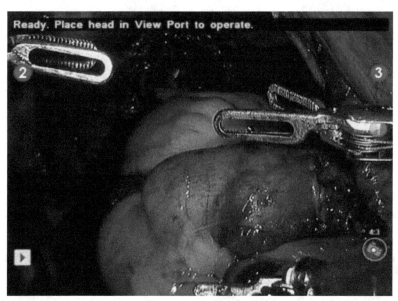

Fig. 21. Completed intracorporeal Studer pouch. (*Archive of Ankara Atatürk Training and Research Hospital, 1st Urology Clinic, Ankara, Turkey*)

Robotic-assisted laparoscopic radical cystoprostatectomy with intracorporeal Studer urinary diversion leads to better wound healing with excellent cosmetic result (Figure 22).

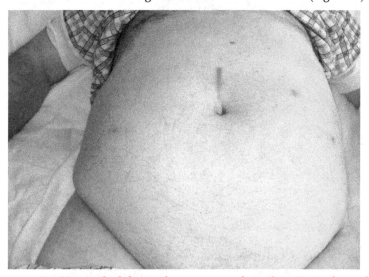

Fig. 22. Postoperative 6th-month abdominal appearance of a male patient who underwent robotic-assisted laparoscopic bilateral neurovascular bundle sparing radical cystoprostatectomy with bilateral extended lymph node dissection and intracorporeal Studer pouch formation for bladder cancer. (*Archive of Ankara Atatürk Training and Research Hospital, 1st Urology Clinic, Ankara, Turkey*)

Patients are discharged after tolerating an oral diet and sufficient ambulation following removal of the lodge drain. A cystography is done by filling the bladder with 200 cc of diluted contrast material on the postoperative 21st-day. When no leakage is seen, urethral catheter is removed. If leakage is detected, urethral catheter is kept for one more week and removed after another cystography.

6.6 Robotic-assisted laparoscopic intracorporeal ileal conduit formation (Canda et al., 2011)

Initially, sigmoid colon is mobilized and left ureter is transposed to the right gutter underneath the sigmoid colon above the vasculature. 20 cm ileal segment including the terminal ileum adjacent to the ceacum is spared and a 15-20 cm of ileal segment is segregated by using tissue staplers.

A Wallace type uretero-ureteric anastomosis is performed as explained above. For inserting the JJ stents into the renal pelves, a feeding tube is passed through the urethra and advanced within the lumen of the ileal segment. Its tip is held close to anastomozed ureteral lumens and JJ stents are passed over a guide wire up to the renal pelves. Then, uretero-ileal anostomosis is performed by using a double armed running 3/0 monocryl suture (Figure 23). Ureteroileal anastomosis is retroperitonealized by using several interrupted sutures in the right gutter laterally.

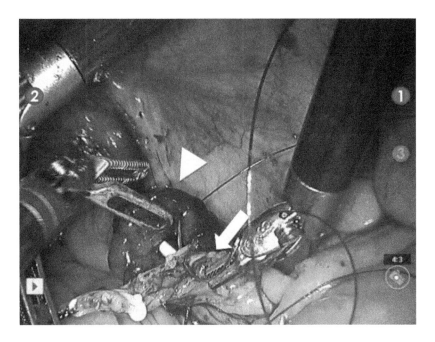

Fig. 23. Uretero-ileal anostomosis with JJ stents and intracorporeal ileal conduit. Arrowhead: ileal conduit, Arrow: Wallace type uretero-ureteric anastomosis. *(Archive of Ankara Atatürk Training and Research Hospital, 1st Urology Clinic, Ankara, Turkey)*

The 8-mm robotic trocar site opening located next to the supraumblical camera port on right is used for ileal conduit stoma following its enlargement. Interrupted 2/0 vicryl sutures are used in order to fix the ileal loop serosa to the anterior rectus sheet. Ileal opening is everted by interrupted 2/0 vicryl sutures to create a nipple type stoma.

Patients are discharged after tolerating an oral diet and sufficient ambulation following removal of the lodge drains.

7. References

Akbulut Z, Canda AE, Atmaca AF, Ozdemir AT, Asil E & Balbay MD. (2010) Robot assisted laparoscopic bilateral nerve-sparing radical cystoprostatectomy: Initial Ankara experience. *J Endourol* 24(Supplement 1):A360:VS8-14.

Akbulut Z, Canda AE, Atmaca AF, Ozdemir AT, Asil E & Balbay MD. (2010) Robot assisted laparoscopic extended pelvic lymph node dissection during radical cystoprostatectomy: Initial Ankara experience. *Eur Urol Suppl* 9(5):521.

Akbulut Z, Canda AE, Atmaca AF, Ozdemir AT, Asil E & Balbay MD. (2010) Robot assisted laparoscopic intracorporeal Studer pouch formation: Initial Ankara experience. *J Endourol* 24(Supplement 1):A359:VS8-12.

Akbulut Z, Canda AE, Ozcan MF, Atmaca AF, Ozdemir AT & Balbay MD. (2011) Robot assisted laparoscopic nerve sparing radical cystoprostatectomy with bilateral extended lymph node dissection and intracorporeal Studer pouch construction: Outcomes of first 12 cases. *J Endourol* In Press.

Canda AE, Atmaca AF, Altinova S, Akbulut Z, Balbay MD. (2011) Robot assisted nerve sparing radical cystectomy with bilateral extended lymph node dissection and intracorporeal urinary diversion for bladder cancer: Initial experience in 27 cases. *BJU Int* Accepted for publication.

Canda AE, Asil E & Balbay MD. (2011) An unexpected resident in the ileum detected during robot assisted laparoscopic radical cystoprostatectomy and intracorporeal Studer pouch formation: Taenia saginata parasite. *J Endourol* 25(2):1-3.

Canda AE, Dogan B, Atmaca AF, Akbulut Z & Balbay MD. (2011) Ureteric duplication is not a contrandication for robot assisted laparoscopic radical cystoprostatectomy and intracorporeal Studer pouch formation. *JSLS* In Press.

Cancer Facts and Figures 2009. Atlanta: American Cancer Society 2009.

Chade DC, Laudone VP, Bochner BH & Parra RO. (2010) Oncological outcomes after radical cystectomy for bladder cancer: open versus minimally invasive approaches. *J Urol* 183(3):862-69.

Clinical Practice Guidelines in Oncology, version 1.2010. Bladder Cancer. National Comprehensive Cancer Network. Available at http://www.nccn.org. Accessed March 15, 2010.

Guru KA, Perlmutter AE, Butt ZM, Piacente P, Wilding GE, Tan W, Kim HL & Mohler JL. (2009) The learning curve for robot-assisted radical cystectomy. *JSLS* 13(4):509-14.

Guru KA, Sternberg K, Wilding GE, Tan W, Butt ZM, Mohler JL, et al. (2008) The lymph node yield during robot-assisted radical cystectomy. *BJU Int.* 102(2):231-4.

Hayn MH, Hussain A, Mansour AM, Andrews PE, Carpentier P, Castle E, Dasgupta P, Rimington P, Thomas R, Khan S, Kibel A, Kim H, Manoharan M, Menon M, Mottrie A, Ornstein D, Peabody J, Pruthi R, Palou Redorta J, Richstone L, Schanne F,

Stricker H, Wiklund P, Chandrasekhar R, Wilding GE & Guru KA. (2010) The learning curve of robot-assisted radical cystectomy: results from the International Robotic Cystectomy Consortium. *Eur Urol.* 58(2):197-202.

Hellenthal NJ, Hussain A, Andrews PE, Carpentier P, Castle E, Dasgupta P, Kaouk J, Khan S, Kibel A, Kim H, Manoharan M, Menon M, Mottrie A, Ornstein D, Palou J, Peabody J, Pruthi R, Richstone L, Schanne F, Stricker H, Thomas R, Wiklund P, Wilding G & Guru KA. (2010) Surgical margin status after robot assisted radical cystectomy: results from the International Robotic Cystectomy Consortium. *J Urol.* 184(1):87-91.

Hellenthal NJ, Hussain A, Andrews PE, Carpentier P, Castle E, Dasgupta P, Kaouk J, Khan S, Kibel A, Kim H, Manoharan M, Menon M, Mottrie A, Ornstein D, Palou J, Peabody J, Pruthi R, Richstone L, Schanne F, Stricker H, Thomas R, Wiklund P, Wilding G & Guru KA. (2011) Lymphadenectomy at the time of robot-assisted radical cystectomy: results from the International Robotic Cystectomy Consortium. *BJU Int.* 107(4):642-6.

Herr H, Lee C, Chang S & Lerner S; Bladder Cancer Collaborative Group. (2004) Standardization of radical cystectomy and pelvic lymph node dissection for bladder cancer: a collaborative group report. *J Urol.* 171(5):1823-8.

Huang GJ & Stein JP. (2007) Open radical cystectomy with lymphadenectomy remains the treatment of choice for invasive bladder cancer. *Curr Opin Urol* 17:369-8.

Huang J, Lin T, Liu H, Xu K, Zhang C, Jiang C, Huang H, Yao Y, Guo Z & Xie W. (2010) Laparoscopic radical cystectomy with orthotopic ileal neobladder for bladder cancer: oncologic results of 171 cases with a median 3-year follow-up. *Eur Urol.* 58(3):442-9.

Kasraeian A, Barret E, Cathelineau X, Rozet F, Galiano M, Sanchez-Salas R & Vallancien G. (2010) Robot-assisted laparoscopic cystoprostatectomy with extended pelvic lymphadenectomy, extracorporeal enterocystoplasty, and intracorporeal enterourethral anastomosis: initial Montsouris experience. *J Endourol.* 24(3):409-13.

Kauffman EC, Ng CK, Lee MM, Otto BJ, Wang GJ & Scherr DS. (2011) Early oncological outcomes for bladder urothelial carcinoma patients treated with robotic-assisted radical cystectomy. *BJU Int.* 107(4):628-35.

Lavery HJ, Martinez-Suarez HJ & Abaza R. (2010) Robotic extended pelvic lymphadenectomy for bladder cancer with increased nodal yield. *BJU Int.* 11. doi: 10.1111/j.1464-410X.2010.09789.x. [Epub ahead of print]

Martin AD, Nunez RN, Castle EP. (2011) Robot-assisted Radical Cystectomy Versus Open Radical Cystectomy: A Complete Cost Analysis. *Urology.* 77(3):621-5.

Menon M, Hemal AK, Tewari A, Shrivastava A, Shoma AM, El-Tabey NA, Shaaban A, Abol-Enein H & Ghoneim MA. (2003) Nerve-sparing robot-assisted radical cystoprostatectomy and urinary diversion. *BJU Int.* 92(3):232-6.

Ng CK, Kauffman EC, Lee MM, Otto BJ, Portnoff A, Ehrlich JR, Schwartz MJ, Wang GJ & Scherr DS. (2010) A comparison of postoperative complications in open versus robotic cystectomy. *Eur Urol.* 57(2):274-81.

Nieder AM, Mackinnon JA, Huang Y, Fleming LE, Koniaris LG & Lee DJ. (2008) Florida bladder cancer trends 1981 to 2004: minimal progress in decreasing advanced disease. *J Urol.* 179(2):491-5

Nix J, Smith A, Kurpad R, Nielsen ME, Wallen EM & Pruthi RS. (2010) Prospective randomized controlled trial of robotic versus open radical cystectomy for bladder cancer: perioperative and pathologic results. *Eur Urol.* 57(2):196-201.

Pruthi RS, Smith A & Wallen EM. (2008) Evaluating the learning curve for robot-assisted laparoscopic radical cystectomy. *J Endourol.* 22(11):2469-74.

Pruthi RS, Nielsen ME, Nix J, Smith A, Schultz H & Wallen EM. (2010) Robotic radical cystectomy for bladder cancer: surgical and pathological outcomes in 100 consecutive cases. *J Urol.* 183(2):510-4.

Rehman J, Sangalli MN, Guru K, de Naeyer G, Schatteman P, Carpentier P & Mottrie A. (2011) Total intracorporeal robot-assisted laparoscopic ileal conduit (Bricker) urinary diversion: technique and outcomes. *Can J Urol.* 18(1):5548-56.

Schumacher MC, Jonsson MN & Wiklund NP. (2009) Robotic cystectomy. *Scand J Surg.* 98(2):89-95

Skinner EC, Stein JP & Skinner DG. (2007) Surgical benchmarks for the treatment of invasive bladder cancer. *Urol Oncol.* 25(1):66-71.

Shamim Khan M, Elhage O, Challacombe B et al: (2010) Analysis of early complications of robotic-assisted radical cystectomy using a standardized reporting system. *Urology.* Sep 7. [Epub ahead of print]

Smith A, Kurpad R, Lal A, Nielsen M, Wallen EM & Pruthi RS. (2010) Cost analysis of robotic versus open radical cystectomy for bladder cancer. *J Urol.* 183(2):505-9.

Stein JP, Cai J, Groshen S & Skinner DG. (2003) Risk factors for patients with pelvic lymph node metastases following radical cystectomy with en bloc pelvic lymphadenectomy: concept of lymph node density. *J Urol.* 170(1):35-41.

6

Robot-Assisted Radical Cystectomy as a Treatment Modality for Patients with Muscle-Invasive Bladder Cancer

Martin C. Schumacher[1,2]
[1]Dept. of Urology, Karolinska University Hospital, Stockholm,
[2]Hirslanden Klinik Aarau,
[1]Sweden
[2]Switzerland

1. Introduction

Over the last two decades open radical cystectomy and urinary diversion have become a widely accepted form of treatment in both men and women with transitional cell carcinoma of the bladder. In the mid-1980s orthotopic urinary diversion with anastomosis to the urethra became an oncologically and functionally acceptable option in appropriately selected male patients. With better understanding of the anatomy and of the continence mechanism, orthotopic urinary diversion was subsequently performed in the early 1990s in female patients[1].

Until today open radical cystectomy is still considered the gold standard treatment for patients with muscle-invasive transitional cell carcinoma of the bladder [2, 3]. This is based on the following observations: First, the best long-term survival rates and lowest local recurrence rates have been reported after radical cystectomy [4 5]. Second, the morbidity and mortality of radical cystectomy have significantly improved during the last decades, and good functional results in patients with orthotopic urinary diversions have been achieved [6 7]. Third, radical cystectomy and pelvic lymph node dissection provides the most accurate tumor staging, thus helps selecting patients for adjuvant treatment protocols [8 9].

Radical cystectomy performed through a laparoscopic approach was first described in 1992 [10]. Since then, laparoscopic radical cystectomy has been reported in over 500 patients and current results suggest that this approach may cause less blood loss, decreased postoperative pain and faster recovery compared to open surgery [11 12]. However, due to the technical difficulty (two-dimensional laparoscopic view, counterintuitive motion, poor ergonomics, and nonwristed instrumentation), the steep learning curve and the lack of long-term oncological results, this treatment has not been adopted by mainstream urology.

The introduction of robot assisted surgery for pelvic laparoscopy, especially in performing radical prostatectomy, has changed the possibilities of performing complicated operations in the small pelvis. Three-dimensional vision with ten-fold magnification and the dexterity provided by the endo-wrist (six degrees of freedom) allows the surgeon to operate the tips of the laparoscopic instruments like an open surgeon [13]. Thus, the surgeon will benefit from a faster learning curve as compared to conventional laparoscopy. Further, these advantages have allowed surgeons to translate standard open surgical procedures to a minimally invasive approach, especially its potential in operating in a narrow pelvis as well as for the reconstruction of the urinary tract.

With the beginning of robot-assisted pelvic surgery a decade ago, radical cystectomy and reconstruction of the urinary tract is currently possible. However, until today, results on robot-assisted radical cystectomy (RARC) are mainly reported from a few centers worldwide. Further, results on RARC with intracorporeal urinary diversion are sparse, as most surgeons perform the reconstructive part outside the abdomen due to technical difficulties and longer operative time.

2. Robot-assisted radical cystectomy

The history of robot-assisted radical cystectomy started with Beecken et al. who was the first to perform a RARC with intracorporeal formation of an ileal orthotopic bladder substitute in 2002 [14]. Operating time was 8.5 hours and blood loss 200ml. At five months post-operatively the oncological and functional result of the reservoir were considered excellent. Menon et al. reported the first series of RARC in 17 patients in 2003 [15]. In their series, an ileal conduit was performed in three patients, a W-pouch in ten, a double chimney in two, and a T-pouch in two cases. Mean operating time for radical cystectomy was 140 min and 120–168 min for the different urinary diversions, which were all performed extracorporeally. Mean blood loss was less than 150 mL, and surgical margins were negative in all cases.

Since then, several case series have been published, however, most RARC series comprise less than 100 cases per center [table 1]. Additionally, our current knowledge on RARC is mainly based on reports from less than twenty different surgical centers worldwide. In order to provide a better overview on the value of RARC, data from a mix of 15 academic and private centers from the USA and Europe are prospectively collected and the results reported by the International Robotic Cystectomy Consortium (IRCC) [16] [17] [18]. Despite increasing evidence that RARC seems as effective as open radical cystectomy, it is still too premature to draw any firm conclusions about the status of RARC.

3. Patient selection

Which patients are suitable for RARC using a minimal invasive approach? As patients planned for radical cystectomy are in general older and have a higher prevalence of smoking-related co-morbidities, pulmonary diseases may cause intraoperative problems. Some of these patients may even not be suitable for robot-assisted interventions because of the need for CO_2 insufflation and the steep Trendelenburg position. The cardiac and respiratory systems are especially vulnerable to the extreme and lengthy head-down position. However, in order to minimize these risks, a 25° Trendelenburg position during radical cystectomy and lymph node dissection is possible without affecting the surgical quality [19]. For the urinary diversion the Trendelenburg position can further be decreased to 15°, thus minimizing potential pulmonary complications.

A question mark regarding contra-indications in selecting patients for RARC remains. Presence of bulky disease, locally advanced disease, or enlarged lymph nodes have been considered relative contra-indications [20] [21]. Khan et al. reported specific surgery-related complications at RARC [22]. They found that patients with multiples intravesical therapies, such as mitomycin or BCG, are more likely to have adhesions between the bladder and the

Author (reference)	No. of pts.	Type of urinary diversion:	extracorporeal intracorporeal	Conversion to open surgery	Mean operative time (min)	Mean perioperative blood loss (ml)	Mean post op. hospital stay (days)	Positive margins (bladder)	No. of lymph nodes removed	Follow-up (months)
Beecken et al, 2003 [14]	1	Orthotopic neobladder	intracorporeal	no	510	200	n. a.	neg.	n. a.	n. a.
Menon et al, 2003 [15]	17	Cystectomy Ileal conduit (3) Orthotopic neobladder (14)	extracorporeal	1 pt	140 260 308	150	n. a.	neg.	x (4 – 27)	n. a.
Hemal et al, 2004 [	24	Ileal conduit (4) Orthotopic neobladder (20)	extracorporeal	no	228 - 348	100 - 300	4 - 5	neg.	3 - 27	n.a.
Galich et al, 2006 [33]	13	Ileal conduit (6) Orthotopic neobladder (5) Indiana pouch (2)	extracorporeal	no	697 (240 – 828)	500 (100 – 1000)	8 (4 – 23)	neg.	n. a.	n. a.
Rhee et al, 2006 [30]	7	Ileal conduit	extracorporeal	no	638 (592 – 684)	479	11 (6 – 16)	neg.	n. a.	n. a.
Abraham et al, 2007 [54]	14	Cystectomy Ileal conduit	extracorporeal	no	410 (340 – 545)	212 (50 – 500)	6 (4 – 7)	1 pt (pT4)	22.3 (13 – 42)	n. a.
Mottrie et al, 2007 [56]	27	Ileal conduit (19) Orthotopic neobladder (8)	extracorporeal	no	340 (150 – 450)	301 (50 – 550)	n. a.	neg.	23 (6 – 37)	10.2
Lowentritt et al, 2008 [38]	4/20#	Ileal conduit (4)	extracorporeal	no	350 (340 – 410)	300 (250 – 500)	5 (3 – 8)	neg.	12 (9 – 16)	n. a.
Murphy et al, 2008 [31]	23	Ileal conduit (19) Orthotopic neobladder (4)	extracorporeal	no	397 (314 – 480)	278 (49 – 507)	12 (8 – 15)	neg.	16 (7 – 25)	17 (4 – 40)
Wang et al, 2008 [32]	32	Ileal conduit (17) Orthotopic neobladder (12) Indiana pouch (3)	extracorporeal	no	390 (210 – 570)	400 (100 – 1200)	5 (4 – 18)	2 pts (pT3 N1)	17 (6 – 32)	n. a.
Woods et al, 2008 [34]	27	Ileal conduit (?) Orthotopic neobladder (?)	extracorporeal	no	400 (225 – 660)	277 (50 – 700)	n. a.	2 pts. (pT4)	12 (7 – 20)	n. a.
Hemal et al, 2008 [55]	6	Ileal conduit (5) Orthotopic neobladder (1)	extracorporeal	no	330	200 (150 – 1000)	9.2	no	12 (4 – 19)	n. a.

n. a. not available, # report on 4 female pts., ≠ one case without urinary diversion, renal failure, ‡ results from pts. < 70 years vs. ≥ 70 years)

Author (reference)	No. of pts.	Type of urinary diversion:	extracorporeal intracorporeal	Conversion to open surgery	Mean operative time (min)	Mean perioperative blood loss (ml)	Mean post op. hospital stay (days)	Positive margins (bladder)	No. of lymph nodes removed	Follow-up (months)
Yuh et al, 2008 [40]	54	n. a.	extracorporeal	2 pts.	n. a.	557	9.1	0 pts. (pTO-pT2) 7 pts. (pT3-pT4)	20 (SD 12) pT0-pT2 15 (SD 7) pT3-pT4	n. a.
Gamboa et al, 2009 [57]	41	Ileal conduit (24) Orthotopic neobladder (17)	intracorporeal	no	498 (320-805)	254 (50-700)	8 (5-37).	2 pts. (pT4)	25 (4-68).	n. a.
Kauffman et al, 2009 [39]	79	Ileal conduit (46) Orthotopic neobladder (33)	extracorporeal	n. a.	378	460	5	6 pts.	18.4	n. a.
Schumacher et al, 2009 [63]	18	Ileal conduit (5) Orthotopic neobladder (13)	intracorporeal	3 pts.	501 (382-750)	525 (200-2200)	12 (6-79)	1 pt. (pT4)	20 (10-42)	25 (4-58)
Richards et al, 2010 [65]	35	Ileal conduit (30) Orthotopic neobladder (5)	extracorporeal	no	530 (458-593)	350 (250-600)	7 (6-9)	1 pt.	16 (11-24)	n.a.
Guru et al, 2010 [52]	26	Ileal conduit (13) Ileal conduit (13)	intracorporeal extracorporeal	no	391 387	315 454	8.8 (5-23) 8.5 (6-14)	1 pt. (pT4)	25 26	n. a.
Pruthi et al, 2010 [68]	100#	Ileal conduit (61) Orthotopic neobladder (38)	extracorporeal (94) intracorporeal (5)	no	276	271	4.9	neg.	19 (8-40)	18.4 (5-44)
Lavery et al, 2010 [66]	15	n. a.	extracorporeal	no	423 (300-506)	160 (50-500)	3.4 (3-7)	neg.	41.8 (18-67)	3
Coward et al, 2011#[22]	99	Ileal conduit (60) Orthotopic neobladder (39)	extracorporeal	no	288 vs. 264	289 vs. 249	4.7 vs. 5.0	neg.	19.5 (8-40) 18.1 (10-37)	n. a.
Khan et al, 2011 [45]	50	Ileal conduit (45) Orthotopic neobladder (5)	extracorporeal	no	361 (240-600)	340 (100 1150)	10 (5-24)	1 pt. (pT4)	17 (11-28)	3
Manoharan et al, 2011 [67]	14	Orthotopic neobladder (14)	extracorporeal	no	310 (± 220)	360 (± 48)	8.5	neg.	12 (± 3)	n. a.
Cha et al, 2011 [72]	85	Ileal conduit Orthotopic Orthotopic neobladder	extracorporeal	no	n. a.	n. a.	n. a.	5.9%	19	18
Schumacher et al, 2011 [35]	45	Ileal conduit (9) Orthotopic neobladder (36)	intracorporeal	3 pts.	477 (325-760)	550 (200-2200)	9 (4-78)	1 pt. (pT4)	22.5 (10-52)	24 (3-77)

Table 1. Contemporary reports/series of robotic-assisted laparoscopic radical cystectomy (RARC) and urinary diversion for TCC of the bladder.

surrounding structures, especially the rectum, rendering dissection difficult. Thus, careful dissection is required in developing the rectovesical plane to avoid injury of the rectum. Prior abdominal surgery, radiotherapy or neoadjuvant chemotherapy may be relative-contraindications for RARC, as these factors can significantly increase the degree of technical difficulty [22] [23].

Patient selection makes a direct comparison between open radical cystectomy series and smaller RARC series difficult. Results from open high-volume centers indicate that approximately two-thirds of patients at radical cystectomy have organ-confined disease, whereas one-third has non-organ-confined disease [24] [25] [26] [27] [28] [29]. In general, the percentage of patients with non-organ-confined disease undergoing RARC is substantially lower than figures reported from major series from open radical cystectomy [table 2] [30] [31] [32] [21, 33-40].

Recent multi-institutional results from the International Robotic Cystectomy Consortium (IRCC) of 527 patients treated with RARC show similar figures regarding the numbers of patients with organ-confined (65%) vs. non-organ-confined (35%) disease, as with open radical cystectomy series [18]. However, data on neoadjuvant chemotherapy were not reported in this series.

4. Surgery-related complications

Although the number of RARC cases reported in the literature is relatively small, the intraoperative complication rate seems comparable to open radical cystectomy series. Nix et al. found in a prospective randomized trial of robotic (n = 21) versus open (n = 20) radical cystectomy no difference in the absolute number of complications (p = 0.279) [41]. Less blood loss was observed in the robotic group (mean 258 mL) compared to the open group (mean 575 mL). Similarly, Wang et al. reported no difference regarding intraoperative complications in their prospective trial between robotic (n = 33) and open radical cystectomy (n = 21) [32]. Again, less blood loss was noted with RARC (mean 400 mL, range 100–1200 mL) compared to open radical cystectomy (mean 750 mL, range 250–2500 mL). Galich et al., in a comparative analysis of early postoperative outcomes following robotic (n = 13) and open (n = 24) radical cystectomy, found no difference between groups regarding surgery-related complications and blood loss [33]. Kauffman et al. collected data on 79 consecutive patients treated with RARC and extracorporeal urinary diversion [42]. In their series, high-grade complications (Clavien III–V) occurred in 16 patients (21%) during the first 3 months postoperatively. Urinary obstruction, intra-abdominal abscess, uro-enteric fistulas, and gastrointestinal bleeding were the most common high-grade complications. The high percentage of overall urinary obstruction (8%) despite extracorporeal urinary diversion without robotic assistance is of concern [42]. Khan et al. reported an 8% ureteric stricture rate, with 6% strictures occurring on the left side in their series of 50 RARC cases [22]. Results from open radical cystectomy series report an uretero-intestinal stricture rate of less than 3% [5]. Performing the anastomosis between the ureters and the urinary diversion outside the abdomen through a small abdominal incision may only be possible with relatively long ureters, thus increasing the risk for ischemic complications. Resection of the ureters at the level where they cross over the common iliac artery minimizes the risk of strictures at the uretero-intestinal anastomosis due to ischemia [43].

Different parameters may affect outcome and risk for surgery-related complications such as age, higher ASA score or previous surgery. Butt et al. did not find a significant association between age, BMI, ASA score and complication rate in their series of 66 RARC cases [44].

Author (reference)	No. of pts.	Age (years)	Organ-confined tumors ≤pT2 (%)	Non-organ-confined tumors > pT2 (%)	Node positive disease (%)	Positive margins (%)	Follow-up (months)
Open radical cystectomy:							
Stein et al, 2001 [24]	1054	66 (range 22 - 93)	669 (64%)	385 (36%)	246 (23%)	1%	122 (range 0 - 336)*
Manoharan et al, 2009 [28]	432	69 (SD ± 9)	262 (60.5%)	170 (39.5%)	90 (21%)	5%	38 (range 1 - 172)
Dotan et al, 2007 [29]	1589	n. a.	858 (54%)	727 (46%)	288 (24%)	4.2%	up to 15 years
Hautmann et al, 2006 [26]	788	65 (SD ± 10)	528 (67%)	260 (33%)	143 (18%)	< 1%	54 (range 0.1 - 223)
Robot-assisted radical cystectomy:							
Galich et al, 2006 [33]	13	70 (range 38 - 88)	7 (54%)	6 (46%)	2 (15%)	0%	n. a.
Rhee et al, 2006 [30]	7	60 (SD ± 9)	6 (86%)	1(14%)	2 (28%)	0%	n. a.
Guru et al, 2008 [36]	58/ 67≠	67 (range 36 - 90)	29 (50%)	29 (50%)	17 (29%)	6 (10.3%)	n. a.
Wang et al, 2008 [32]	32	70 (range 41 - 84)	23 (72%)	9 (28%)	6 (19%)	2 (6%)	n. a.
Murphy et al, 2008 [31]	23	65 (SD ± 9.4)	17 (74%)	6 (26%)	2 (8.7%)	0%	17 (range 4 - 40)
Dasgupta et al, 2008 [37]	20	66 (range 36 - 77)	15 (75%)	5 (25%)	2 (10%)	0%	23 (range 7 - 44)
Lowentritt et al, 2008 [38]	4/ 20#	69.5 (SD ± 10.5)	1 (25%)	3 (75%)	1 (25%)	0%	n. a.
Woods et al, 2008 [34]	27	67 (range 49 - 80)	n. a.	n. a.	9 (33%)	2 (7.4%)	n. a.
Yuh et al, 2008 [40]	54	67	19 (35%)	35 (65%)	n. a.	7 (13%)	n. a.
Kauffman et al, 2009 [39]	79	71 (SD ± 11)	47 (59%)	32 (41%)	12 (15%)	6 (7.6%)	26.4
Pruthi et al, 2010 [68]	100	65.5 (range 33 - 86)	87 (87%)	13 (13%)	20 (20%)	0%	18.4 (range 5 - 44)
Schumacher et al, 2011 [35]	45	60.6 (range 37 – 79)	35 (77.8%)	10 (22.2%)	9 (20%)	1 (2.2%)	24 (range 3 – 77)

n. a. not available; * 91 % of pts with FU > 3 years; # results on 4 female cases; ≠58 pats eligible for analysis

Table 2. Patient characteristic of contemporary robotic-assisted radical cystectomy (RARC) and open radical cystectomy series for TCC of the bladder.

Similar, Coward et al. did not find worse outcomes in terms of complications when comparing older patients (≥ 70 years) with higher ASA scores vs. younger patients (< 70 years) treated with RARC [45].

Schumacher et al. assessed the surgery-related complications at RARC with total intracorporeal urinary diversion during their learning curve [35]. A total of 45 patients were pooled in 3 consecutive groups of 15 cases each to evaluate the complications according to the Clavien classification [46]. Overall, fewer complications were observed between the groups over time, with a significant decrease in late versus early complications (P = 0.005 and P = 0.058). However, the early Clavien grade III complications remained significant (27%) and did not decline with time; thus indicating the complexity of the intracorporeal urinary diversion. Khan et al., assessed early surgery-related complications using also the Clavien Classification [22]. Early complications were observed in 34% of patients. Clavien grade IIIa/b complications were seen in 29% of their patients. Both series have somehow a lower complication rate compared to the 64% complication rate from a large series of 1142 open radical cystectomy patients from the Memorial-Sloan-Kettering Cancer Center (MSKCC) [47]. The higher percentage of non-organ-confined tumors in the open series from MSKCC may be one factor to explain this difference in favor of the robotic approach.

Hayn et al., from the IRCC assessed whether previous robotic surgical experience affects on the implementation and execution of robot-assisted radical cystectomy [17]. They found that previous robot-assisted radical prostatectomy (RARP) case volume might affect the operative time, blood loss, and lymph node yield at RARC. In addition, surgeons with increased RARP experience operated on patients with more advanced tumors. Previous RARP experience, however, did not appear to affect the surgical margin status.

5. Lymphadenectomy

Pelvic lymphadenectomy at radical cystectomy is the standard treatment for patients with muscle-invasive bladder cancer. Radical cystectomy series report that approximately 25% of patients initially staged T1–T4 N0 M0 who undergo lymphadenectomy have lymph node metastases; and the absolute number of positive nodes removed affects survival [9 48].

It has been stated that, as a guideline, removal of >20 nodes per patient should be the aim [48]. Others have reported an improved cancer-specific survival rate of 65% when ≥ 16 nodes were retrieved compared to 51% when < 16 nodes were retrieved [49]. Whereas some experts do recommend that at least 10 nodes should be removed at pelvic lymph node dissection [50] [51]. While assessing the lymph node counts obtained after lymph node dissection at radical cystectomy from various institutional series, huge differences in node count are noted. Median node count has been reported to vary from 8 to 80, and is also affected by the extent of a pelvic lymphadenectomy [9 24 52 53 47 48 54 55 56 57 58]. Interindividual variances, sending separate or en-bloc nodal packages, and the pathologic work-up of the specimens may explain differences in reporting on the number of nodes removed/detected by the pathologist [58 59]. Other factors such as the commitment of the surgeon in performing a lymph node dissection or selecting patients for more or less extensive lymphadenectomy may explain differences in nodal count [60].

Controversy still persists regarding the boundaries and terminology used in lymph node dissection. Mills et al. describe a *standard* lymph node dissection that includes removal of nodal tissue up to and including the common iliac bifurcation, including the internal iliac vessels, presacral area, obturator fossa, external iliac vessels, and distal part of the common iliac artery [61]. In order to avoid injury to the hypogastric nerves, nodes medial to the ureter (proximal half of the common iliac artery, aortic bifurcation) are not removed. In contrast, Stein et al. define an *extended* lymph node dissection as including all nodal tissue in the boundaries of: the aortic bifurcation and common iliac vessels (proximally); the genitofemoral nerve (laterally); the circumflex iliac vein and lymph node of Cloquet (distally); the hypogastric vessels (posteriorly), including the obturator fossa, pre-sciatic nodes bilaterally; and the presacral lymph nodes anterior to the sacral promontory [62].

Data on lymph node yield and oncological outcome in RARC series are still limited, however, node counts are similar to open radical cystectomy series [21 31 35 34 36 63]. Earlier reports from various RARC series describe mostly the boundaries of a *limited* (obturator fossa only) or *standard* template with less than a median of 20 nodes removed [63]. A recent report by Pruthi et al. performing an *extended* lymph node dissection, described a median node yield of 28 nodes (range 12–39) [64]. Schumacher et al. found similar node counts in their series of 45 patients with a mean of 22.5 nodes (range 10 - 52) removed [35]. Applying a template up to the aortic bifurcation resulted in a mean of 32 nodes removed. Richards et al. compared lymph node counts from 35 open radical cystectomy cases to their first 35 RARC cases [65]. Median total lymph node yield was similar between groups, with 15 nodes (range 11 - 22) in the open cystectomy group compared to 16 nodes (range 11 - 24) in the RARC group. Lavery et al, reported in their first 15 RARC cases undergoing an extended pelvic lymphadenectomy up to the aortic bifurcation a mean nodal yield of 41.8 nodes (range 18 - 67) [66]. Kauffmann et al. applying a similar template at RARC found a mean of 19.1 nodes (range 0 - 56) removed [42]. Evaluating the number of nodes removed from different institutions, the IRCC reported that at RARC 82.9% underwent a pelvic lymphadenectomy, which resulted in a mean of 17.8 nodes (range 0 - 68) removed [18]. According to these reports, it seems that robotic lymphadenectomy applying an *extended* lymph node dissection template, if indicated, up to the aortic bifurcation is technically feasible with intraoperative morbidity similar to open series [63].

6. Urinary diversion

The first case of RARC with intracorporeal urinary diversion was performed by Beecken et al. in 2002 [14]. Operative time was 8.5 hours, and therefore attention was turned towards extracorporeal urinary diversion in order to decrease operative times. Menon et al. were the first to describe their technique of extracorporeal diversion, using a 5–8 cm mid-line incision [15]. Until today, the majority of urinary diversions in conjunction with RARC are done extracorporeally [table 1] [67]. However, standardization of the intracorporeal procedure and decreasing operative times might turn the interest towards this approach [19 68]. We have previously reported our results in a series of 18 patients treated with RARC and totally intracorporeal urinary diversion, later, results in 45 patients were published [19 35]. Mean operative time was 476 min (range 325–760) and mean blood loss 669 mL (range 200–2200) [35]. Whether there is an advantage of performing the complete procedure intracorporeally or not is less clear. At least in female patients, the specimen can be removed through an incision via the vaginal wall, thus avoiding a mid-line incision. The technical difficulties in performing the urinary diversion totally intracorporeally have so far prevented its wide-spread adoption. Results reported by Schumacher and co-workers indicate at least at the beginning of their learning curve increased surgery-related complications using an intracorporeal urinary diversion approach [35]. Rehman et al. reported on 9 patients treated with RARC and totally intracorporeal confection of an ileal conduit [69]. One postoperative iatrogenous necrosis of the ileal conduit, probably caused by retraction of the organ bag occurred.

7. Oncologic outcome

To objectively assess oncological outcomes in patients treated either with open radical cystectomy or RARC for bladder cancer one needs to focus on: long-term cancer control, surgical quality (positive margins), tumor spillage, and port site metastasis.

Today, the highest long-term survival rates were reported for open radical cystectomy with an extended lymph node dissection. Stein et al. reported 5-year and 10-year recurrence-free survival rates of 68% and 60%, respectively, among 1,054 patients treated with radical cystectomy and extended lymph node dissection with curative intent [24]. For lymph node-negative, organ-confined disease, 5-year and 10-year recurrence-free survival rates were 85% and 82%. Similar results have been reported from other high-volume centers performing open radical cystectomy [25 26 27 28 29].

Whether the same cancer control rates equivalent to results from open radical cystectomy series can be achieved with RARC is still unknown; to date there are no long-term data available [70]. Median time to any recurrence after radical cystectomy is approximately 12 months, whereas 86% of recurrences occur within 3 years [24]. The mean follow-up in the current RARC series ranged from 3 to 77 months [tables 1 and 2]. However, in all of these RARC series median follow-up is short (<24 months), and reported survival data in which all patients have passed at least a 12 months follow-up do not exist.

The surgical quality at radical cystectomy independent of the surgical approach is essential for optimal local cancer control. Thus, negative margins must be achieved to avoid local tumor recurrence, which ultimately results in the death of the patient. Positive surgical margins have been reported to be 5% or less in high-volume open radical cystectomy series [25 26 27 28 29]. The incidence of positive margins at RARC ranged from 0% to 13% [21 30 31 32 34 36 37 38 39 40 71 72]. Guru et al, reported a 10.3% positive margin rate at RARC, whereas Yuh et al. found 13% positive margins in their patients [36 40]. Whether this high positive margin rate is attributable to the learning curve in these series is not clear. Data from the IRCC showed an overall 7% positive margin rate in their pooled 496 patients [17]. For patients with pathologic stage ≤ T3, 3.7% had a positive margin, whereas for patients with pathologic stage T3 or T4, 16% had a positive margin. The authors found with increasing surgical experience at RARC an improvement of their positive margin rate [17].

Port site metastasis in urological malignancies are of concern; they do occur, albeit infrequently. The etiology of port site metastasis is unknown. Port site metastasis has been reported after RARC and laparoscopic radical cystectomy for bladder cancer [73 74].

8. Post-operative recovery

Perioperative pathophysiology and care suggest that a multitude of factors contribute to postoperative morbidity, length of hospital stay, and convalescence in patients undergoing surgery [75]. Radical cystectomy is still associated with significant perioperative morbidity — this despite the implementation of accelerated postoperative recovery programs, or so-called "fast-track" surgery [76]. Comparison between historical cystectomy series and recent studies regarding post-operative recovery are difficult, as the concept of "fast-track" surgery has only been adopted by the urologic community during the last decade.

In order to reduce perioperative morbidity at cystectomy, Pruthi and co-workers have implemented and continuously improved the perioperative management in their 362 patients [77]. Reported findings from the last 100 (open and RARC) of these 362 cystectomy cases showed favorable return of bowel function (mean time to flatus 2.2 days, and mean time to bowel movements 2.9 days), the majority of patients being discharged after a mean of 5 days. Readmission was observed in 12% of patients, and the most common reasons for readmission were urinary tract infection (3%), gastrointestinal disorders (2%), and deep venous thrombosis (2%). The same group has published a randomized trial and assessed perioperative outcomes in patients treated with open versus robotic radical cystectomy [41]. Patients undergoing robotic cystectomy had longer operative times (4.2 versus 3.5 hours; $p <$ 0.001) and less blood loss (258 versus 575 mL; $p < 0.001$) than did patients with open cystectomy. Further, patients in the robotic group demonstrated a faster return of bowel activity (median time to flatus 2.3 days versus 3.2 days, and time to bowel movement 3.2 days versus 4.3 days). Hospital stay did not differ between groups (robotic 5.1 days, open 6.0 days; $p = 0.239$). Patients in the robotic group required significantly less analgesia than did patients with the open approach ($p = 0.019$). Similar results have been reported by Ng et al., comparing 104 open cystectomy with 83 RARC cases [78]. The robotic group demonstrated decreased blood loss (460 mL versus 1172 mL; $p < 0.0001$) and shorter length of hospital stay (5.5 days versus 8 days; $p < 0.0001$) than did the open cystectomy group. Wang et al., comparing open radical cystectomy with RARC patients, reported reduced blood loss, faster return to regular diet, and shorter hospital stay in the robotic group [32]. One may argue that fewer non-organ-confined tumors (28%) in the RARC group may have influenced their results compared to 57% non-organ-confined tumors in the open group. A recent study by Coward et al. found similar results regarding time to flatus (median 2 days) and time to bowel movements (median 3 days) after RARC in their series [45].

Despite the presumed advantages of less postoperative pain, faster return of bowel movements, shorter hospital stay, and overall quicker recovery over open surgery, the exact role of laparoscopy in improving perioperative outcomes remains unclear.

9. Quality of life

Quality of life (QoL) and postoperative recovery after surgery are important factors with direct financial implications for the health care system. Karvinen et al. reported on the effect of exercise and QoL in survivors of bladder cancer [79]. Findings from their study indicate that exercise is positively associated with QoL and the ability to perform physical activity results in increased QoL. If patients are able to return more quickly to preoperative levels with minimally invasive surgery, i.e. robotic surgery, they might be able to initiate exercise sooner, which in turn improves their QoL.

Yuh et al. evaluated QoL in a small single-center study after RARC [20]. Despite some inheriting limitations of the study design, QoL appeared to return to base-line by 3 months after RARC, and improved further at 6 months. The authors postulated that short-term improvement in QoL might also have positive implications regarding initiating adjuvant treatment protocols in these patients. Further studies are required to assess the physical and psychological implications of robotic surgery on QoL in patients undergoing radical cystectomy.

Functional results have been reported after open nerve-sparing radical cystectomy and orthotopic bladder substitution, however, reports from RARC series assessing continence and potency rates are sparse [7] [80].

10. Costs

The introduction of new and costly technologies into daily clinical practice has been criticized, especially during periods of economic uncertainty. With the introduction of expensive robotic technology cost-effectiveness has become more important. For robot-assisted radical prostatectomy some studies have shown volume-dependant cost advantages [81] [82]. Less information on cost-analysis is available for RARCS.

Smith et al., from North Carolina, US, performed a cost analysis at their institution between robotic and open radical cystectomy [83]. The financial costs of robotic and open radical cystectomy were categorized into operating room and hospital components, and further divided into fixed and variable costs for each. Variable costs were related to several factors, such as length of hospital stay. For each procedure the means of 20 cases were used to perform a comparative cost analysis. Based on their results, robotic cystectomy is associated with an overall higher financial cost of $1,640.

Martin et al. performed a detailed cost-analysis for open radical cystectomy vs. RARC cases [84]. They found that the most critical parameters for increased costs were operative time and hospital stay, which favored the robotic approach at their institution. Further, they stated that the real cost advantages are mostly seen when indirect costs are considered, such as treatment of perioperative complications or readmission rates due to complications.

Costs are difficult to measure and comprise other factors than just the perioperative period. Thus, earlier return to normal activity and reduced sick-leave might be important factors justifying these additional costs offered by the robotic approach.

11. Conclusions

Based on the current literature RARC is evolving rapidly as an alternative technique to open surgery in patients requiring radical cystectomy and urinary diversion. Lymph node yield and perioperative outcomes are similar to open radical cystectomy series; however, long-term oncological results are unknown. Several small prospective or randomized single-center trials showed comparable results between RARC and open cystectomy. However, the surgical procedure is technically demanding, especially when performing the urinary diversion totally intracorporeal. It is advisable to concentrate this type of surgery to high-volume centers where robotic expertise and technology is available.

12. References

[1] Stein JP, Penson DF, Wu SD, Skinner DG. Pathological guidelines for orthotopic urinary diversion in women with bladder cancer: a review of the literature. J Urol 2007;178:756-60.

[2] Stein JP, Skinner DG. Radical cystectomy for invasive bladder cancer: long-term results of a standard procedure. World J Urol 2006;24:296-304.

[3] Stein JP. Improving outcomes with radical cystectomy for high-grade invasive bladder cancer. World J Urol 2006;24:509-16.

[4] Stein JP, Skinner DG. Results with radical cystectomy for treating bladder cancer: a 'reference standard' for high-grade, invasive bladder cancer. BJU Int 2003;92:12-7.

[5] Hautmann RE, Volkmer BG, Schumacher MC, Gschwend JE, Studer UE. Long-term results of standard procedures in urology: the ileal neobladder. World J Urol 2006;24:305-14.

[6] Leissner J. [Lymphadenectomy for bladder cancer. Diagnostic and prognostic significance as well as therapeutic benefit]. Urologe A 2005;44:638-44.

[7] Studer UE, Burkhard FC, Schumacher M, et al. Twenty years experience with an ileal orthotopic low pressure bladder substitute--lessons to be learned. J Urol 2006;176:161-6.

[8] Stein JP. The role of lymphadenectomy in patients undergoing radical cystectomy for bladder cancer. Curr Oncol Rep 2007;9:213-21.

[9] Dhar NB, Klein EA, Reuther AM, Thalmann GN, Madersbacher S, Studer UE. Outcome after radical cystectomy with limited or extended pelvic lymph node dissection. J Urol 2008;179:873-8; discussion 8.

[10] Parra RO, Andrus CH, Jones JP, Boullier JA. Laparoscopic cystectomy: initial report on a new treatment for the retained bladder. J Urol 1992;148:1140-4.

[11] Haber GP, Campbell SC, Colombo JR, Jr., et al. Perioperative outcomes with laparoscopic radical cystectomy: "pure laparoscopic" and "open-assisted laparoscopic" approaches. Urology 2007;70:910-5.

[12] Basillote JB, Abdelshehid C, Ahlering TE, Shanberg AM. Laparoscopic assisted radical cystectomy with ileal neobladder: a comparison with the open approach. J Urol 2004;172:489-93.

[13] Wiklund NP. Technology Insight: surgical robots--expensive toys or the future of urologic surgery? Nat Clin Pract Urol 2004;1:97-102.

[14] Beecken WD, Wolfram M, Engl T, et al. Robotic-assisted laparoscopic radical cystectomy and intra-abdominal formation of an orthotopic ileal neobladder. Eur Urol 2003;44:337-9.

[15] Menon M, Hemal AK, Tewari A, et al. Nerve-sparing robot-assisted radical cystoprostatectomy and urinary diversion. BJU Int 2003;92:232-6.

[16] Hellenthal NJ, Hussain A, Andrews PE, et al. Surgical margin status after robot assisted radical cystectomy: results from the International Robotic Cystectomy Consortium. J Urol 2010;184:87-91.

[17] Hayn MH, Hussain A, Mansour AM, et al. The learning curve of robot-assisted radical cystectomy: results from the International Robotic Cystectomy Consortium. Eur Urol 2010;58:197-202.

[18] Hellenthal NJ, Hussain A, Andrews PE, et al. Lymphadenectomy at the time of robot-assisted radical cystectomy: results from the International Robotic Cystectomy Consortium. BJU Int 2010;107:642-6.

[19] Schumacher MC, Jonsson MN, Wiklund NP. Robotic cystectomy. Scand J Surg 2009;98:89-95.

[20] Yuh B, Butt Z, Fazili A, et al. Short-term quality-of-life assessed after robot-assisted radical cystectomy: a prospective analysis. BJU Int 2009;103:800-4.

[21] Pruthi RS, Nielsen ME, Nix J, Smith A, Schultz H, Wallen EM. Robotic radical cystectomy for bladder cancer: surgical and pathological outcomes in 100 consecutive cases. J Urol 2010;183:510-4.

[22] Khan MS, Elhage O, Challacombe B, Rimington P, Murphy D, Dasgupta P. Analysis of early complications of robotic-assisted radical cystectomy using a standardized reporting system. Urology 2011;77:357-62.

[23] Haber GP, Crouzet S, Gill IS. Laparoscopic and robotic assisted radical cystectomy for bladder cancer: a critical analysis. Eur Urol 2008;54:54-62.

[24] Stein JP, Lieskovsky G, Cote R, et al. Radical cystectomy in the treatment of invasive bladder cancer: long-term results in 1,054 patients. J Clin Oncol 2001;19:666-75.

[25] Madersbacher S, Hochreiter W, Burkhard F, et al. Radical cystectomy for bladder cancer today--a homogeneous series without neoadjuvant therapy. J Clin Oncol 2003;21:690-6.

[26] Hautmann RE, Gschwend JE, de Petriconi RC, Kron M, Volkmer BG. Cystectomy for transitional cell carcinoma of the bladder: results of a surgery only series in the neobladder era. J Urol 2006;176:486-92; discussion 91-2.

[27] Yossepowitch O, Dalbagni G, Golijanin D, et al. Orthotopic urinary diversion after cystectomy for bladder cancer: implications for cancer control and patterns of disease recurrence. J Urol 2003;169:177-81.

[28] Manoharan M, Ayyathurai R, Soloway MS. Radical cystectomy for urothelial carcinoma of the bladder: an analysis of perioperative and survival outcome. BJU Int 2009;104:1227-32.

[29] Dotan ZA, Kavanagh K, Yossepowitch O, et al. Positive surgical margins in soft tissue following radical cystectomy for bladder cancer and cancer specific survival. J Urol 2007;178:2308-12; discussion 13.

[30] Rhee JJ, Lebeau S, Smolkin M, Theodorescu D. Radical cystectomy with ileal conduit diversion: early prospective evaluation of the impact of robotic assistance. BJU Int 2006;98:1059-63.

[31] Murphy DG, Challacombe BJ, Elhage O, et al. Robotic-assisted laparoscopic radical cystectomy with extracorporeal urinary diversion: initial experience. Eur Urol 2008;54:570-80.

[32] Wang GJ, Barocas DA, Raman JD, Scherr DS. Robotic vs open radical cystectomy: prospective comparison of perioperative outcomes and pathological measures of early oncological efficacy. BJU Int 2008;101:89-93.

[33] Galich A, Sterrett S, Nazemi T, Pohlman G, Smith L, Balaji KC. Comparative analysis of early perioperative outcomes following radical cystectomy by either the robotic or open method. JSLS 2006;10:145-50.

[34] Woods M, Thomas R, Davis R, et al. Robot-assisted extended pelvic lymphadenectomy. J Endourol 2008;22:1297-302.

[35] Schumacher MC, Jonsson MN, Hosseini A, et al. Surgery-related Complications of Robot-assisted Radical Cystectomy With Intracorporeal Urinary Diversion. Urology 2011;77:871-6.

[36] Guru KA, Sternberg K, Wilding GE, et al. The lymph node yield during robot-assisted radical cystectomy. BJU Int 2008;102:231-4; discussion 4.

[37] Dasgupta P, Rimington P, Murphy D, et al. Robotic assisted radical cystectomy: short to medium-term oncologic and functional outcomes. Int J Clin Pract 2008;62:1709-14.

[38] Lowentritt BH, Castle EP, Woods M, Davis R, Thomas R. Robot-assisted radical cystectomy in women: technique and initial experience. J Endourol 2008;22:709-12.

[39] Kauffman EC, Ng CK, Lee MM, et al. Critical analysis of complications after robotic-assisted radical cystectomy with identification of preoperative and operative risk factors. BJU Int 2009;105:520-7.

[40] Yuh B, Padalino J, Butt ZM, et al. Impact of tumour volume on surgical and pathological outcomes after robot-assisted radical cystectomy. BJU Int 2008;102:840-3.

[41] Nix J, Smith A, Kurpad R, Nielsen ME, Wallen EM, Pruthi RS. Prospective randomized controlled trial of robotic versus open radical cystectomy for bladder cancer: perioperative and pathologic results. Eur Urol 2010;57:196-201.

[42] Kauffman EC, Ng CK, Lee MM, et al. Critical analysis of complications after robotic-assisted radical cystectomy with identification of preoperative and operative risk factors. BJU Int 2010;105:520-7.

[43] Schumacher MC, Scholz M, Weise ES, Fleischmann A, Thalmann GN, Studer UE. Is there an indication for frozen section examination of the ureteral margins during cystectomy for transitional cell carcinoma of the bladder? J Urol 2006;176:2409-13; discussion 13.

[44] Butt ZM, Fazili A, Tan W, et al. Does the presence of significant risk factors affect perioperative outcomes after robot-assisted radical cystectomy? BJU Int 2009;104:986-90.

[45] Coward RM, Smith A, Raynor M, Nielsen M, Wallen EM, Pruthi RS. Feasibility and Outcomes of Robotic-assisted Laparoscopic Radical Cystectomy for Bladder Cancer in Older Patients. Urology 2011.

[46] Dindo D, Demartines N, Clavien PA. Classification of surgical complications: a new proposal with evaluation in a cohort of 6336 patients and results of a survey. Ann Surg 2004;240:205-13.

[47] Shabsigh A, Korets R, Vora KC, et al. Defining early morbidity of radical cystectomy for patients with bladder cancer using a standardized reporting methodology. Eur Urol 2009;55:164-74.

[48] Karl A, Carroll PR, Gschwend JE, et al. The impact of lymphadenectomy and lymph node metastasis on the outcomes of radical cystectomy for bladder cancer. Eur Urol 2009;55:826-35.

[49] Leissner J, Hohenfellner R, Thuroff JW, Wolf HK. Lymphadenectomy in patients with transitional cell carcinoma of the urinary bladder; significance for staging and prognosis. BJU Int 2000;85:817-23.

[50] Stein JP, Cai J, Groshen S, Skinner DG. Risk factors for patients with pelvic lymph node metastases following radical cystectomy with en bloc pelvic lymphadenectomy: concept of lymph node density. J Urol 2003;170:35-41.

[51] Herr H, Lee C, Chang S, Lerner S. Standardization of radical cystectomy and pelvic lymph node dissection for bladder cancer: a collaborative group report. J Urol 2004;171:1823-8; discussion 7-8.

[52] Guru K, Seixas-Mikelus SA, Hussain A, et al. Robot-assisted intracorporeal ileal conduit: Marionette technique and initial experience at Roswell Park Cancer Institute. Urology 2010;76:866-71.

[53] Hemal AK, Abol-Enein H, Tewari A, et al. Robotic radical cystectomy and urinary diversion in the management of bladder cancer. Urol Clin North Am 2004;31:719-29, viii.

[54] Abraham JB, Young JL, Box GN, Lee HJ, Deane LA, Ornstein DK. Comparative analysis of laparoscopic and robot-assisted radical cystectomy with ileal conduit urinary diversion. J Endourol 2007;21:1473-80.

[55] Hemal AK, Kolla SB, Wadhwa P. First case series of robotic radical cystoprostatectomy, bilateral pelvic lymphadenectomy, and urinary diversion with the da Vinci S system. J Robotic Surg 2008;2:35-40.

[56] Mottrie A, Caprpentier P, Schatteman P, et al. Robot-assisted laparoscopic radical cystectomy: initial experience on 27 consecutive patients. J Robotic Surg 2007;1:197-201.

[57] Gamboa AJ, Young JL, Dash A, Abraham JBA, Box GN, Ornstein DK. Pelvic lymph node dissection and outcomes of robot-assisted radical cystectomy for bladder carcinoma. J Robotic Surg 2009;3:7-12.

[58] Bochner BH, Cho D, Herr HW, Donat M, Kattan MW, Dalbagni G. Prospectively packaged lymph node dissections with radical cystectomy: evaluation of node count variability and node mapping. J Urol 2004;172:1286-90.

[59] Ather MH, Alam ZA, Jamshaid A, Siddiqui KM, Sulaiman MN. Separate submission of standard lymphadenectomy in 6 packets versus en bloc lymphadenectomy in bladder cancer. Urol J 2008;5:94-8.

[60] Kulkarni GS, Finelli A, Lockwood G, et al. Effect of healthcare provider characteristics on nodal yield at radical cystectomy. Urology 2008;72:128-32.

[61] Mills RD, Fleischmann A, Studer UE. Radical cystectomy with an extended pelvic lymphadenectomy: rationale and results. Surg Oncol Clin N Am 2007;16:233-45.

[62] Stein JP, Quek ML, Skinner DG. Lymphadenectomy for invasive bladder cancer. II. technical aspects and prognostic factors. BJU Int 2006;97:232-7.

[63] Schumacher MC, Jonsson MN, Wiklund NP. Does extended lymphadenectomy preclude laparoscopic or robot-assisted radical cystectomy in advanced bladder cancer? Curr Opin Urol 2009;19:527-32.

[64] Pruthi RS, Wallen EM. Robotic-assisted laparoscopic pelvic lymphadenectomy for bladder cancer: a surgical atlas. J Laparoendosc Adv Surg Tech A 2009;19:71-4.

[65] Richards KA, Hemal AK, Kader AK, Pettus JA. Robot assisted laparoscopic pelvic lymphadenectomy at the time of radical cystectomy rivals that of open surgery: single institution report. Urology 2010;76:1400-4.

[66] Lavery HJ, Martinez-Suarez HJ, Abaza R. Robotic extended pelvic lymphadenectomy for bladder cancer with increased nodal yield. BJU Int 2010.

[67] Manoharan M, Katkoori D, Kishore TA, Antebie E. Robotic-assisted radical cystectomy and orthotopic ileal neobladder using a modified Pfannenstiel incision. Urology 2011;77:491-3.

[68] Pruthi RS, Nix J, McRackan D, et al. Robotic-assisted laparoscopic intracorporeal urinary diversion. Eur Urol 2010;57:1013-21.

[69] Rehman J, Sangalli MN, Guru K, et al. Total intracorporeal robot-assisted laparoscopic ileal conduit (Bricker) urinary diversion: technique and outcomes. Can J Urol 2011;18:5548-56.

[70] Chade DC, Laudone VP, Bochner BH, Parra RO. Oncological outcomes after radical cystectomy for bladder cancer: open versus minimally invasive approaches. J Urol 2010;183:862-69.

[71] Guru KA, Kim HL, Piacente PM, Mohler JL. Robot-assisted radical cystectomy and pelvic lymph node dissection: initial experience at Roswell Park Cancer Institute. Urology 2007;69:469-74.

[72] Cha EK, Wiklund NP, Scherr DS. Recent advances in robot-assisted radical cystectomy. Curr Opin Urol 2011;21:65-70.

[73] El-Tabey NA, Shoma AM. Port site metastases after robot-assisted laparoscopic radical cystectomy. Urology 2005;66:1110.

[74] Stolla V, Rossi D, Bladou F, Rattier C, Ayuso D, Serment G. Subcutaneous metastases after coelioscopic lymphadenectomy for vesical urothelial carcinoma. Eur Urol 1994;26:342-3.

[75] Kehlet H, Dahl JB. Anaesthesia, surgery, and challenges in postoperative recovery. Lancet 2003;362:1921-8.

[76] Olbert PJ, Baumann L, Hegele A, Schrader AJ, Hofmann R. [Fast-track concepts in the perioperative management of patients undergoing radical cystectomy and urinary diversion: review of the literature and research results]. Urologe A 2009;48:137-42.

[77] Pruthi RS, Nielsen M, Smith A, Nix J, Schultz H, Wallen EM. Fast track program in patients undergoing radical cystectomy: results in 362 consecutive patients. J Am Coll Surg 2010;210:93-9.

[78] Ng CK, Kauffman EC, Lee MM, et al. A comparison of postoperative complications in open versus robotic cystectomy. Eur Urol 2009;57:274-81.

[79] Karvinen KH, Courneya KS, Venner P, North S. Exercise programming and counseling preferences in bladder cancer survivors: a population-based study. J Cancer Surviv 2007;1:27-34.

[80] Mottrie A, Schatteman P, Fonteyne E, Rotering J, Stockle M, Siemer S. [Robot-assisted laparoscopic radical cystectomy]. Urologe A 2008;47:414, 6-9.

[81] Lotan Y, Cadeddu JA, Gettman MT. The new economics of radical prostatectomy: cost comparison of open, laparoscopic and robot assisted techniques. J Urol 2004;172:1431-5.

[82] Scales CD, Jr., Jones PJ, Eisenstein EL, Preminger GM, Albala DM. Local cost structures and the economics of robot assisted radical prostatectomy. J Urol 2005;174:2323-9.

[83] Smith A, Kurpad R, Lal A, Nielsen M, Wallen EM, Pruthi RS. Cost analysis of robotic versus open radical cystectomy for bladder cancer. J Urol;183:505-9.

[84] Martin AD, Nunez RN, Castle EP. Robot-assisted Radical Cystectomy Versus Open Radical Cystectomy: A Complete Cost Analysis. Urology;77:621-5.

7

Current Trends in Urinary Diversion in Men

S. Siracusano, S. Ciciliato, F. Visalli, N. Lampropoulou and L. Toffoli
Department of Urology – Trieste University
Italy

1. Introduction

Prior to the introduction of the ileal conduit more than four decades ago, the options for urinary diversion after cystectomy were extremely limited. Direct cutaneous anastomoses of the collecting system (cutaneous pyelostomies, ureterostomies) offered patients a short-term diversion, but the benefits were outweighed by significant complications: recession or stenosis of the stoma. The first choice of diversion was the ureterosigmoidostomy with or without antireflux technique. Then it fell in popularity and was replaced with continent/non-continent uretero-ileo-cutaneous diversions. Only in the last years the continent orthotopic neobladder has been widely employed as first procedure choice. At present, patients can be offered a non-continent cutaneous diversion, a continent cutaneous diversion or an orthotopic neobladder urinary reconstruction (ONR).

2. Surgical indications

Urinary diversion is necessary in patients who undergo cystectomy.
The choice of a specific urinary diversion should be performed on the basis of the mental status of the patient, renal function and overall health (Table1).
The main surgical indications to perform a urinary diversion or a bladder replacement using transposed intestinal segments are bladder cancer, neurogenic bladder dysfunction, idiopathic detrusor overactivity and chronic inflammatory conditions (such as interstitial cystitis, tuberculosis, schistosomiasis and postradiation bladder contraction) [1].
If surgical cystectomy is indicated due to invasive bladder cancer the choice for replacing the lower urinary tract function rests between conduit diversion, bladder replacement or continent diversion [2].
In patients affected by neurogenic bladder dysfunction due to congenital or acquired disorders (e.g. Neural tube defect or spinal cord injured patients) the main indications for such surgery is represented by intractable incontinence, deteriorating renal function and high bladder pressures. The choices would include either bladder reconstruction, replacement or continent diversion [3].
Equally in subjects with severe idiopathic detrusor overactivity, if conservative measures fail the surgical therapy which may involve transposition of intestinal segments into the urinary tract (e.g. Clam enterocystoplasty) can provide effective treatment for some patients [4].

Finally in patients affected by idiopathic interstitial cystitis with a failure of all conservative treatments the surgical choices range from ileal conduit diversion to orthotopic neobladder reconstruction (ONR). In this context in case of bladder tuberculosis resulting in intolerable frequency, pain, urgency and haematuria with a small and incapable bladder the surgical therapy ranges from ileal conduit diversion to augmentation cystoplasty [5].

Choice of urinary diversion

At present urologists have a variety of urinary diversions using different types of bowel segments based on an individual patient's need and desire. In the past the ureterosigmoidostomy and the rectal neobladder as described by Mouclaire were the earliest forms of continent urinary diversion however, due to the rate of complications, these surgical solutions are at present abandoned. The ileal conduit remains the most common form of non-continent urinary diversion practiced worldwide today and it is the standard to which all other urinary diversions are compared [6]. Continent cutaneous diversions using detubularized colonic segments requiring timed intermittent self-catheterization. These diversions gained popularity in the 1980s and are still applied today in patients for whom an ONR is not indicated. In this way the ONR represents the most innovative surgical solution of the last thirty years because it seems to offer a satisfactory quality of life.

Urinary diversions used today in patients undergoing radical cystectomy can be categorized into three basic categories as follows : I) bowel conduits II) continent cutaneous stomal reservoirs using colonic segments III) orthotopic neobladder reconstruction (ONR) [7]. On the basis of the above reported classification we will restrict our focus on the ileal conduit, on the continent cutaneous diversions and the ONR by the use of ileal bowel.

The ileal conduit is the simplest and most commonly performed urinary diversion for which the longest follow-up is available and due to the short operative time it is often applied in patients with significant medical comorbidities in an attempt to minimize postoperative complications and the need for reoperation [8].

The continent urinary diversion involves the creation of a low pressure reservoir of good capacity using a detubularised intestinal segments as described by Kock [9]. In this setting several techniques can be used to maintain continence adopting the principle of the nipple valve and one of the most popular type is the flap valve by the use of the appendix implanted into the reservoir as described by Mitrofanoff [10]. In this surgical technique the distal end of the continence channel is brought out as a stoma through the abdominal wall for clean intermittent self-catheterisation, thus avoiding the use of a stoma bag but requiring the ability of the patient to catheterize the stoma.

In ONR the most used intestinal segment is the ileum due to its easy and ductile use while colonic segments although they had already been employed at the beginning of the "ONR era" they showed a higher number of late complications in comparison with ileum segments [11].

Patients selection criteria: Absolute and relative contraindications

The primary goals of urinary diversion are to provide the best local cancer control, to reduce the potential range of complications and to guarantee the best quality of life for the patient. The decision process is complex and involves consideration of issues related to cancer stage and location, medical comorbidities, technical surgical issues, treatment needs, and patient desires related to quality-of-life and lifestyle (Table 2). In this setting, patients should be aware that intraoperative pathological findings could modify the type of urinary diversion planned, as in the case of a short mesentery or cancer-related issues such as positive urethral margin, or gross extravesical disease precluding a negative surgical margin. For this reason, all patients planned for an ONR should have a stoma site marked preoperatively by an enterostomal therapist and at the same time have read and accepted the informed consent for an alternative urinary diversion [7,12,13].

In this way an absolute contraindication to continent diversion of any type is compromised renal function that results from long-standing obstruction or chronic renal failure, with serum creatinine levels above 150 to 200 mol/L.

In patients with borderline renal function, creatinine clearance should be evaluated because at least a creatinine clearance of 60 mL/min is recommended for continent diversions [14]. A severe hepatic dysfunction is also a contraindication for continent diversion [15] because the reabsorption and recirculation of urinary metabolites require normal liver function [16-17-20]. In fact the interposition of intestine in the urinary tract results in a marked increase in the absorption of urinary ammonia into the portal circulation resulting in a metabolic adaptation in a normal functioning liver without a hyperammonemia with a consequent altered mental status [19].

Regarding related contraindications, we know that these are steadily decreasing. However some, such as mental impairment, external sphincter dysfunction or recurrent urethral stricture, deserve serious consideration.

Notably, old age is not a contraindication for ONR. Older patients, as part of the informed consent, need to be aware that they have a greater incidence of enuresis or nocturnal incontinence than do younger men, but age by itself should not be a contraindication. In this context, physiologic rather than chronologic age must be taken into consideration [20]. Although urinary continence rates are somewhat lower in patients over 70 years of age, satisfactory continence rates and functional outcomes can be obtained. [21,22].

Obesity does not preclude orthotopic diversion and in some cases an orthotopic diversion may be advantageous because of the difficulty of constructing an optimal stoma for a urostomy appliance with conduits and the difficulty in negotiating a catheter through a thick abdominal wall for catheterization of a continent cutaneous pouch. In addition, large fluctuations in patient weight can change the angle of the originally constructed pouch making it difficult to catheterize [23].

Satisfactory functional outcomes with ONR after cystectomy have been reported in carefully selected patients who have received previous definitive, full dose pelvic irradiation [24,25]. However, these are technically complex and demanding procedures with a high risk for perioperative complications [26]. Common complications reported in post-radiation surgical series include ureteral stricture in up to 32% of patients, prolonged incontinence in up to 44%, stomal problems in up to 39%, and fistulas in up to 7%. Reoperations to address these complications occur in 8% to 69% of patients and the most common reasons for reoperation include stomal revisions, ureteral anastomotic revisions, and procedures to correct incontinence and repair of fistulas [24,27].

Patients with compromised intestinal function, particularly inflammatory bowel disease, may be better served by an incontinent bowel conduit. A thorough evaluation of the colon by a contrast enema, sigmoidoscopy, or colonoscopy is recommended when planning to use large bowel segments for the urinary diversions to rule out colonic pathology such as diverticulosis, inflammatory bowel disease, or occult colon cancer, which would prevent their use. A family or personal history of colon cancer or familial polyposis may predispose the patient to developing an adenocarcinoma in a colonic urinary reservoir segment and should be taken into consideration during the diversion selection process [28,29].

In conclusion the goal of patient counseling about urinary diversion should be to determine the method that is the safest for cancer control, that has the fewest complications over both the short and the long term and that provides the easiest adjustment for patients' lifestyle, thereby supporting the best quality of life [7]. The ileal conduit is still the best urinary diversion method in many patients who have bladder cancer with associated chronic medical disease or certain surgical factors that render other urinary diversion techniques difficult to carry out. Finally we believe that all patients are potentially candidates for an ONR although the main problem is to identify patients for whom an ONR may be not indicated.

Bowel Segment	Primary Indication
Gastric	Children requiring diversion (extrophy,pelvic radiation); Renal insufficiency
Jejunum	Pelvic radiation; Deficient ureteral length; Compromised viability of other small or large bowel
Ileum or ileal-colic reservoirs	Malignancies requiring removal of the bladder; Severe hemorrhagic cystitis; Incontinence
Colon (ureterosigmoidostomy)	Children requiring diversion (extrophy, pelvic radiation); No other bowel segment alternative
Transverse colon conduit	Malignancies requiring removal of the bladder; Small bowel not practical

Table 1. Indications for use of bowel segments in urinary diversion [1,6]

Absolute contraindications
Impaired renal function
Impaired hepatic function
Inadequate intellectual capacity
Positive apical urethral margin (for neobladder)
Unmotivated patient
Relative contraindications
Advanced age
Need for adjuvant chemotherapy
Prior pelvic radiation
Bowel disease (especially inflammatory bowel disease)
Urethral pathology
Local disease and high risk of local recurrence

Table 2. Absolute and Relative Contraindications for Continent Cutaneous/Orthotopic Neobladder Urinary Diversions [1,6]

3. Non continent cutaneous diversions: Surgical aspects and postoperarative complications

The ileal and the colon conduit represent the non-continent cutaneous urinary diversions. The ileal conduit has been the mainstay of urinary diversion over the past forty-five years and, in authors' opinion, it remains the first choice against all other compared urinary diversions. It consists of diverting urine to a short intestinal segment brought out through the anterior abdominal wall. The ileal resection can induce malabsorption of bile salts and vitamin B_{12}. The colon conduit was less employed because of resulted in electrolyte abnormalities and was more amenable to antireflux ureteral implantation techniques. The non-refluxing technique is employed for a better maintenance of upper urinary tract integrity.

Ileal conduit

Ureteroileal urinary diversion is the most common method of non-continent urinary diversion. The basic technique for creation of the ileal loop has not changed significantly since the original description by Seiffer 1935. The procedure was subsequently popularized by Bricker.

The patient is placed in supine position and a vertical midline or paramedian incision from the symphysis pubis to the umbilicus or beyond is required for good exposure [30].

The ureters are identified and transected approximately 3 or 4 cm above the bladder and then they are minimally mobilized taking care to preserve the surrounding adventitia and fat. The conduit is constructed using an ileal segment 15 to 20 cm long that is isolated approximately 20 cm proximal to the ileocecal valve [31,32,33].

Once the appropriate length of bowel is selected and isolated, the mesentery is divided proximally and distally and individual mesenteric blood vessels are ligated. The bowel is divided, thus isolating the segment selected for conduit construction. The continuity of the small intestine is reestablished, allowing for normal bowel function. The base of the conduit is closed and the ureters are reimplanted directly, creating an antirefluxing ureteroileal anastomosis.

Ureteral stents (small-diameter, multichannel, silicone catheters) are placed through the ureteral anastomosis, the conduit and into the pelvis to facilitate urinary drainage while the anastomosis is healing [33-34].The conduit is usually positioned in the right lower quadrant of the abdomen in an isoperistaltic direction [32].

To create the stoma, a small circle of skin is excised at the premarked site. And the underlying cylinder of fat is removed. The fascia is incised in a cruciate fashion. The end of the conduit is brought through the lateral aspect of the rectus abdominis muscle and anchored to the fascia, and the stoma is then formed [34]. The stoma should protrude, without tension approximately 2,5-3 cm above the skin surface. A Rutzen bag can be applied to the stoma on the fifth or sixth postoperative day with complete comfort for the patient [34].

Jejunal conduit

Jejunal conduit urinary diversion is used rarely, since many better alternatives are available. However, jejunal conduits have been used in cases in which there has been significant ileal and colonic disease caused by previous irradiation and inflammatory bowel disease or there has been loss of the middle and distal ureter [35].

As is discussed later, electrolyte disturbances can occur after incorporation of intestinal segments into the urinary tract; these are more common when the jejunum is used for conduit construction. In approximately 40% of patients with jejunal urinary conduits, hyponatremic, hyperkalemic, hypochloremic metabolic acidosis and azotemia develop [36]. The jejunum is unable to maintain large solute gradients, so large amounts of water and solute pass through the jejunal wall. Sodium and chloride are rapidly excreted into the conduit, and potassium is passively absorbed [36-37].

Aldosterone is produced, resulting in reabsorption of hydrogen and excretion of potassium into the distal tubule of the kidney and consequent acidosis and movement of potassium from the body's intracellular stores. As water is lost into the conduit, extracellular fluid volume is reduced, as is the glomerular filtration rate. The renin-angiotensin system is activated, which further stimulates aldosterone secretion. Urea may be absorbed from the jejunal lumen, which (with dehydration) contributes to azotemia [36]. As with other bowel segments incorporated into the urinary tract, the length of jejunum should be as short as possible to reduce metabolic abnormalities. The ureters are brought out from the retroperitoneum below the ligament of Treitz. An appropriate segment of jejunum is identified and isolated and it is important to preserve an adequate blood supply to the segment. In contrast to the ilal conduit, the isolated jejunum should lie above the reanastomosed jejunum. The proximal end of the conduit is directed towards the retroperitoneum and the conduit is oriented in an isoperistaltic direction. The ureters are anastomosed to the jejunum, with placement of stents to reduce early postoperative electrolyte abnormalities. The mesenteric window is closed using nonasorbable sutures. The stoma is created in the same way as described for an ileal conduit and is usually located in the right upper quadrant [38].

Colon conduit

There are several advantages to using the large bowel for the construction of urinary conduits: nonrefluxing ureterointestinal anastomoses are easily performed, possibly abrogating the deleterious effects of reflux on the upper urinary tracts [37-39].

In the colon conduit stomal stenosis is uncommon because of the wide diameter of the large bowel but limited absorption of electrolytes occurs; the blood supply to the transverse and sigmoid colon is abundant [39]. Either the transverse or the sigmoid colon can be used, allowing for placement of the conduit high or low in the abdomen, depending on the integrity and condition of the ureters. Use of the transverse colon for conduit construction is especially well suited for patients who have received extensive pelvic irradiation or when the middle and distal ureters are absent [37,39].

The blood supply of the transverse colon is based on the middle colic artery.

The greater omentum is separated from the superior surface of the transverse colon, and a segment of bowel, usually 15 cm in length, is selected for the conduit [39]. Short mesenteric incisions are made, and the colon is divided proximally and distally. Once the conduit is isolated, bowel continuity is reestablished. The proximal end of the conduit is closed and fixed in the midline posteriorly. The ureters are brought through small incisions in the posterior peritoneum and reimplanted into the base of the conduit [39]. The stoma may be positioned on either the patient's right or left side.

A sigmoid conduit is constructed in a similar manner. Great care should be taken to preserve the blood supply by carefully selecting a segment with a good blood supply and by making short mesenteric incisions. The conduit is positioned lateral to the reapproximated sigmoid colon. Ureteral reimplantation and stoma construction are completed [39].

The ureters can be reimplanted into the large intestine either in a way that prevents reflux or by anastomosis directly into the bowel. Ureteral reflux is prevented by constructing a short tunnel (approximately 2-3 cm in length) of bowel mucosa, through which the distal ureter runs [37,39]. Frequently, this is accomplished by incising the tenia of the large bowel for a distance of 3-4 cm. The incision is carried through the muscular fibers of the bowel wall, sparing the mucosa. A small elliptic segment of mucosa is removed, and a mucosa-to-mucosa anastomosis is performed between the ureter and the mucosa of the bowel. The muscularis of the tenia is repositinated over the ureter to create the tunnel [39].

Cutaneous ureterostomy

This surgical technique is based on the simple bilateral ureterostomy or alternatively on the transureteroureterostomy. From a technical point of view the first surgical solution is easier and faster than the transureteroureterostomy. In particular, in order to carry out of a transureteroureterostomy with cutaneous ureterostomy the ureters are isolated with care to preserve the blood supply. A retroperitoneal course anterior to the great vessels for the least dilated is created [40,41]. If only a single ureter is obstructed, a simple stoma can be created by sewing the end of the ureter flush with the skin at the stoma site. Another option, when the ureter is narrow, is to create a V-flap stoma. If both ureters are dilated, a single stoma can be created by suturing the ureters together, everting them and anastomosing the ends to the skin. When a single ureter is dilated, transureterostomy with retroperitoneal passage of the smaller ureter to the controlatereral side is combined with the cutaneous ureterostomy [38].

Postoperative complications

Complications occurring after urinary diversion are generally a product of surgical technique, the underlying disease process and its treatment, the age of the patient, and the length of follow-up. Postoperative complications are divided into early and late.

Early complications (occurring in approximately 10% of patients) are wound infection, followed by ureteroileal leakage, intestinal obstruction, intestinal fistula and acute pyelonephritis [30].

Late complications (10-20% of patients) include metabolic disorders, stomal stenosis, cronic pyelonephritis, and calculi [30].

Metabolic and nutritional disorders

Fluid, electrolyte, nutrient, and waste product excretion or absorption normally occurs across the intestinal wall. The extent of absorption or excretion is dependent on the concentration of these substances in the lumen or blood and on which segment of bowel is in contact with them.

Metabolic abnormalities may occur when intestinal segments are interposed into the urinary tract [33].

The pathogenesis and nature of metabolic abnormalities occurring after incorporation of the ileum or colon into the urinary tract differ from those associated with jejunal conduits [35]; when such segments are used, sodium and chloride are absorbed across the bowel surface. Chloride is absorbed in slight excess of sodium, resulting in a net loss of bicarbonate into the bowel lumen. Preexisting renal failure contributes to the development and severity of the disorder, as does a large bowel surface area and long contact time. Hyperchloremic acidosis is more common in patients who undergo ureterosigmoidostomy than in patients who undergo simple conduit construction using either the ileum or the colon, because of the larger surface area and longer contact time with urine associated with ureterosigmoidostomies [42].

Hyperchloremic metabolic acidosis may manifest clinically as weakness, anorexia, vomiting, Kussmaul breathing, and coma. One potential long-term complication of chronic acidosis may be decreased bone calcium content and osteomalacia [36].

Bile salts are important for fat digestion and uptake of vitamins A and D. Bile salt metabolism may be altered after ileal resection [43].

Resecton of small segments of the ileum may be associated with mild malabsorption and steatorrhea owing to increased concentrations of bile salts delivered to the colon.

The increased concentration of such salts leads to decreased colonic absorption of water and electrolytes [35].The distal ileum is important for reabsorption of bile acidis, the use of this part of intestine for uncontinent urinary diversion causes abnormal high concentrations of bile acids in the colon leading to diarrhea due to the altered sodium absorption [43].

Vitamin B12 deficiency may occur as a result of resecting the terminal ileum to resconstruct the lower urinary tract. The signs of vitamin B 12 deficiency include megaloblastic macrocytic anemia and neurologic injury, which become permanent if allowed to persist [33,35,42,44].

Stomal complications

Stoma related complications occurred in 15% of patients with the most frequent being parastomal hernia, stenosis and various skin irritations or fungal infections [32,33]. The majority of stoma related complications occurred within the first 5 years after surgery [32].

Stomal stenosis can lead to conduit elongation and upper-tract obstruction. This condition can be diagnosed relatively easily by catheterizing the stoma and measuring the residual urine volume. It is corrected by revision of the stoma [42].

Skin irritation or infections are most common in procedures in which an appliance is worn and there is prolonged contact of the skin with urine. Some patients' skin may be sensitive to adhesive agents [30].

Urinary tract infection and pyelonephritis

Pyelonephritis occurs in approximately 12% of patients who have undergone urinary diversion. The infectious complications occurred at a median of 1.8 years after surgery [45].

Treatment is based on a properly collected urine sample for culture. A urine sample should not be collected from the pouch; rather, the pouch should be removed, the stoma cleansed with an antiseptic, and a catheter advanced gently through the stoma.

If infection has occurred in a patient with a simple conduit, the volume of residual urine within the conduit should be recorded. Obstruction and stasis of urine within the reconstructed urinary tract are risk factors for the development of infection [32].

Although many patients with preexisting dilation of the upper urinary tract show improvement or resolution of the dilation after urinary diversion or bladder substitution, progressive renal deterioration as manifested by hydronephrosis or an increasing serum creatinine level (or both) occur in a certain percentage of patients who undergo these procedures [42]. The incidence of either complication increases after 10 years. Pyelographic evidence of upper urinary tract deterioration has been noted in up to 50% of patients who have undergone urinary diversion at an early age.

Recurrent upper urinary tract infection and high-pressure ureteral reflux and obstruction, usually in combination, contribute to the likelihood of renal deterioration.

Calculi

Calculi occur in approximately 8% of patients who undergo urinary diversion, at a median of 2.5 years after surgery [33].

Such patients have several risk factors for the development of various calculi.

Nonabsorbable staples, mesh, or suture material used to construct conduits or reservoirs may act as a nidus for stone formation [33].

Colonization in either conduits or reservoirs is common, whereas symptomatic infection is much rarer.

Certain bacteria can contribute to stone formation; some bacteria commonly found in the urinary tract, including: Proteus, Klebsiella, and Pseudomonas species, produce urease, a urea-splitting enzyme that contributes to the formation of ammonia and carbon dioxide.

Hydrolysis of these products results in an alkaline urine supersaturated with magnesium ammonium phosphate, calcium phosphate, and carbonate apatite crystals.

Management of such infection-related stones requires stone removal, resolution of infection, and, often, use of adjunctive agents to complete stone dissolution [33].

The likelihood of stone formation is increased by the development of systemic acidosis, as described previously. Prolonged contact of the urine with the intestinal surface facilitates the exchange of chloride for bicarbonate [33].

Bicarbonate loss results in systemic acidosis and hypercalciuria. The combination of hypercalciuria and alkaline urine predisposes a patient to the development of calcium calculi. In addition, the terminal ileum is responsible for bile salt absorption; if this portion of the intestine is used for conduit or bladder reservoir construction, excess bile salts in the intestine may bind calcium and result in increased absorption of oxalate, which may lead to the development of oxalate-containing calculi [36].

Hypocitraturia may also be a risk factor for stone disease in patients undergoing bladder replacement [36].

Excess conduit length, urine stasis, and dehydration make the development of calculi more likely.

4. Orthotopic neobladder reconstruction (ONR): Surgical aspects and postoperative complications

In 1979, Camey and Le Duc published their clinical experience with ONR. This orthotopic bladder substitute has evolved into the most ideal form of urinary diversion available today and should be considered the gold standard with which other forms of diversion are compared. Before 1990, the orthotopic substitution was reserved for male patients with invasive bladder cancer while the same surgical approach was considered contraindicated in the female subjects because the urethra was removed during cystectomy to assure adequate oncological results. It was also believed that the female patient would be unable to maintain the continence mechanism if orthotopic diversion was performed after cystectomy. Actually, it has been shown that the urethra can be saved in the most women undergoing cystectomy for bladder cancer without compromising the oncological results [46].

Models of ONR

Radical cystectomy is the standard treatment for localized muscle-invasive bladder cancer. Different types of intestinal segments have been used for urinary diversion, including stomach, ileum, colon in humans and animals. However, the terminal ileum is most often used for bladder substitution. Therefore, the ideal diversion should be fully continent, cosmetically impeccable, allowing easy and complete emptying within socially acceptable intervals, and preserve renal function [47].

-   In Camey II orthotopic substitution a total of 65 cm of ileum is isolated, with an area of the ileum identified to reach the region of the urethra in a tension-free manner. After the integrity of the bowel is restored, the mesenteric trap is closed, and the isolated portion of ileum is opened along the antimesenteric border for the entire length, except the area previously identified for urethral anastomosis. In this region, the ileal incision is directed toward the mesenteric border. The ileum is then placed in a transverse U orientation. The medial borders of the U are sutured together with a running absorbable suture. A fingertip opening is made in the preselected area for the ileourethral anastomosis, the entire ileal plate is brought down to the pelvis, and urethroenteric anastomosis is performed. The ureteroileal anastomosis is then performed by a Le Duc technique. The reservoir is completed by folding the ileal plate and suturing with a running absorbable suture. The ends of the U are anchored to the pelvic floor to reduce tension [48].

-   The ileal neobladder developed by Hautmann was an ileal reservoir with a "W configuration" that wanted to guarantee a reduction of nighttime incontinence. A segment of terminal ileum of approximately 70 cm is selected. The bowel is reconstituted, and the mesenteric trap is closed. The ileal section that reaches the urethra most easily is identified and marked with a traction suture along the antimesenteric border. The isolated bowel segment is then arranged in either an M or W shape and is incised. The entire segment is opened along the antimesenteric border except for a 5-cm section along the traction suture, where the incision is directed toward the anterior mesenteric border to make a U-shaped flap. This facilitates anastomosis of the neobladder to the urethra. The four limbs of the M or W are then sutured to one another with a running absorbable suture. In the center of the previously developed flap, a segment of the ileal wall is excised. The ileourethral anastomosis is then performed with the sutures tied from "inside" the neobladder. Once the ileal neobladder is situated in the pelvis and the urethral sutures are tied, the ureters are implanted from inside the neobladder through a small incision in the ileum at a convenient site as reported by Abol-Enein (Fig.1) or in monolateral fashion as described by Siracusano [49]. The remaining portion of the anterior wall is then closed with a running absorbable suture.

-   The Studer ileal bladder substitute uses a portion of terminal ileal segment: 54 to 60 cm is isolated approximately 25 cm proximal to the ileocecal valve. Bowel continuity is restored, and the ends of the isolated segment are closed with a running absorbable suture. The distal 40-cm segment of ileum is placed in a U shape and opened along the antimesenteric border. The ureters are split and anastomosed in an end-to-side fashion to the proximal afferent tubular portion of ileum. The two medial borders of the U-shaped ileum are then oversewn with a running absorbable suture. The bottom of the U is folded over between the two ends of the U. After the lower half of the anterior wall

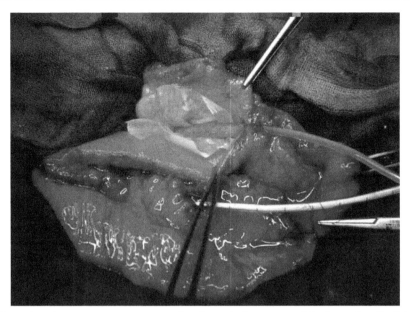

Fig. 1. Spatulated ureters are anastomosed to intestinal mucosa of the lateral wall of the trough. The ureters are anastomosed on 8 Fr anti-reflux double "J" stents (By Siracusano Eur Urol 38 : 313, 2000)

and part of the upper half are closed, a finger is introduced through the remaining reservoir opening to determine the most caudal part of the neobladder. A hole is cut out in this dependent portion of ileum, away from the suture line, which allows urethral anastomosis. The urethroenteric anastomosis is performed, and the remaining portion of the reservoir is then closed [50].

- The Kock ileal reservoir utilizes intussuscepted nipple valves for both the afferent and efferent limbs to prevent urinary reflux. A total of 61 cm of terminal ileum is isolated. 22-cm segments are placed in a U configuration and opened adjacent to the mesentery. The more proximal 17-cm segment of ileum will be used to make the afferent intussuscepted nipple valve. The posterior wall of the reservoir is then formed by joining the medial portions of the U with a continuous running suture. A 5- to 7-cm antireflux valve is made by intussusception of the afferent limb with the use of Allis forceps clamps. The afferent limb is fixed with two rows of staples placed within the leaves of the valve. The valve is fixed to the back wall from outside the reservoir. After completion of the afferent limb, the reservoir is completed by folding the ileum on itself and closing it (anterior wall). The most dependent portion of the reservoir becomes the neourethra. Ureteroileal anastomosis is performed first, and urethroenteric anastomosis is completed in a tension-free, mucosa-to-mucosa fashion [51].

- The "vescica ileale padovana" (VIP) is a modified form of Camey II with a more spherical reservoir. A portion of terminal ileum 40 cm long is isolated approximately 20 cm proximal to the ileocecal valve and opened along the antimesenteric border. The distal 10-cm segment is intended to constitute a tunnel for ileal-urethral anastomosis, while the proximal 30-cm segment of ileum is folded in a jellyroll fashion to produce a posterior plate. The pouch is then closed anteriorly [52].

- The T pouch ileal neobladder is a variant of Koch ileal reservoir but with a new, safe and simple antireflux technique. The T pouch is constructed from a 44-cm segment of terminal ileum placed in a V formation with a more proximal 8- to 10-cm segment of ileum used to form the antireflux limb. The entire mesentery remains intact to provide excellent viability. Windows of Deaver are opened (with Penrose drains placed into each window) in the distal 3 to 4 cm of the isolated afferent limb. The blood supply remains intact to this afferent ileal segment. A series of interrupted silk sutures are used to approximate the serosa of the adjacent 22-cm limbs (cephalad portion), with the passage of sutures through the corresponding window of Deaver. After the silk suture is passed through the window of Deaver, it is placed at a corresponding site on the adjacent 22-cm segment and then brought back through the same window of Deaver and tied down. The anchored portion of afferent limb is tapered on the antimesenteric border. The ileal segments are opened adjacent to the mesentery beginning at the apex and carried upward to the ostium of the afferent limb. Once the incision reaches the ostium of the afferent limb, it is directed to the antimesenteric border and then carried upward. This provides excellent ileal flaps to cover the tapered afferent ileal segment that is anchored into the serous trough. The ostium of the afferent segment is sutured to the ileal flaps. The ileal flaps are then brought over and oversewn to cover the tapered afferent ileal segment. This completes the posterior wall of the reservoir and forms the antireflux flap-valve mechanism. The reservoir is folded and closed in the opposite direction from which it was opened. The ureteroileal anastomosis is performed to the proximal portion of the afferent ileal segment. The anterior suture line is stopped just short of the right side. Then the result will be anastomosed to the urethra [53].

- The surgeons of Turin University propose an operative technique of a new Y-shaped ileal neobladder reconstruction. The procedure is performed with the isolation of 40cm of ileum, 15-20cm before the ileocecal valve. The isolated segment is arranged in a Y-shape with two central segments of 14cm and two limbs of 6cm. The two central segments are brought together and detubularized, with a nonabsorbable mechanical stapler inserted through an opening made at the lowest point of the neobladder. The Y-neobladder is anastomosed to the urethra with five sutures in 2-0 polyglycolic acid, over a 22F silastic catheter. The ureters, resected above the crossing with the iliac vessels and spatulated anteriorly, are anastomosed to the dorsal aspect of the two limbs with 5.0 polyglycolic acid sutures, using the direct Nesbit technique. Ureteral stents, previously placed, are brought out through the distal portions of each chimney and then through the anterior abdominal wall. The two limbs are fixed to the psoas muscles [54].

- In relation to the use of colon for carrying out ONR we report Mansson's technique and the pouches described by the Mainz School and by Reddy respectively.

In particular Mansson proposes an orthotopic neobladder substitution using a right colon segment (Mansson pouch). The entire right colon and cecum are isolated, and a transverse ileocolonic anastomosis is performed to provide bowel continuity. The ileal stump at the ileocecal valve is closed with a running absorbable suture. The colonic segment is then opened along the anterior taenia, leaving the proximal 2 to 3 inches of cecum intact. An appendectomy is performed, and the ureters are implanted in an antireflux fashion within the reservoir. The colon is then folded in a Heineke-Mikulicz manner and closed with a running absorbable suture. The ureterocolonic anastomosis is then performed [55].

- The surgeons of Mainz Institute describe a surgical procedure with a segment of both ileum and right colon (Mainz pouch). A 10- to 15-cm segment of cecum, in continuity with a 20- to 30-cm segment of ileum, is isolated. An ascending ileocolostomy is performed. The entire segment of bowel is opened along the antimesenteric border, sacrificing the ileocecal valve. The bowel is placed in a W configuration, with the first limb of the W represented by cecum and the middle two limbs represented by ileum. The adjacent three limbs are sutured together with an absorbable suture, forming the posterior plate of the reservoir. At the cephalic portion of the cecum, tunneled ureterocolonic anastomosis is performed. A buttonhole incision is made in the cecum at the base of the reservoir, and a ureterocolonic anastomosis is performed. After this, the reservoir is closed side to side with absorbable suture [56].
- Reddy and Lange describe an orthotopic reconstruction with sigmoid segment (Reddy pouch). A 35-cm portion of descending colon and sigmoid is isolated and arranged in a U configuration. The medial taenia of the U is incised down to an area just short of the urethral anastomosis. The incised medial limbs of the U are then brought together with an absorbable suture. Ureteral implantation is performed in a tunnel antireflux fashion. A small button of colon is removed from the most dependent portion of the reservoir, and the urethroenteric anastomosis is performed. The reservoir is then closed side to side [57].

Complications

The patients may incur early and late complications as previously reported in non continent cutaneous diversions. The early post-operative complications may be identified as enterocolitis, acute pyelonephritis or lymphorrhoea. Therefore, chronic urinary retention, stricture of neobladder-urethra anastomosis, urosepsis secondary to bilateral hydronephrosis and neobladdder stones are the main late complications for this form of surgery [58]. Finally the utilization of small bowel for urinary diversion may interfere with the physiological renal acid and salt regulation while osteoporosis and osteomalacia might theoretically develop from a persistent hypokalemic, hyperchloremic acidosis.

5. Conclusions

For many years the ileal conduit and the ureterosigmoidostomy were considered the primary choice for urinary diversion following cystectomy. In the last twenty years the surgical procedures of urinary tract reconstruction after bladder removal have evolved from simply urinary diversions and protecting the upper tract to creating a socially and psychologically more acceptable quality of life. Nevertheless at present there is no optimal surgical urinary diversion for all patients but surgical solutions that must be applied to each type of patient.

6. References

[1] Ghulam Nabi, June D Cody, Norman Dublin, Samuel McClinton , James MO N'Dow, David E Neal, Robert Pickard, Sze M Yong. Urinary diversion and bladder reconstruction/replacement using intestinal segments for intractable incontinence or following cystectomy Cochrane Database of Systematic Reviews, 2009

[2] Manoharan M and AM Nieder: "surgical management: cystectomy and urinary diversion" pp348-360 in Urological Oncology, VH Nargund, D Raghavan, HM Sandler Ed, Springer-Verlag London ltd 2008.

[3] Stein R, Wiesner C, Beetz R, Schwarz M, Thüroff JW. Urinary diversion in children and adolescents with neurogenic bladder: the Mainz experience. Part I: Bladder augmentation and bladder substitution--therapeutic algorisms. Pediatr Nephrol. 2005;20(7):920-5

[4] Lewis DK, Morgan JR, Weston PM, Stephenson TP. The "clam": indications and complications. British Journal of Urology 1990;65:488–91.

[5] Benchekroun A, Lachkar A, Soumana A, Farih MH, Belahnech Z, Marzouk M, Faik M. Urogenital tuberculosis. 80 cases. Ann Urol, 1998;32(2):89-94.

[6] Bricker EM: Bladder substitution with isolated small intestine segments; a progress report. Am Surg 1952;18:654-664.

[7] Dipen J. Parekh and S. Machele Donat Urinary Diversion: Options,Patient Selection, and Outcomes Semin Oncol 2007;34:98-109,

[8] Turnbull RB Jr: Intestinal stomas. Surg Clin North Am 1958; 38:1361-1372,

[9] Kock NG, Nilson AE, Nilsson LO, Norlen LJ, Philipson BM. Urinary diversion via a continent ileal reservoir: clinical results in 12 patients. Journal of Urology 1982;128(3):469–75

[10] Sumfest JM, Burns MW, Mitchell ME. The Mitrofanoff principle in urinary reconstruction. J Urol. 1993;150, 1975-1878

[11] Hautmann RE: Urinary diversion: Ileal conduit to neobladder. J Urol 2003; 169:834-842,

[12] Henna as a durable preoperative skin marker. Henna as a durable preoperative skin marker. World J Surg. 2011;35(2):311-5

[13] Bass EM, Del Pino A, Tan A, Pearl RK, Orsay CP, Abcarian H. Does preoperative stoma marking and education by the enterostomal therapist affect outcome? Dis Colon Rectum. 1997;40(4):440-2

[14] Mills RD, Studer UE: Metabolic consequences of continent urinary diversion. J Urol 1999;161:1057-1066.

[15] Mills RD, Studer UE: Metabolic consequences of continent urinary diversion. J Urol 1999; 161:1057-1066.

[16] Koch MO, McDougal WS, Thompson CO: Mechanisms of solute transport following urinary diversion through intestinal segments: An experimental study with rats. J Urol 1991; 146:1390-1394.

[17] Koch MO, McDougal WS, Flora MD: Urease and the acidosis of urinary intestinal diversion. J Urol 1991;146:458-462.

[18] McDougal WS, Koch MO: Accurate determination of renal function in patients with intestinal urinary diversions. J Urol 1986; 135:1175-1178.

[19] Kaveggia FF, Thompson JS, Schafer EC, et al: Hyperammonemic encephalopathy in urinary diversion with urea-splitting urinary tract infection. Arch Intern Med 1990;150:2389-2392.

[20] Studer UE, Hautmann RE, Hohenfellner M, Mills RD, Okada Y, Rowland RG, et al. Indications for continent diversion after cystectomy and factors affecting long-term results. Urol Oncol 1998; 4:172-82

[21] Steven K, Poulsen AL: The orthotopic Kock ileal neobladder: Functional results, urodynamic features, complications and survival in 166 men. J Urol 2000;164:288-295.

[22] Elmajian DA, Stein JP, Esrig D, et al: The Kock ileal neobladder: Updated experience in 295 male patients. J Urol 1996; 156:920-925.

[23] Colwell JC, Fichera A: Care of the obese patient with an ostomy. J Wound Ostomy Continence Nurs 2005; 32:378-383.

[24] Gheiler EL, Wood DP Jr, Montie JE, et al: Orthotopic urinary diversion is a viable option in patients undergoing salvage cystoprostatectomy for recurrent prostate cancer after definitive radiation therapy. Urology 1997; 50:580-584.

[25] Bochner BH, Figueroa AJ, Skinner EC, et al: Salvage radical cystoprostatectomy and orthotopic urinary diversion following radiation failure. J Urol 1998; 160:29-33.

[26] Lebret T, Herve JM, Barre P, et al: Urethral recurrence of transitional cell carcinoma of the bladder. Predictive value of preoperative latero- montanal biopsies and urethral frozen sections during prostatocystectomy. Eur Urol 1998; 33:170-174.

[27] Chang SS, Alberts GL, Smith JA Jr, et al: Ileal conduit urinary diversion in patients with previous history of abdominal/pelvic irradiation. World J Urol 2004; 22:272-276.

[28] Albertini JJ, Sujka SK, Helal MA, et al: Adenocarcinoma in a continent colonic urinary reservoir. Urology 1998; 51:499-500.

[29] Pickard R: Tumour formation within intestinal segments transposed to the urinary tract. World J Urol 2004; 22:227-234.

[30] Oneeka W, Vereb M, Libertino J. Noncontinent urinary diversion. Urol Clin North Am. 1997; 24: 735-743

[31] Gburek B.M,Lieber M.M, Blute M.L. Comparison of studer ileal neobladder and ileal conduit urinary diversion with respect to perioperative outcome and late complications.J Urol. 1998; 160: 721-723

[32] Madersbacher S, Schmidt J, Eberle M.J, Thoeny H.C, Burkhard F, Hochreiter W, Studer E. Long-term outcome of ileal conduit diversion. J Urol. 2003; 169: 985-990.

[33] Shimko M, Tollefson M, Umbreit E, Farmer S, Blute M, Frank I. Long-Term Complications of Conduit Urinary Diversion. J Urol. 2011; 185: 562-567

[34] Bricker E. Bladder substitution after pelvic evisceration. J Urol. 2002; 167:1140-1145

[35] Hautmann R. Urinary diversion: ileal conduit to neobladder. J Urol. 2003; 169:834-842.

[36] Hall C, Koch M, McDouglas S. Metabolic Consequences of Urinary Diversion Through Intestinal Segment. Urol Clin North Am. 1991; 18: 725-735.

[37] Carroll P et all. Urinary Diversion & Bladder Substitution. Smith's General Urology 17th edition. Mc GrawHill.

[38] DownsT et all. Noncontinent and Continent Cutaneous Urinary Diversion. Urologic Oncology 2005. Elsevier.

[39] Richie J. Sigmoid Conduit Urinary Diversion. Urol Clin North Am. 1986; 13: 225-231.

[40] Beland G, laberge I. Cutaneous transureterostomy in children. J Urol. 1975; 114:588-590.

[41] Rainwater L, Leary F, Rife C. Transureteroureterostomy with cutaneous ureterostomy: a 25-year experience. J Urol. 1991; 146:13-15.

[42] Nieuwenhuijzen J, Vries R, Bex A, van der Poel H, Meinhardt W, Antonini N, Horenblas S. Urinary Diversion after Cystectomy: The Association of Clinical factors, Complications and Functional Results of Four Different Diversions. Eur Urol. 2008; 53:834-844.

[43] Olofsson G, Fjalling M, Kilander A, Ung k, Jonsson O. Bile acid malabsorption after continent urinary diversion with an ileal reservoir. J Urol. 1998; 160:724-727

[44] Terai A, Okada Y, Shichiri Y, Kakehi Y, Terachi T, Arai Y, Yoshida O. Vitamin B 12 Deficency in patients with Urinary Intestinal Diversion. Int J Urol. 1997; 4:21-25.

[45] Fitzgerald J, Malone M, Gaertner R, Zinman L. Stomal construction, complication, and reconstruction. Urol Clin North Am. 1997; 24: 729-733.

[46] Campbell-Walsh. *Urology.* (2007) Saunders IX Edition, Volume I

[47] Granberg CF et al. *Functional and oncological outcomes after orthotopic neobladder reconstruction in women.* BJU Int 2008; 102; 1551-1555

[48] Barre PH et al. *Update on the Camey II procedure.* World J Urol 1996; 14(1): 27-8

[49] Siracusano S. et Al. *Modified Ghoneim's technique using single serous-lined extramural orthotopic ileal W-bladder.* Eur Urol 2000; 38 : 313-5,

[50] Studer UE et al. *Orthotopic ileal neobladder.* BJU Int (2004) 93(1): 183-93

[51] Ghoneim MA et al. *An appliance-free, sphincter-controlled bladder substitute: the urethral Kock pouch.* J Urol 1987; 138(5): 1150-4

[52] Novara G et al. *Functional results following vescica ileale Padovana (VIP) neobladder: midterm follow-up analysis with validated questionnaires.* Eur Urol 2010; 57(6): 1045-51

[53] Stein JP et al. *The T pouch: an orthotopic ileal neobladder incorporating a serosal lined ileal antireflux technique.* J Urol 1998; 159(6): 1836-42

[54] Fontana D et al. *Y-neobladder: an easy, fast, and reliable procedure.* Urology. 2004; 63(4): 699-703

[55] Månsson W et al. *Continent urinary tract reconstruction - the Lund experience.* BJU Int. 2003; 92(3): 271-6

[56] Thuroff JW et al. *The Mainz pouch (mixed augmentation ileum 'n zecum) for bladder augmentation and continent urinary diversion. 1985.* Eur Urol 2006; 50(6): 1142-50

[57] Reddy PK. *The colonic neobladder.* Urol Clin North Am 1991; 18(4): 609-14

[58] Wyczolkowski M et al. *Studer orthotopic ileal bladder substitute construction – surgical techniqueand complication management: one center and 12-year experience.* Adv Med Sci 2010; 55(2); 146-15

Part 4

Future Treatments

8

The H19-IGF2 Role in Bladder Cancer Biology and DNA-Based Therapy

Imad Matouk[1,2,*] et al
[1]Department of Biological Chemistry, Institute of Life Sciences,
The Hebrew University of Jerusalem, Jerusalem
[2]Department of Biology, Science and Technology, Alquds Abu-Dis University, Jerusalem
Israel

1. Introduction

The H19-IGF2 locus within the imprinted cluster of the human chromosome 11, has been implicated in a variety of disorders and cancer pre-disposition including bladder cancer. BBN induced bladder cancer model in rats has identified both H19 and IGF2 among differentially expressed genes that are induced in response to carcinogen exposure.

In this chapter, the role of both H19 and IGF2 genes in cancer will be handled in general with special focus on bladder cancer. Although IGF2 role in human cancers is relatively well established, recent data from our laboratory and others have just revealed a critical role for H19 RNA in the process of tumorigenicity including that of the bladder. H19 functions as a stress modulator, being induced by hypoxia, and a survival factor that is involved in several fundamental processes of tumorigenesis. Furthermore, we uncovered a molecular mechanism that integrates H19, p53 and HIF1-α to hypoxic stress response. Placing the H19 gene product in this deadly circuit undoubtedly will have major impacts in its utility as a target for cancer gene therapy.

Regulatory sequences of both H19 and IGF2 have already been used to successfully target expression of a toxic protein, diphtheria toxin A (DT-A), in carcinoma cells in culture, in several xenograft, orthotopic animal models, and in chemically induced BBN model of bladder cancer. In case of H19, it is successfully used in patients with bladder carcinoma for a period of over 5 years and recently a clinical trial phase I/IIa using this therapeutic approach has been successfully completed. It is also successfully used in other types of human cancers but will not be handled in the current chapter.

We will discuss also novel approaches, to create a new family of plasmids. In one approach a cytotoxic gene is driven by two different regulatory sequences, selected from the cancer-specific promoters H19, IGF2-P3 and IGF2-P4 carried on a single construct. In a second

* Naveh Evantal[1], Doron Amit[1], Patricia Ohana[1], Ofer Gofrit[3], Vladimir Sorin[1], Tatiana Birman[1],
Eitan Gershtain[1] and Abraham Hochberg[1]
[1]Department of Biological Chemistry, Institute of Life Sciences,
The Hebrew University of Jerusalem, Jerusalem, Israel
[2]Department of Biology, Science and Technology, Alquds Abu-Dis University, Jerusalem, Israel
[3]Department of Urology, Hadassah Hebrew University Medical Center, Jerusalem, Israel

approach a single promoter is used to drive two cytotoxic genes having synergistic effect on a single construct. Both approaches show superior tumor growth inhibition activity, in preclinical studies of bladder cancer.

Bladder Cancer is the fourth most common cancer in men accounting for about 7% of all cancer cases and 3% of all cancer related mortality. Each year, more than 50,000 new patients are diagnosed with bladder cancer in the USA and about 10,000 die from this disease (Jemal et al., 2010). Carcinogens activity on a susceptible epithelium is believed to be the cause of bladder cancer. Many industrialized chemicals are causally related; benzidine, βnapthylamine, 4-aminobiphenyl, etc. However, the commonest cause of bladder cancer nowadays, is by far cigarette smoking accounting for about half of all bladder cancers (Burch et al., 1989). Whether bladder cancer arises from a single transformed cell (clonogenic theory) or from multiple transformed cells (field change theory), is still under debate.

Painless hematuria is the hallmark of bladder cancer. This dramatic symptom urgently brings the patient to see a doctor. Therefore, most bladder tumors are diagnosed during the lifetime of the patient. Bladder tumors can also present with irritative urinary symptoms (urinary urgency, frequency and dysuria). Bladder tumors can be diagnosed by ultrasonography, intravenous urography, or computerized tomography. The resolution of these radiologic techniques is low, and only a 5 to 10 mm lesion can be detected. Cystoscopy done by inserting an optical instrument into the bladder can diagnose bladder tumors as small as 1mm. Urinary cytology is an important adjunct to cystoscopy, especially for the diagnosis of the flat lesion carcinoma in-situ (CIS).

Most bladder tumors arise from the epithelial lining the urinary system-the transitional epithelium (urothelium), and are therefore, transitional cell carcinomas (or urothelial carcinomas). Bladder cancer is a heterogeneous disease with wide variations in molecular pathogenesis, morphology and prognosis. They are classified according to their depth of invasion into the bladder wall (stage) and according to the degree of histological anaplasia (grade).

As in most other types of cancer, it is believed that 4-6 DNA hits are required for malignant transformation (Duggan et al., 2004). These include deletions, mutations and loss of heterozygosity (LOH) of genetic material that carries tumor suppressor genes or proto-oncogenes, and epigenetic changes such as CpG methylations that modify gene expression. There are at least 2 major pathogenic pathways leading to 2 completely different bladder cancers. One pathway leads a low grade, papillary bladder cancer (about 75% of all bladder tumors). This type of tumor has a proliferative ability but no ability to invade the epithelial lamina propria and muscle of the bladder, to metastasize and to kill the patient. The second pathway leads to a high grade, solid tumor that has an invasive and metastatic potential (about 15% of the tumors). Possibly, there is a third pathway that leads to a high grade papillary tumor (about 10% of the tumors) (Goebell &Knowles, 2010). While low grade tumors tend to recur but almost never endanger the life of the patient, high grade tumors are often lethal.

It is believed that low grade tumors develop following this pathway: Urothelial hyperplasia→ urothelial atypia →low grade TCC. The most prominent molecular change in this group is mutation in FGFR3, found up to 88% of these tumors (van Rhijn et al., 2002). In most cases these are activation mutation that probably supports tumor proliferation by stimulating the RAS-MAPK pathway. The frequency of FGFR3 mutations in high grade tumors is much lower. Activation of the phosphatidylinositol 3–kinase (PI3K) pathway by a wide range of mechanisms is also typical to low grade tumors (Goebell &Knowles, 2010).

High grade bladder tumors develop following this pathway: Urothelial atypia →dysplasia → CIS →Invasive TCC→metastatic disease. The most prominent molecular changes in high grade tumors involve inactivation of the p53 and RB pathways. p53, whose activity is augmented in the presence of DNA damage, arrests cells at G1-S checkpoint by inducing the transcription of the CDK inhibitors-p21/Waf1, and GADD45. Then the cell may either correctly repair its DNA or undergo apoptosis. Deletions or mutations in the p53 pathway are found in about 70% of the high-grade tumors.

The Retinoblastoma gene codes for an 110kDa nuclear phosphoprotein acting as a tumor suppressor that also arrest cells at G1. It is often mutated by a truncating mutation of the carboxyl terminal. Mutations or deletions in Rb gene are found in 30% of the patients with advanced bladder cancers. They result in uncontrolled cellular proliferation even without mitogenic signals. Hypermethylation of the Rb promoter region can have the same effect. Similarly, loss of the cyclin dependent kinase inhibitor p16 either by mutation, deletion, or by promoter hypermethylation, as documented in 20-45% of the bladder cancers prevents Rb activation by hyper-phosphorylation, or leads to uncontrolled cell cycle progression (Schultz, 1998).

Epithelial to mesenchymal transition (EMT) is an important process typical to high grade tumors. It is characterized by down regulation of the adhesion molecule E-cadherin and of proteins associated with cell polarity along with up regulation of fibronectin, vimentin and matrix metalloproteases (MMPS). EMT is induced by cytokines like the TGFβ and is associated with increased invasion, migration and angiogenesis.

Alterations in chromosome 9 are the most common cytogenetic findings in bladder cancer. Of these, the most common are deletions and LOH in the short arm, home of the tumor suppressor genes and cell-cycle regulators CDKN2A (encoding for p16 and p14[ARF]) and CDKN2B (encoding for p15). In a rather consistent manner high grade tumors demonstrate LOH of 3p, 8p, 13q, and 17p, while low grade tumors demonstrate LOH of chromosome 9 only (Knowles et al., 2001).

Animal models are critical in the understanding of bladder cancer pathogenesis and in the quest for new treatments. Most animal models in bladder cancer are in rodents. Although various models exist, we'll focus on carcinogen induced bladder cancer model.

1.1 Carcinogen induced bladder cancer in mice and rats

In this model, the rodent is given a carcinogen, most commonly in the drinking water. BBN (N -butyl-N- (4-hydroxybutyl) nitrosamine) is a carcinogen given to the rodents in a concentration of 0.05% in the drinking water. It induces bladder tumors in 95% of the rodents after 25 weeks of administration (Okada et al., 1975). The tumors produced by the carcinogen resemble human bladder cancer in histology, etiology, and in kinetics (25 rat weeks equal 10 human years- the believed incubation period of human bladder cancer). Molecular events occurring during chemical carcinogenesis can be followed (Ariel et al., 2004). Tumor development and the response to novel treatments can be assessed non-invasively, without scarifying the animal using ultrasonography (Gofrit et al., 2006). The main disadvantages of this model are necessity to handle a carcinogen and the long period required for tumor production.

In our lab we used this model to "fish up" genes involved in bladder tumorigenesis using microarray analyses. We identified both H19 and IGF2 among differentially expressed genes that are induced in response to carcinogen exposure (Elkin et al., 1998, Ariel et al., 2004)

In the following sections we will present the role of both H19 and IGF2 genes in tumorigenicity. Then we will discuss pre-clinical and clinical data for the successful treatment of bladder cancer by DNA-based drug developed in our laboratory based on both the H19 and IGF2 regulatory sequences to drive the expression of a toxic protein, diphtheria toxin A (DT-A). This approach also proved to be successful in other cancer types; ovarian (Mizrahi et al., 2010), prostate (submitted) in human patients, and pre-clinically under development in glioblastoma (under preparation), lung (Hasenpusch et al., 2011), and colorectal liver metastasis (Ohana et al., 2005). This chapter will focus only on bladder cancer. Pre-clinical data using novel approaches for the treatment of bladder cancer with improved cytotoxic effect will be presented as well.

2. The H19-IGF2 locus and tumorigenesis

The IGF2 and H19 genes are both located on the short arm of chromosome 11 and are reciprocally imprinted. Genomic imprinting of the IGF2 and H19 genes has been shown to play a role in the regulation of the IGF2 and H19 expressions during embryonic development and in cancer. The role of genomic imprinting in tumor development is not well understood and it is beyond the scope of this chapter. Over-expressions of H19 and IGF2 genes in many tumors may or may not be associated with loss of imprinting.

2.1 The pivotal role of H19 RNA in tumorigenesis

H19 is an oncofetal gene that expresses only RNA and not protein, being expressed in the embryo, repressed in the adult, and re-expressed in a variety of human tumors, for review (Matouk et al., 2005). *H19* is emerging as one of the key players in cancer biology. We and others have demonstrated an essential role of H19 RNA in tumor development, and the association and contribution of H19 RNA with various aspects of tumorigenic process. This contradicts the initial proposal that H19 gene product has a tumor suppressive activity (Hao et al., 1993).

Our strategy to delineate the role of H19 RNA in tumor development is based on determining if tumor development is dependent on H19 expression through both over-expression and knockdown approaches in different tumor models including bladder cancer. To shed light into its mechanism of action our strategy is based on identifying upstream effectors and also downstream targets by applying the global gene expression profiling to identify genes modulated by both H19 over-expression and knockdown. Here again bladder cancer model is included.

Our results, supported by results from others, reveal that H19 RNA harbors oncogenic properties, enhancing the development of carcinogenesis. In this section we'll present major findings that support this issue and highlight its relevance to bladder cancer where possible.

2.1.1 H19 RNA is essential for human tumor growth

Although H19 over-expression sometimes associated with loss of imprinting have been reported in a large arrays of human cancers, direct evidence of its tumorigenic role was lacking. Using two cell line models including bladder carcinoma, we provided evidences, that H19 is critical for tumor development. Our in vivo results show that bladder carcinoma formed from UMUC3 cells in which the H19 RNA have been knocked down , induce a very significant retardation of tumor growth. Similar results were reproduced using other carcinoma model (Matouk et al., 2007).

Moreover we showed that ectopic H19 expression enhances the tumorigenic potential of bladder carcinoma cells in vivo. Tumors induced from T24P bladder carcinoma cell line ectopically over-expressing H19 RNA, differ significantly in their growth properties and growth kinetics in vivo relative to the control, and are well vascularized with evidences of tumor hemorrhage (Matouk et al., 2007). H19 RNA also enhances entry to S-phase of the cell cycle of bladder cancer cells under serum starved condition, but not under normal cell culture condition (Ayesh et al., 2002). Further supports for the tumorigenic properties have been reported in other cancer models. H19 over-expression of ectopic origin confers a proliferative advantage for breast epithelial cells in a soft agar assay and in several combined immunodeficient mice (Lottin et al., 2002). c-Myc induces the expression of the H19 RNA. c-Myc binds to the E-boxes near the imprinting control region to facilitate histone acetylation and transcriptional initiation of the H19 gene, to potentiate tumorigenesis (Barsyte-Lovejoy et al., 2006). The H19 is reported to be a target gene for the hepatocyte growth factor (HGF), further signifying the potential role of H19 RNA in hepatocellular carcinoma development (Adriaenssens et al, 2002). Furthermore, H19 RNA is important for entry into S-phase after serum starvation recovery by E2F binding to its promoter (Berteaux et al, 2005). Recently, it was reported that the Retinoblastoma tumor suppressor gene is a target gene for miR-675 which is produced from exon-1 of the H19 gene (Tsang et al., 2010).

2.1.2 H19 is induced by hypoxia – the P53 brakes and the HIF-1α engine

It is well established that every solid tumor encounters hypoxic regions beyond certain diameters. Hypoxia is a major trigger for tumor angiogenesis, metastasis, chemo-resistance and also associated with poor prognosis at least in some types of human cancers. All of these conditions as discussed below are associated with an increase of H19 RNA expression. Over-expression of *H19* RNA, is accompanied with up-regulation of a 95 kDa membrane glycoprotein (p95) observed in a variant of breast and lung carcinomas that are multi- drug resistance (Doyle et al., 1996). Moreover, results show that the level of H19 RNA is elevated in the multidrug resistance variant of HCC cell lines. Here doxorubicin resistance phenotype is related to H19 over-expression (Tsang et al., 2007).

H19 provides a novel and clinically useful diagnostic marker for prognosticating human bladder carcinoma. More striking is the predictive value of H19 for tumor recurrence. We have found that in transitional cell carcinoma of the bladder with tumors that express H19 in most cells have shorter median disease-free survivals (Ariel et al., 2000).

We have identified downstream targets modulated by H19 over-expression in the T24P bladder carcinoma cell line (Ayesh et al., 2002); comparing the m-RNA levels of many genes between cells containing high levels of H19 RNA (from H19 expressing plasmid) to that of the same cells lacking H19 RNA, showed a clear preference towards genes promoting cellular migration, angiogenesis and metastasis.

All of these observations prompted us to explore the effect of hypoxia on H19 expression and to delineate the mechanism of action involved. Indeed, under hypoxic conditions, we have reported that in bladder carcinoma cell lines T24P and UMUC3, and hepatocellular carcinoma cell line Hep3B the H19 RNA is significantly elevated (Matouk et al., 2007).

Following these initial studies we screened about thirty different carcinomas cell lines of different lineages and origins for their ability to induce H19 RNA in hypoxic stress (Matouk et al., 2010). We observed very different patterns of response to hypoxia. To gain insight into the possible mechanism associated with the H19 response to hypoxia, we searched for a common denominator among these cell lines.

It is well established today that the tumor suppressor signaling pathway of p53 can be activated by stress signals such as hypoxic stress and can either trans-activate or trans-repress its target genes to influence the cellular response. The key processes regulated by p53 pathway include cell cycle arrest, apoptosis, DNA repair, senescence, metastasis and angiogenesis, depending on cell types, nature of the inducer, cell intrinsic environment, and the activities of other signal transduction pathways. These observations suggests a possible association between the status of p53 (wild type or mutant) and H19 responsiveness to hypoxic stress. Moreover the involvement of the wild type tumor suppressor gene p53 in the down regulation of the H19 promoter activity which lacks a p53 consensus site and a TATA box was previously shown by (Dugimont et al., 1998). Taking all of these observations into account and the availability of IARC TP53 mutation database, we explored the possible involvement of p53 in determining H19's behavior in hypoxic response.

We recently demonstrated a tight correlation between *H19* RNA elevation by hypoxia and the status of the p53 tumor suppressor. In cells harboring wild type p53 (p53^{wt}) *H19* RNA is not induced upon hypoxia, whereas in cells carrying a mutated p53 (p53^{mt}) the *H19* message is significantly induced most strongly in p53-null cells. Furthermore through both over-expression and knockdown approaches we identified HIF1-α as the factor that is responsible for H19 elevation under hypoxic stress (Matouk et al., 2010).

H19 functions, consequently, as a stress modulator and a survival factor and is involved in several fundamental processes, including epithelial-mesenchymal transition (EMT), malignant transformation, cell-cycle transition, metastasis and neo-angiogenesis. EMT is an important process on the way to the malignant phenotype; notably- H19 up-regulation occurs in the stroma as well as in the epithelium. In the metastatic tumor stage, which bears a striking similarity to the embryonic stage, H19 involvement appears to be essential: adherent and cohesive cells lose their anchorage, migrate under stressful conditions to remote sites and replicate with neovascular support. Thus, H19 is a central figure in the cancer embryonic shift (Matouk et al., 2008).

In the light of our study, a molecular mechanism that integrates H19, p53 and HIF1-α to hypoxic stress response is uncovered. As hypoxia readily occurs in the majority of solid tumors driving critical steps in tumor development and metastasis and resistance to therapeutic modalities, placing the H19 gene product in this deadly circuit undoubtedly will have major impacts in its utility as a target for cancer gene therapy. Indeed a DNA-based drug depending on H19 regulatory sequence and diphtheria toxin is now in clinical trial with promising results (Ohana et al., 2004, Sidi et al., 2008, Mizrahi et al., 2010). We'll concentrate on bladder cancer.

2.1.3 Targetted therapy for bladder cancer mediated by a plasmid expressing DTA under the control of H19 regulatory sequences – clinical data

During the past few years we have developed a DNA based therapy strategies for treating tumors expressing H19 RNA. The successful development of anti-tumor gene therapy depends on the use of a combinatorial approach aimed at targeted delivery and specific expression of effective anti-tumor agents. We exploit the unique H19 transcriptional regulatory sequences for directing tumor-selective expression of toxins. For this purpose we use non-viral vectors due to their potential to circumvent the main disadvantage of adenoviral vectors, caused by immune responses directed against adenovirus proteins which limit their ability to be administered iteratively. As a toxic gene, we used the diphtheria toxin A chain (DT-A), which has suitable properties for achieving efficacious cancer cell killing. DT-A peptide catalyzes ADP-ribosylation at the dipthamide residue of the cellular translation elongation factor 2 (eEF-2), inhibiting protein synthesis and causing cell death. While a very low level of DT-A expression suffices for cell killing, DT-A released from the lysed cells is not able to enter the neighboring cells in the absence of the DT-B chain.

All preclinical studies needed to set up the stage for using this approach to treat bladder cancer patients will not be handled in this chapter, and are reviewed elsewhere (Matouk et al., 2005).

Clinical studies

The goals of treatment are to reduce tumor recurrence, decrease the risk of disease progression, avoid cystectomy (bladder sparing treatment), and improve survival. Preventing progression to muscle invasive disease is of key importance because even with aggressive treatment, including radical cystectomy, as few as 50% of patients with muscle invasive disease will survive 5 years (Dalbagni et al., 2001).

The primary factors that influence risk of disease progression include: 1. the number of tumors at primary diagnosis; 2. recurrence rate in a previous period or an early recurrence at 3 months after the first resection; 3. size of the tumor (tumors larger than 3 cm are more likely to recur than smaller tumors); and stage and grade of the tumor.

The initial clinical development plan for DTA-H19/PEI for bladder cancer is in the intermediate-risk patient population who has failed prophylactic therapy with either BCG or chemotherapy. In the Phase 1/2a study, the safety and preliminary efficacy was examined in this population. Having determined that the highest dose tested in this trial, the 20 mg dose of DTA-H19, was well tolerated and elicited complete responses in 2 of 5 evaluable patients, the Phase 2b clinical protocol will assess the safety of this regimen in a larger patient population as well as the efficacy in a marker tumor clinical trial design.

Compassionate Use in Bladder Cancer. Two patients had recurrent superficial TCC of the bladder and had failed multiple courses of Bacille Calmette-Guérin (BCG) and chemotherapy, and two additional patients that underwent nephrourectomy due to a diagnosis of recurrent superficial TCC that showed BCG intolerance.

The investigations in the first two bladder cancer patients demonstrated that intravesical instillation of DTA-H19/PEI is safe up to a dose of 5 mg in a single administration or a cumulative dose of 70 mg intravesically. No local or systemic adverse effects considered attributable to DTA-H19 treatment were observed throughout treatment. In addition, DTA-H19 DNA was not detectable in the circulation by PCR analysis of blood samples taken after the first and second week of treatment, and 2 hours after plasmid administration. DTA-H19 DNA was detectable in a tumor biopsy taken 18 hours after intravesical administration and in voided urine for 1 week after treatment. Tumor regression (75% reduction in marker tumor size) was observed in marker tumors of both patients. One of the 2 compassionate patients was treated over a nearly 5 year period with 22 intravesical administrations of either a 2 mg or 4 mg dose of DTA-H19/PEI for a cumulative dose of 70 mg of plasmid DNA. Treatments were well tolerated, and although the marker tumor persisted, it did not increase in size, stage or grade during the 14-month period before it was finally resected along with one other new low grade papillary tumor. No increase in stage or grade of TCC was observed.

The patient that had a nephroureterectomy due to a diagnosis of high-grade TCC in the renal pelvis was treated with 6 weekly 10 mg injections of DTA-H19/PEI via the left nephrostome at a total volume of 15 ml each. After completion of the 6 plasmid infusions the patient underwent nephroscopy that revealed the following: renal pelvis with no presence of tumors and several papillary tumors on the left bladder wall in the trigon. Findings were biopsied, analyzed, and diagnosed as low grade TCC. Four months later, the patient underwent nephrography during which no tumors were observed. Urine cytology confirmed the absence of tumor cells.

There were no significant events or side effects throughout the patient's treatments. Overall, this was a good tumor response in a patient with only one kidney who was considered to be anephric and with dialysis during the last year. The treatment was well-tolerated by the patient, and there was no evidence of any negative systemic or urinary tract effect. During the treatments, the patient was fully functional, continued to work, and did not suffer any effect to his quality of life (QOL). The second patient that had nephroureterectomy had multiple recurrences with the appearance of multi-focal lesions in the bladder. The patient underwent additional resection of a number of lesions that were localized inside and on the walls of the bladder. Since the patient was not a candidate to receive BCG treatment due to his compromised immune system, and after being refractory to Mitomycin C or Synergo, and refusal to undergo cystectomy, he was offered treatment with DTA-H19/PEI. He was treated with 20 mg of DTA-H19/PEI twice a week for the period of 4 weeks and once a week for another 2 weeks. Cytoscopy conducted at the end of the treatment showed an improvement in the number of lesions and in the general appearance of the bladder. The histological diagnosis of the biopsy showed low grade Ta.

Phase 1/2a Clinical Trial in Conventional Treatment Refractory Bladder Cancer Patients. A Phase 1/2a clinical trial was designed to determine the maximum tolerated dose (MTD) and assess the safety and preliminary efficacy of 5 different doses (2 mg, 4 mg, 6 mg, 12 mg, and 20 mg of DTA-H19) of DTA-H19/PEI given as 6 intravesical infusions into the bladder of patients with superficial bladder cancer (stages Ta and carcinoma *in situ* (CIS)) who had failed intravesical therapy with BCG. Patients had a diagnosis of superficial Stage Ta or CIS, grade 1 or 2 superficial bladder cancer that was confirmed by histopathology and that expressed H19 which was shown by *in situ* hybridization (ISH). Treatments were given weekly for 3 weeks followed 1 week later by safety and disease assessments, then another 3 weekly instillations were performed. Each dose cohort received the same dose for all treatments. Doses were escalated if none of the first 3 patients in the preceding dose cohort experienced a dose-limiting toxicity (DLT) after the first 3 weekly intravesical treatments. A DLT was defined as any grade 3 or greater toxicity by the National Cancer Institute Common Terminology Criteria for Adverse Events (NCI-CTCAE) that was considered to be related to the investigational product during the first 3 weekly intravesical treatments. Prior to initiating treatment, papillary tumors were resected leaving a single marker tumor. Videocystoscopy was performed 4, 8, and 12 weeks after the start of treatment for a safety evaluation of the bladder and also to record the presence or absence of the marker tumor and any other lesions suspicious for TCC of the bladder. If the marker tumor was still present at the Week 12 assessment, it was to be resected. If any new lesions were observed at Week 12, they were also to be resected. Patients whose disease had not progressed (i.e., no new tumors, increase in the size of the marker tumor by at least 50%, or increase in stage or any grade 3) were offered continued once monthly treatments and follow-up for up to 1 year.

A total of 18 patients were enrolled in this study. No DLTs were observed in this study. As the highest dose of product tested was the 20 mg dose of DTA-H19/PEI, this dose was considered the MTD for this study. The most frequently reported adverse events (AEs) considered at least possibly related to investigational products for any dose cohort were mild to moderate in severity and were most commonly renal and urinary disorders.

Of the 18 patients evaluable for tumor response at Week 12, a total of 4 patients had a complete response (CR) [complete disappearance of the marker tumor and no recurrence) including 2 of the 3 patients in the 2 mg dose cohort, and 2 of 6 patients in the 20 mg dose cohort. In addition, 2 patients (one in each of the 2 mg and 12 mg dose groups) had an incomplete partial response [IPR - complete disappearance of the marker tumor but with new tumor(s) occurring] suggesting that DTA-H19/PEI did have an effect on these marker tumors as well. Other responses included 1 partial response (PR - reduction in size of marker tumor by 50% and no new tumors present) (12 mg dose cohort) and 5 patients with SD (marker tumor still present but has not increased in size by more than 50% and no new tumors) (3 patients in the 4 mg dose cohort, 1 patient in the 12 mg dose cohort, and 1 patient in the 20 mg dose cohort). Thus, in this small study, there was evidence of tumor ablation over the dose range from 2 to 20 mg of DTA-H19/PEI. The 20 mg dose of DTA-H19/PEI was selected for evaluation in the Phase 2b clinical trial because this dose had an acceptable safety profile, showed objective tumor responses, and as the mechanism of action of DTA-H19/PEI is tumor-specific cytotoxicity, theoretically the highest safe dose has the greatest likelihood of an efficacious outcome.

2.2 Insulin-like growth factor 2 (IGF2) and tumorigenesis

IGF2 expression is driven by four different promoters (P1-P4) that produce 4 different transcripts all of which give rise to the same mature protein, a 67-amino acid polypeptide. The four promoters are activated in a development-dependent and tissue-specific manner. In fetal liver, promoters P2–P4 are active, of which P3 is the most active promoter, and promoter P1 is inactive. However, in liver tissue, shortly after birth, the IGF2 promoter P1 is exclusively active. The imprinting of the human IGF2 gene is promoter-specific. The P2, P3 and P4 promoters display monoallelic activity in embryonic, neonatal and postnatal liver specimens, whereas in adult, P1 is transcribed from both alleles.

The IGF2 peptide is a member of the insulin-like growth-factor family and is known to play an important role in the growth and differentiation of various tissues (Rechler 1990). This family also includes IGF1, insulin and relaxin. IGF2 is released to the extracellular fluid where it interacts with different cell membrane receptors and binding proteins. IGF2 binds three different types of receptors: IGF type 1 (IGF-1R), insulin receptor (IR) and IGF-2/mannose 6-phospate receptors (IGF-2R/M6P). The receptors, however, differ completely in structure and function (Yu and Rohan 2000). Ligand binding to IGF-1R and IR mediates mitogenic and anti-apoptotic effects. IGF-2R/M6P has tumor suppressor function and it mediates IGF2 degradation (Morison and Reeve 1998, Randhawa and Cohen 2005).

IGF2 can promote different functions depending on the cell type in which it is acting, and is a strong mitogen for a wide variety of cancer cell lines. It acts on the cell division cycle (DNA replication and mitosis) and on the cell growth (cellular enlargement), possibly by interfering with control cell checkpoint proteins. Moreover, IGF2 functions as an anti-apoptotic agent. For example, it blocks c-Myc and SV40 T-antigen induced apoptosis in Raf-1 fibroblast cells (Ishii et al., 1993, Morali et al., 2000).

The mitogenic and metabolic actions of IGF2 in embryonic development and tumorigenesis are mediated by the IGF-1R and/or IR-A and are tightly regulated at different levels. These levels include the IGF-receptors availability, IGF2 interaction with its receptors and binding proteins (IGFBPs) and its degradation following internalization of the IGF2 after binding to its receptor, especially IGF-2R. Moreover, the IGF2 mRNA and protein levels are regulated by different ways. Any abnormality at one or more of these levels can be correlated to tumorigenesis. Over-expression of growth factors, or their receptors is a common event in malignancy and provides the underlying mechanisms for one of the hallmarks of cancer, namely uncontrolled proliferation (Hanahan and Weinberg 2000).

Transgenic mice, over-expressing the IGF2 gene, developed spontaneous tumors at a high frequency (Bates et al., 1995, Moorehead et al., 2003, Rogler et al., 1994), suggesting that over-expressed IGF2 may be involved not only in the progression of tumors but also in the initiation of neoplasia. IGF2 over-expression is significantly correlated to the increased tumor progression and proliferative activity as well as to decreased patient survival (Kawamoto et al., 1998, Rogler et al., 1994, Takanami et al., 1996)

Several mechanisms can potentially result in IGF2 over-expression in cancer, including, loss of imprinting (LOI) of the maternal allele, loss of heterozygosity (LOH) with paternal duplication, amplification of the IGF2 gene and abnormally activated signaling pathway leading to transcriptional up-regulation of the active alleles reviewed by (Hahn et al., 2000). IGF2 imprinting is relaxed in many different types of tumors, including bladder cancer (Byun et al., 2007).

The link between IGF2 and metastasis may be the basis for the identification of IGF2 and IGF-IR as predictors of poor outcome in many types of cancer.

In the rat model of bladder cancer induced by BBN, we observed over-expression of igf2 in the tumor, relative to the low level of expression in the normal tissue (Ariel et al., 2004).

Moreover we detected high levels of IGF2 mRNA expression from P3, P4 or both promoters in TCC samples. Whereas normal bladder samples showed no expression from either promoter. The human IGF2-P3 and IGF2-P4 promoters are highly active in bladder carcinoma. We showed that these constructs were able to selectively kill tumor cell lines and inhibit tumor growth in-vitro and in-vivo in accordance to the transcriptional activity of the above-mentioned regulatory sequences, when they are used to drive the expression of DTA (Ayesh et al., 2003, Amit et al., 2011).

3. Double promoter vectors: Novel approaches for the treatment of bladder cancer with improved cytotoxic effect

3.1 Double promoter DTA-expressing vectors

We have shown that IGF2 or H19 are significantly expressed in 50-84% of human bladder carcinoma respectively (Elkin et al, 1995) but not in normal bladder. Whereas combined expression (e.g. H19 and IGF2-P3/P4) was detected at high levels in nearly 100% of human bladder cancer samples. By that proving that the double promoter vectors are suitable for treating all bladder cancer patients. P3 and P4 were able to express the DTA in tumor cells in vitro, and inhibited tumor growth of mice heterotopic model, proving that both promoters could be used successively, in addition to H19 promoter, as part of the double promoter constructs (Ayesh et al., 2003, Amit et al., 2010, Amit et al., 2011).

Double promoter expressing vectors were created, carrying on a single construct two separate DNA sequences expressing the diphtheria toxin A-fragment (DTA), from two different regulatory sequences, selected from cancer-specific promoters H19, IGF2-P3 and IGF2-P4. This novel approach, create a new family of plasmids regulated by two regulatory sequences, which in their natural genome position are both proximately located and are reciprocally imprinted.

These vectors were then used to transfect and to eradicate tumor cells in culture or to inhibit tumor growth (*in vivo*), in heterotopic and orthotopic CD1 nude mice, bladder tumor models.

The activity of the double promoter vectors was tested and compared to the activity of the single promoter vectors. The double promoter vectors exhibited superior activity compared to the single promoter vectors. Furthermore, an augmented-than-additive activity was exhibited, compared to combination activity of the single promoter vectors, in cell lines and in heterotopic bladder cancer mice (Amit et al., 2010, Amit et al., 2011).

3.2 A single promoter driving two cytotoxic genes with synergistic effect

Because it is unlikely that gene transfer reaches every cell of a cancer, DNA based therapy approaches are thought to require the induction of a 'bystander' effect. An interesting approach for this purpose is cytokine DNA based therapy. TNF-α is a multifunctional and immuno-regulatory cytokine that exhibits direct tumor cell cytotoxicity, possesses anti-angiogenic properties, and enhances antitumor immunity by activating immune cells such as dendritic cells and T cells. Systemic delivery of the TNF-α protein has had limited success clinically because of severe dose limiting toxic effects. This limitation can be overcome by the use of a gene delivery approach, combined with a tumor specific promoter to express TNF-α in the tumor tissue.

In this approach, an enhanced cytotoxic effect could be achieved that could also overcome the resistance developed by tumor cells to either one of the toxin. It was reported that several cell lines – none are bladder cancer- are resistant to Diphtheria toxin and therefore would not be affected by the pH19-DTA vector. Adding TNF-α to the existing system was in agreement with supporting evidence of some publications showing a synergistic effect in cell cytotoxicity mediated by TNF-α and diphtheria toxin. This was shown on ovarian cancer cell lines- sensitive or resistant to both diphtheria toxin and TNF-α and on renal cell carcinoma cell lines (Morimoto et al., 1991, Mizutani et al., 1994). Using a construct in which both TNF-α and DTA expressions are driven by H19 tumor specific promoter, would overcome the dose limiting toxic effects of the systemic delivery of TNF-α protein.

So, we investigated a plasmid carrying, in addition to DTA, the gene for human hTNF-α. The pH19-TNF-IRES-DTA plasmid was built while the construct carries a viral IRES sequence (from the ECMV virus) 3' of the TNF. This IRES construct is 619 pb long and responsible the synthesis of DTA from the m-RNA transcript.

3.2.1 Synergistic effect in the killing activity of DTA and TNF in vitro using different cell line models

In vitro the cytotoxic effect in cells treated with the pH19-TNF-IRES-DTA plasmid was determined by luciferase assay (Ohana et al., 2004). To test for potency of this construct, cells were also treated with a plasmid carrying either the DTA or TNF under the control of the H19 promoter. Cells from human, mouse and rat origin expressing H19 RNA were co-transfected with 2 µg/well of LucSV40 and the indicated concentrations of pH19-DTA, pH19-TNF or pH19-TNF-IRES-DTA plasmids. Luciferase activity was determined and compared to that of cells transfected with LucSV40 alone (**Figure 1**). In order to rule out the possibility of a false positive result due to the combined plasmid's structure effect, we reversed the TNF sequence in the pH19-TNF-IRES-DTA plasmid to eliminate the expression of TNF (pH19-TNFrev-IRES-DTA). The killing potency of the pH19-TNF-IRES-DTA plasmid was significantly higher compared to the pH19-DTA plasmid alone, even at very low concentrations. As the concentrations got higher the difference was diminished (**Figure 1**).

It should be noted that the use of the pH19-DTA plasmid alone was sufficient to cause a substantial decrease in luciferase activity, leading to 80-90% decrease in high concentrations, whereas the use of pH19-TNF alone showed little decrease, if any, and in some cases even an increase. When expressed in conjunction with the DTA domain, it clearly enhances cell death.

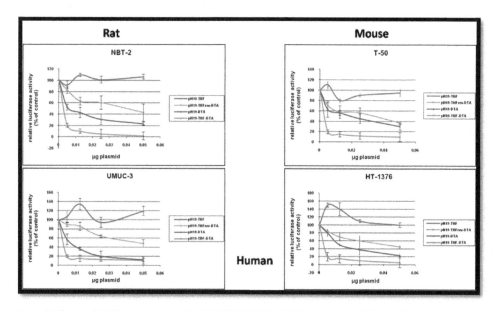

Fig. 1. Enhanced killing activity of pH19-TNF-IRES-DTA vector in different bladder carcinoma cell lines.

The killing potential of the pH19-DTA (blue), pH19-TNF (pink) or pH19-TNF-IRES-DTA(orange) vectors in human UMUC-3 and HT-1376, mouse T-50 and rat NBT-II was measured as a reduction of luciferase activity induced by LucSV40. Cells were co-transfected with 2 µg/well of LucSV40 and the indicated concentrations of pH19-DTA, or pH19-TNFα, or pH19-TNF-IRES-DTA. The pH19-TNFrev-IRES-DTA(green) served as a control.

3.2.2 In-vivo tumor growth inhibition by the pH19-DTA, pH19-TNF or pH19-TNF-IRES-DTA vectors in a carcinogen rat bladder cancer model

In vivo we utilize the carcinogen (BBN) induced rat bladder cancer model. Rats were treated with the above mentioned plasmids used in the in-vitro studies. An additional control plasmid carrying the gene of Luciferase under the regulation of the H19 promoter (pH19-Luc) was included.

The therapeutic plasmid was given at two different times in order to investigate the correlation of the treatment efficiency to the severity and invasiveness of the disease. In the first, the plasmid treatments started after the rats received BBN for 20 weeks. By this time, the rats had developed visible tumors is their bladders. In the second, the plasmid treatment started only 16 weeks after the beginning of BBN administration in which tumors were visible only by histopathological examination.

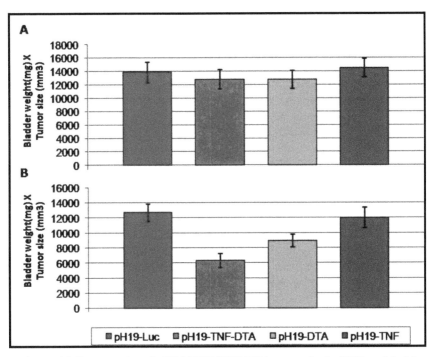

Fig. 2. Enhanced killing activity of pH19-TNF-IRES-DTA vector in the BBN rat bladder cancer model depending on time schedule of the treatments.

Tumor index (volume X weight) of rat's bladders as measured after treatment with three injections of pH19-DTA(green), pH19-TNF(brown) or pH19-TNF-IRES-DTA(red), and pH19-Luc(blue). A. Results of tumor index of rat's bladders which started treatments after 20 weeks. B. Results of tumor index of rat's bladders which started treatments after 16 weeks.

Each rat, in both experiments and in each group, received intravesical injection of 50 µg of the plasmid administered 3 times with an interval of 3 days between treatments. Four days after the last treatment, all rats were sacrificed and bladders were removed, weighed, photographed, excised and taken either for histological analysis or for DNA/RNA preparation. Tumor index was derived as mentioned. **Figure 2** shows the results of the in vivo experiments, where rats were treated from these two time points and onward.

We decided to try and estimate the tumor's volume by picturing each tumor at several angles, allowing us to use image analysis software in order to receive a reasonable estimation. This was multiplied by the bladder's weight in order to give us a new, more comprehensive index of the tumor's status. It can be seen in the results that when starting the treatments after 20 weeks of BBN administration, virtually no effect is achieved in any of the plasmids. On the other hand, starting the treatments after 16 weeks showed a remarkable inhibition of tumor progression compared to the control. When administrated with pH19-DTA the tumor was delayed by approximately 30%, while when using the pH19-TNF-IRES-DTA vector about 50% inhibition was measured. No effect was seen when pH19-TNF was used. These results suggest that when treatment begins in an early stage it can be a highly potent one.

4. Concluding remarks and future perspectives

Our ability to understand the biology of bladder cancer at the molecular level utilizing the ever growing biotechnologies is an important step for understanding a wide range of signaling events in both healthy cells and in the context of carcinogenesis. Substantial progress has been made in this avenue. Many new genes that are involved in bladder carcinogenesis have been identified. It is clear the H19-IGF2 locus is playing a central role in this aspect. As the role of IGF2 in embryogenesis and tumorigenesis is relatively well understood, H19 as a stress modulator is recently emerging to be involved in several fundamental processes of tumorigenesis including that of the bladder. Yet the exact molecular mechanisms that integrate H19 to such diverse events and circuits that are malfunctioning in cancer need further investigations.

In our lab, different regulatory sequences, selected from cancer-specific promoters of H19, IGF2-P3 and IGF2-P4 linked to the potent toxin (DTA), have been successfully used to drive cytotoxicity to cancer cells in vitro, in vivo, in different tumor models, and more importantly in bladder cancer patients, at least in the case of H19, with promising results. Similar approaches are also used in other types of human cancers including ovarian, hepatocellular, and pancreatic cancers and are clinically encouraging. Preclinically, this approach also shows promising results in lung cancer, glioblastoma and colorectal cancer metastasis to the liver. We are working on novel approaches to increase the cytotoxicity of the therapeutic plasmids, and to increase the numbers of patients that can benefit from this therapy. Furthermore, and given the central role of hypoxia and also p53 in the resistance of conventional therapeutic options and the involvement of the IGF2-H19 locus, we are developing sequential treatments of the therapeutic plasmids with conventional chemotherapeutic drugs with encouraging results. Moreover, the preclinical utility of short interfering RNA to knockdown both H19 and IGF2 is under development.

5. Acknowledgement

We thank BioCancell Therapeutic for financial support. Additional support was provided through the grant from Phillip Morris.

6. References

Adriaenssens, E. Lottin, S. Berteaux, N. Hornez, L. Fauquette, W. et al. (2002) Cross-talk between mesenchyme and epithelium increases H19 gene expression during scattering and morphogenesis of epithelial cells. *Exp Cell Res* 275:215-229.

Amit, D. & Hochberg, A. (2010) Development of targeted therapy for bladder cancer mediated by a double promoter plasmid expressing diphtheria toxin under the control of H19 and IGF2-P4 regulatory sequences. *J Transl Med.* 8:134-152.

Amit, D. Tamir, S. Birman, T. Gofrit, ON. & Hochberg, A. (2011) Development of targeted therapy for bladder cancer mediated by a double promoter plasmid expressing diphtheria toxin under the control of IGF2-P3 and IGF2-P4 regulatory sequences. *Int J Clin Exp Med.* 4:91-102.

Ariel, I. Sughayer, M. Fellig, Y. Pizo, G. Ayesh, S. et al. (2000) The imprinted H19 gene is a marker of early recurrence in human bladder carcinoma. *Mol Pathol* 53: 320-323.

Ariel, I. Ayesh, S. Gofrit, O. Ayesh, B. Abdul-Ghani, R. et al. (2004) Gene expression in the bladder carcinoma rat model. *Mol Carcinog* 41: 69-76.

Ayesh, B. Matouk, I. Ohana, P. Sughayer, MA. Birman, T. et al. (2003) Inhibition of tumor growth by DT-A expressed under the control of IGF2 P3 and P4 promoter sequences. *Mol Ther.* 2003 7:535-41.

Ayesh, S. Matouk, I. Schneider, T. Ohana, P. Laster, M. et al. (2002) Possible physiological role of H19 RNA. *Mol Carcinog* 35: 63-74.

Barsyte-Lovejoy, D. Lau, SK. Boutros, PC. Khosravi, F. Jurisica, I. et al. (2006) The c-Myc oncogene directly induces the H19 noncoding RNA by allele-specific binding to potentiate tumorigenesis. *Cancer Res* 66: 5330-5337.

Bates, P. Fisher, R. Ward, A. Richardson, L. Hill, DJ. Et al. (1995) Mammary cancer in transgenic mice expressing insulin-like growth factor II (IGF-II). *Br J Cancer* 72: 1189-1193.

Berteaux, N. Lottin, S. Monte, D. Pinte, S. Quatannens, B. et al. (2005) H19 mRNA-like noncoding RNA promotes breast cancer cell proliferation through positive control by E2F1. *J Biol Chem* 280: 29625-26636.

Burch, JD. Rohan, TE. Howe, GR. Risch, HA. Hill, GB. et al. (1989) Risk of bladder cancer by source and type of tobacco exposure: a case-control study. *Int J Cancer* 44: 622-628.

Byun, HM. Wong, HL. Birnstein, EA. Wolff, EM. Liang, G. et al. (2007) Examination of IGF2 and H19 loss of imprinting in bladder cancer. *Cancer Res* 67: 10753-10758.

Clemmons, DR. Busby, WH. Arai, T. Nam, TJ. Clarke, JB. et al. (1995) Role of insulin-like growth factor binding proteins in the control of IGF actions. *Prog Growth Factor Res* 6: 357-366.

Dalbagni, G. et al. (2001) Cystectomy for bladder cancer: a contemporary series. *J Urol* 165: 1111-1116.

Doyle, LA. Yang, W. Rishi, AK. Gao, Y. & Ross, DD. (1996) H19 gene overexpression in atypical multidrug-resistant cells associated with expression of a 95-kilodalton membrane glycoprotein. *Cancer Res* 56: 2904-2907.

Duggan, BJ. Gray, SB. McKnight, JJ. Watson, CJ. Johnston, SR. et al. (2004) Oligoclonality in bladder cancer: the implication for molecular therapies. *J Urol* 171: 419-25.

Dugimont, T. Montpellier, C. Adriaenssens, E. Lottin, S. Dumont, L. et al. (1998) The H19 TATA-less promoter is efficiently repressed by the wild-type tumor suppressor gene product p53. *Oncogene* 16: 2395-2401.

Elkin, M. Shevelev, A. Schulze, E. Tyckocinsky, M. Cooper, M. et al. (1995) The expression of the H19 and IGF-2 genes in human bladder carcinoma. *FEBS Lett* 374: 57-61.

Elkin, M. Ayesh, S. Schneider, T. de Groot, N. Hochberg, A. et al. (1998) The dynamics of the imprinted H19 gene expression in the mouse model of bladder carcinoma induced by N-Butyl-N-(4-hydroxybutyl)nitrosamine.*Carcinogenesis*19:2095-99

Goebell, PJ. & Knowles, MA. (2010) Bladder cancer or bladder cancers? Genetically distinct malignant conditions of the urothelium. *Urol Oncol* 28: 409-28.

Gofrit, ON. Birman, T. Dinaburg, A. Ayesh, S. Ohana, P. et al. (2006) Chemically induced bladder cancer--a sonographic and morphologic description. *Urology* 68: 231-235.

Hahn, H. et al. (2000) Patched target Igf2 is indispensable for the formation of medulloblastoma and rhabdomyosarcoma. *J Biol Chem* 275: 28341-28344.

Hanahan,D. & Weinberg, RA. (2000) The hallmarks of cancer. *Cell* 100: 57-70.

Hao, Y. Crenshaw, T. Moulton, T. Newcomb, E. & Tycko, B. (1993) Tumor-suppressor activity of H19 RNA. *Nature* 365: 764-767.

Hasenpusch, G. Pfeifer, C. Aneja, MK. Wagner, K. Reinhardt, D. et al. (2011) Aerosolized BC-819 Inhibits Primary but Not Secondary Lung Cancer Growth. *PLoS One* 6: e20760.

Ishii, DN. Glazner, GW. & Whalen LR. (1993) Regulation of peripheral nerve regeneration by insulin-like growth factors. *Ann N Y Acad Sci* 692: 172-182.

Jemal, A. Siegel, R. Xu, J. & Ward, E. (2010) Cancer statistics, 2010. *CA Cancer J Clin.* 60: 277-300.

Kawamoto, K. Onodera, H. Kan, S. Kondo, S. & Imamura, M. (1999) Possible paracrine mechanism of insulin-like growth factor-2 in the development of liver metastases from colorectal carcinoma. *Cancer* 85: 18-25.

Liu, Y. Lehar, S. Corvi, C. Payne, G. & O'Connor, R. (1998) Expression of the insulin-like growth factor I receptor C terminus as a myristylated protein leads to induction of apoptosis in tumor cells. *Cancer Res* 58: 570-576.

Lottin, S. Adriaenssens, E. Dupressoir, T. Berteaux, N. Montpellier, C. et al. (2002) Overexpression of an ectopic H19 gene enhances the tumorigenic properties of breast cancer cells. *Carcinogenesis* 23:1885-95.

Matouk, I. Ohana, P. Ayesh, S. et al. (2005) The oncofetal H19 RNA in human cancer, from the bench to the patient. *Cancer Therapy* 3: 249-266.

Matouk, IJ. deGroot, N. Mezan, S. Ayesh, S. Abu-Lail, R. et al. (2007) The H19 non-coding RNA is essential for human tumor growth PloS ONE 2 : e845.

Matouk, IJ. Ohana, P. Galun, E. & Hochberg, A. (2008) The pivotal role of the oncofetal H19 RNA in human cancer, A new hope. Gene therapy and cancer research focus. Nova publisher. 241-260.

Matouk, IJ. Mezan, S. Mizrahi, A. Ohana, P. Abu-Lail, R. et al. (2010) The oncofetal H19 RNA connection: hypoxia, p53 and cancer. *Biochim Biophys Acta.* 1803:443-51.

Mizrahi, A. Czerniak, A. Ohana, P. Amiur, S. Gallula, J. et al. (2010) Treatment of ovarian cancer ascites by intra-peritoneal injection of diphtheria toxin A chain-H19 vector: a case report. *J Med Case Reports.* 4:228.

Mizutani, Y. Bonavida, B. & Yoshida, O. (1994) Cytotoxic effect of diphtheria toxin used alone or in combination with other agents on human renal cell carcinoma cell lines. *Urol Res.* 22:261-6.

Moorehead, RA. Sanchez, OH. Baldwin, RM. & Khokha, R. (2003) Transgenic overexpression of IGF-II induces spontaneous lung tumors: a model for human lung adenocarcinoma. *Oncogene* 22: 853-857.

Morali, OG. Jouneau, A. McLaughlin, KJ. Thiery, JP. & Larue, L. (2000) IGF-II promotes mesoderm formation. *Dev Biol* 227:133-45:

Morimoto, H. Safrit, JT. & Bonavida, B. (1991) Synergistic effect of tumor necrosis factor-alpha- and diphtheria toxin-mediated cytotoxicity in sensitive and resistant human ovarian tumor cell lines. *J Immunol* 147:2609-16.

Morison, IM. & Reeve, AE. (1998) Insulin-like growth factor 2 and overgrowth: molecular biology and clinical implications. *Mol Med Today* 4: 110-115.

Ohana, P. Schachter, P. Ayesh, B. Mizrahi, A. Birman, T. et al. Regulatory sequences of H19 and IGF2 genes in DNA-based therapy of colorectal rat liver metastases. *J Gene Med.* 3:366-74.

Ohana, P. Gofrit, O. Ayesh, S. Al-Sharef, W. Mizrahi, A. et al. (2004) Regulatory sequences of the H19 gene in DNA based therapy of bladder cancer. *Gene Therapy Molecular Biology* 8: 181-192.

Okada, M. Suzuki, E. & Hashimoto, Y. (1976) Carcinogenicity of N-nitrosamines related to N-butyl-N-(4-hydroxybutyl) nitrosamine and N,N,-dibutylnitrosamine in ACI/N rats. *Gann* 67: 825-34.

Randhawa, R. & Cohen, P. (2005) The role of the insulin-like growth factor system in prenatal growth. *Mol Genet Metab* 86: 84-90.

Rogler, CE. Yang, D. Rossetti, L. Donohoe, J. Alt, E. et al. (1994) Altered body composition and increased frequency of diverse malignancies in insulin-like growth factor-II transgenic mice. *J Biol Chem* 269: 13779-13784.

Schulz, WA. (1998) DNA methylation in urological malignancies. *Int J Oncol* 13: 151-67.

Shapiro, A. Kelley, DR. Oakley, DM. Catalona, WJ. & Ratliff, TL. (1984) Technical factors affecting the reproducibility of intravesical mouse bladder tumor implantation during therapy with Bacillus Calmette-Guerin. *Cancer Res* 44: 3051-4.

Sidi, AA. Ohana, P. Benjamin, S. Shalev, M. Ransom, JH. et al. (2008) Phase I/II marker lesion study of intravesical BC-819 DNA plasmid in H19 over expressing superficial bladder cancer refractory to bacillus Calmette-Guerin. *J Urol.*180:2379-83.

Takanami, I. Imamuma, T. Hashizume, T. Kikuchi, K. Yamamoto, Y. et al. (1996) Insulin-like growth factor-II as a prognostic factor in pulmonary adenocarcinoma. *J Surg Oncol* 61: 205-208.

Tsang, WP. & and Kwok, TT. (2007) Riboregulator H19 induction of MDR1-associated drug resistance in human hepatocellular carcinoma cells. *Oncogene* 26: 4877-4881.

Tsang, WP. Ng, EK. Ng, SS. Jin, H. Yu, J. et al. (2010) Oncofetal H19-derived miR-675 regulates tumor suppressor RB in human colorectal cancer. *Carcinogenesis.* 31:350-8.

van Rhijn, BW. Montironi, R. Zwarthoff, EC. Jöbsis, A. & van der Kwast, TH. (2002) Frequent FGFR3 mutations in urothelial papilloma. *J Pathol.* 198:245-51.

Yu, H. & Rohan, T. (2000) Role of the insulin-like growth factor family in cancer development and progression. *J Natl Cancer Inst* 92: 1472-1489.

Part 5

Basic Science Research and Bladder Cancer

9

Intracellular Arsenic Speciation and Quantification in Human Urothelial and Hepatic Cells

Ricarda Zdrenka, Joerg Hippler, Georg Johnen,
Alfred V. Hirner and Elke Dopp
University of Duisburg-Essen, Ruhr-University Bochum, University Hospital Essen
Germany

1. Introduction

Arsenic can be found in nearly every part of the geosphere. It is viewed as the most harmful toxin in drinking water worldwide. At many places on earth the drinking water contains concentrations above 10 μg/l, which significantly exceed the tolerable value recommended by the WHO (World health organization [WHO], 2001). This is considered as a health threat for millions of people, especially in Bangladesh, Vietnam, and Latin America, where the geogenic origin has already been proved (Ng et al., 2003). The sources of this considerable arsenic occurrence (Fig. 1) are geogenic (erosion), mining activities, and geothermal waters (Smedly & Kinniburgh, 2002).

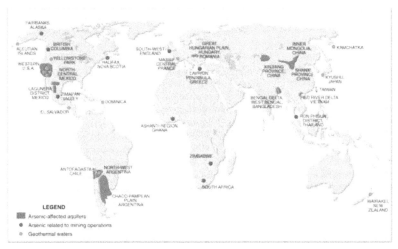

Fig. 1. Map of arsenic affected aquifers (Smedly & Kinniburgh, 2002)

The main arsenic species detected in drinking water are arsenite and arsenate. But the geothermal waters (Hot Spots) in the Yellostone Nationalpark, USA, predominantly contain several mg/l of methylated thioarsenicals such as mono-, di-, tri-, and tetrathioarsenate, as well as methylated arsenoxy- and -thioanions (Planer-Friedrich et al., 2007). In the surrounding atmosphere 0.5 – 200 mg/m³ of volatile arsenic species can be detected, which have been identified, among others, as $(CH_3)_2AsCl$, $(CH_3)_3As$, $(CH_3)_2AsSCH_3$, and CH_3AsCl_2 (Planer-Friedrich et al., 2006).

A second important source of arsenic is the air, whereas only one third of the occurring arsenic is of natural origin. Further anthropogenic sources are ore mining, smelteries, and the combustion of fossil fuels [Lozna & Biernat, 2008].

Among polluted air and contaminated drinking water also the human diet is of importance. For example, high doses of arsenic can be detected in fish, seafood, and algae, so that in 2004 the Food Agency of the UK warned against the consumption of Hijiki (hijikia fusiforme, black sea weed) (Food Standards Agency of the UK, 2004) as it contains inorganic arsenic up to 100 mg/kg. High arsenic concentrations can be found in the urine of the consumers (Nakjima et al., 2006). Francesconi published in 2010 the detection of up to 50 different arsenic compounds in fish and seafood, whereas their toxicity still is widely unknown (Francesconi, 2010).

Especially rice and rice products exhibit considerable noxious effects as they contain high doses of toxic inorganic arsenic (Meharg et al., 2008; Signes-Pastor et al., 2009; Sun et al., 2009) and form the nutrition base especially of the Asian people. But not only the rice from Asia but also the rice from the middle of the USA is contaminated with arsenic, the latter sustaining its contaminant not basically from natural sources but from pesticides anciently used on the cotton plantations. Finally DDT was introduced replaced arsenic in biocides (Hirner & Hippler, 2011). Fig. 2 summarises the several pathways of the human exposure to arsenic.

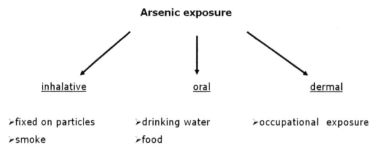

Fig. 2. Pathways of human exposure to arsenic (Dopp, 2007)

Chronic low-dose exposure may cause various diseases including bladder and other cancers. After ingestion arsenic is distributed to several organs, where it undergoes biotransformation. In 2005 Hayakawa et al. suggested a metabolic pathway (Fig. 3) for arsenic in rat liver tissue homogenate. Hereby arsenic-glutathione complexes are formed, which are then methylated by arsenic methyltransferase (Cyt19) and S-adenosyl-L-methionine (SAM) (Hayakawa et al., 2005).

This biotransformation of arsenic is generally regarded as a detoxifying process. Nevertheless, the trivalent arsenic intermediates and metabolites such as MMA(III) (monomethylarsonous acid) and DMA(III) (dimethylarsinous acid) are considered the most cyto- and genotoxic species (Dopp et al., 2010a). The liver is the main site of arsenic metabolism, and the renal route is the most important excretion pathway. A number of human studies have revealed that predominantly monomethylarsonic acid (MMA(V)) and dimethylarsinic acid (DMA(V)) can be detected in urine samples of arsenic-exposed individuals. Furthermore, Aposhian et al.

detected concentrations of about 50 nM MMA(III) in the urine of an arsenic-exposed human population in Romania (Aposhian et al., 2000). Studies in rats have shown that ingestion of DMA(V) causes bladder cancer (Wei et al., 1999) after chronic exposure. Subsequent experiments indicated that a large number of secondary arsenic metabolites are formed and renally excreted. For example, thiolated arsenicals such as dimethylmonothioarsonic acid (DMMTA(V)) were detected in the urine of DMA(V)-exposed rats (Yoshida et al., 1998). It is still unknown, however, which of the various arsenic metabolites is responsible for the development of bladder cancer. The metabolism of arsenic is of great importance for toxicological studies. As summarised by Dopp et al. (2010b) and Hirner & Rettenmeier (2010), the cyto- and genotoxic effects are highly dependent on the particular arsenic species, its cellular uptake, and its intracellular metabolism. For example, the toxicity of MMA(III) is 20 times greater than that of As(III) (Styblo et al., 2002; Bredfeldt et al., 2006).

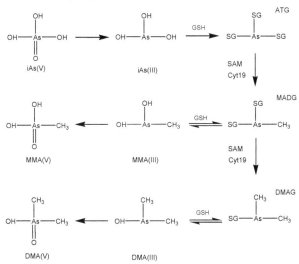

Fig. 3. Mechanism of arsenic biomethylation according to Hayakawa (Hayakawa et al., 2005)

Acute arsenic toxicity causes abdominal pain, nausea and faintness, vomiting, diarrhoea, and seizures (Gorby & Albuquerque, 1988). In contrast, chronic arsenic toxicity is less conspicuous. Characteristic symptoms are Mees' lines and hyperkeratosis predominantly at palms and soles of the feet. Furthermore, vascular diseases and peripheral neuropathy, and diabetes mellitus may occur (Smith et al., 2000). Until now, more than 60 million people in Bangladesh and India are still at risk of arsenic induced diseases due to arsenic concentrations of 10 - 50 µg/l or even higher (Chakraborti et al., 2004).

Moreover, chronic arsenic exposure is also associated with an increased risk of cancer. Especially arsenic induced lung cancer, as well as skin, kidney, and bladder cancer were reported (Chiou et al, 1995; Chen et al., 2010; Tseng, 2007).

The mechanisms of arsenic toxicity are only poorly understood. The structural likeness of arsenate and phosphate (Fig. 4), which is called molecular mimicry, results for example in the use of the same cellular transporters. Furthermore, there are plenty of biomolecules known, in which arsenate replaces phosphate, such as arsenosugars, arsenolipids and arsenobetaine (Rosen et al., 2011).

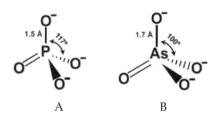

A   B

Fig. 4. Molecular mimicry of phosphate (A) and arsenate (B) (Rosen et al., 2011, modified)

The relevance of this molecular mimicry is pointed out in the study of Wolfe-Simon et al. (2011), reporting that phosphate can be substituted by arsenate in macromolecules of a bacterium, strain GFAJ-1 of the Halomonadaceae, isolated from Mono Lake, CA. However, these data are currently controversially discussed in the literature. Hereby few points have to be considered, first the rapid hydrolysis of arsenate esters, and second the notably altered three dimensional structure of macromolecules like DNA (Rosen et al., 2011).

One generally accepted mechanism for arsenic toxicity is the generation of reactive oxygen species (ROS). While ROS physiologically occur during cellular respiration or aerobic metabolism they also can result from exposure to oxidants. Already low levels of As(III) and MMA(III) are reported to generate ROS and therefore cause oxidative stress (Eblin et al., 2008; Wnek et al., 2009). These highly reactive radicals are discussed to exhibit their toxicity via induction of DNA damage, formation of DNA adducts, or alteration of DNA methylation and histone modifications (Wnek et al., 2009), and finally leading to carcinogenesis (Kitchin & Ahmad, 2003; Huang et al., 2004). In addition, arsenic is known to interfere with nucleotide and base excision repair at very low, non-cytotoxic concentrations and was observed for both trivalent and pentavalent metabolites. Hereby, MMA(III) and DMA(III) were reported to exhibit the strongest effects (Hartwig et al., 2003). One key mechanism is the inactivation of poly (ADP-ribose) polymerase (PARP) already at extremely low, environmentally relevant concentrations (Hartwig et al., 2002; Hartwig et al., 2003). Wnek et al. (2009) reported that the relative PARP activity was significantly reduced during chronic exposure of immortalised human urothelial cells (UROtsa) to 50 nM MMA(III). After removal of MMA(III) PARP activity increased again. Trivalent arsenic species are known to attach to zinc-binding structures generally found in DNA repair enzymes leading to alteration or inhibition of those proteins and finally the loss of genomic integrity (Kitchin & Wallace, 2008). In contrast, former studies report the insensitivity of isolated and purified DNA repair enzymes against inhibition by arsenic (Hu et al., 1998). This leads to the assumption that there are different modes of action for arsenic inhibited DNA repair, on the one hand by directly targeting DNA repair proteins, and on the other hand by altered signal transduction or gene expression.

Another mechanism of arsenic induced carcinogenesis is the altered cytoplasmic and nuclear signal transduction, modifying proteins involved in cell proliferation, differentiation, and apoptosis (Wnek et al., 2009). Hereby ROS were detected to be one key mechanism for the influence of As(III) and MMA(III) on the mitogen-activated protein kinase (MAPK) signaling pathway leading to consistent changes in cellular signalling (Eblin et al., 2008). The persistence of MMA(III)-induced altered cellular functions even after the removal of arsenic exposure point to lasting genomic or epigenetic changes and thus the highly carcinogenic potential of arsenic and its metabolites.

Furthermore, not only the molecular changes in the genome of arsenic exposed tissue and the altered signal transduction are of interest, but also the resulting phenotypical alterations. For the medical treatment of cancer it is of great interest whether the tumour has metastatic potential. Therefore, the tumour requires invasive growth into the surrounding tissue and the blood vessels. For example, the decrease of E-cadherin expression on the cellular surface is necessary for the detachment from the original tumour, and the increased expression of integrins is an important requirement for the attachment in the surrounding tissues like cells or extracellular matrix.

To better understand the underlying mechanisms of arsenic toxicity and carcinogenicity, further studies have to be carried out to correlate genotypic and metabolic effects with phenotypical alterations, especially under chronic exposure conditions. Therefore, it is important to detect and analyse intracellular arsenic species and their metabolic products. In own studies we have investigated the cellular uptake of arsenic species in non-methylating human urothelial (UROtsa) and methylating human hepatic cells (HepG2) and have speciated and quantified the intracellularly detected arsenic. Induced genotoxic effects in UROtsa cells were measured with the Alkaline Comet Assay and the malignant transformation after chronic arsenic treatment was assayed by using the Colony Formation Assay and the Migration and Invasion Assay. Our latest results are presented here.

2. Experimental

2.1 Cell culture

Studies were carried out using the human immortalized urothelial cell line UROtsa (generous gift from Prof. M. Styblo, University of North Dakota, USA). The UROtsa cells were maintained in Earle's minimal essential medium (MEM) (CC-PRO, Oberdorla, Germany) enriched with 10 % FBS (fetal bovine serum; GIBCO, Darmstadt, Germany), 0.5 % Gentamycin (CC-Pro GmbH, Oberdorla, Germany) and 1 % L-glutamine (CC-Pro GmbH, Oberdorla, Germany).

For comparison of a methylating and non-methylating cell line, HepG2 cells (human liver cells, methylating cells) were used as a second cell line. HepG2 cells were obtained from ATCC (HB 8065; ATCC, Manassas, VA, USA) and cultured in Earle's minimal essential medium (MEM) (CC-PRO, Oberdorla, Germany) enriched with 10 % FBS (GIBCO, Darmstadt, Germany), 0.5 % Gentamycin (CC-Pro GmbH, Oberdorla, Germany), 1 % L - glutamine (CC-Pro GmbH, Oberdorla, Germany), 1 % non essential amino acids (CC-Pro GmbH, Oberdorla, Germany) and 1 % sodium pyruvate (CC-Pro GmbH, Oberdorla, Germany).

All cells were grown under typical cell culture conditions (37 °C, 5 % CO_2, humidified incubator) and medium was replaced every 2 – 3 days. Cells were grown to 75 - 80 % confluence. For subculture the cells were washed with PBS (Phosphate buffered saline; GIBCO, Darmstadt, Germany) and UROtsa and HepG2 cells were detached using 0.25 % trypsine containing 0.1 % EDTA (2-[2-[bis(carboxymethyl)amino]ethyl-(carboymethyl) amino]acetic acid (CC-Pro GmbH, Oberdorla, Germany)) and finally split into ¼ and transferred into new flasks.

For chronic treatment 300,000 UROtsa cells were seeded into 75 cm² flasks and fed with 25 ml medium containing 50 nM, 75 nM, or 100 nM MMA(III), respectively. UROtsa cells fed with medium without any arsenic compound served as negative control. Once a week the cells were subcultured and fed with fresh exposure medium and 4 days later the exposure medium was replaced again. For cell detachment 0.25 % trypsin without EDTA (CC-Pro GmbH, Oberdorla, Germany) was used to prevent the complexation of arsenic.

2.2 Intracellular arsenic speciation and quantification

The following methodology (Hippler et al., 2011) was used for intracellular arsenic speciation and quantification: Cells were seeded into 150 cm² flasks and grown to confluence before experiments were performed. Both cell lines (UROtsa and HepG2) were incubated for five minutes to 24 hours in fresh growth medium containing 5 µM MMA(III) (exposure medium). The negative control consisted of cells incubated in fresh medium without any arsenic compound and subsequently they were handled the same way as the exposed cells. Additionally, a second negative control was trypsinised for cell counting.

After incubation the exposure medium was withdrawn and stored at -80°C. Cells were washed with 10 ml PBS and 10 ml Ampuwa (sterile deionised water). For the next washing step 10 ml 0.1 mM DMPS (2,3-bis(sulfanyl)propane-1-sulfonic acid) were used to remove traces of extracellular uncombined arsenic ions. The last washing step with 10 ml PBS was carried out to remove the residues of DMPS before lysis (Fig. 5.). All washing solutions were retained and stored at -80 °C until arsenic speciation analysis.

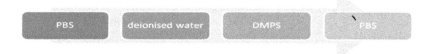

Fig. 5. Washing process prior the intracellular arsenic speciation and quantification: Exhaustive cell washing ensures the removal of all extracellular arsenic residues after the exposure (Hippler et al., 2011, modified).

The cell lysis was performed using the Precellys®24 tissue homogeniser (Peqlab Biotechnologie GmbH, Erlangen, Germany) as a tool for mechanical lysis. Therefore the cells were first detached from the culture flasks using a cell scraper and transferred to 0.5 ml tubes containing ceramic beads with a diameter of 1.4 mm (Peqlab Biotechnologie GmbH, Erlangen, Germany). Exhaustive homogenisation was obtained within three intervals of 20 seconds and 6500 rpm. Final centrifugation using a MiniSpin plus centrifuge at 14.000 x g (Eppendorf AG, Hamburg, Germany) assured a complete separation of the cell lysates from membranes and other solid, insoluble cellular structures. This non-soluble fraction of each sample was then digested using Proteinase K until the pellet was dissolved. Further oxidation with hydrogen peroxide (30 %) assured the release of arsenic from peptides and other cellular molecules.

After exposure, lysis and centrifugation all solutions and samples were stored at -80 °C. The cell lysates were thawed immediately before HPLC-ICP/MS analysis. Depending on the arsenic content of the samples, 1 to 25 µl were injected onto the HPLC-column.

For quantification a multi-As species standard containing 2 pg to 200 pg As(III), MMA(III), DMA(V), MMA(V), DMA(III), and As(V) was injected. Peak areas were obtained by monitoring transient signals for As at m/z 75 in non-collision cell mode at dwell times of 100 ms. The linearity of the external calibration resulted in an excellent calibration (e.g. MMA(V): r^2 = 0.9999; DMA(V): r^2 = 0.999). Limits of detection were approximately 3 pg As, varying slightly depending on the arsenic species. Table 1 presents the conditions for the high performance liquid chromatography (HPLC) and inductive coupled plasma mass spectrometry (ICP/MS). For reproduction the whole experiment was performed twice.

HPLC conditions		ICP/MS conditions	
HPLC Column	Phenomenex Luna 3μ C18(2) 100 Å	Forward power (RF)	1580 W
Column temperature	30 °C	Plasma gas rate (cool gas flow)	15 L Argon min^{-1}
Eluent flow rate	0.5 ml min^{-1}	Carrier gas flow rate	~ 0.8 L min^{-1}
Injection volume	1 – 25μl	Make-up gas flow rate	~ 0.25 L min^{-1}
		Sample depth	5.7 mm
Eluent:		Spray chamber	Quarz, cooled, 2 °C
Malonic acid	2 mM		
Tetrabutylammonium hydroxide (TBAH)	6 mM	Isotopes monitored	^{73}As, ^{35}Cl, ^{77}(^{40}Ar^{37}Cl)^{34}S, ^{71}Ga, ^{73}Ge, ^{115}In, ^{103}Rh
Methanol	5 v/v %		
Water	95 v/v %		
pH	6.0		

Table 1. Conditions for the high performance liquid chromatography (HPLC) and inductive coupled plasma mass spectrometry (ICP/MS) (Hippler et al., 2011, modified)

2.3 Alkaline Comet Assay

For detection of genotoxic effects caused by arsenic exposure, the Alkaline Comet Assay was used. This assay detects single and double strand breaks of the DNA by single cell gel electrophoresis. Therefore UROtsa cells were seeded with a density of 100,000 cells / 2 ml medium into each well of a 24-well-plate and incubated over night. For exposure cell culture medium was removed and 2 ml of the exposure medium containing the arsenic compounds As(III) (arsenite), As(V) (arsenate), MMA(III) (monomethylarsonous acid), MMA(V) (monomethylarsonic acid), DMA(V) (dimethylarsinous acid) and TMAO (trimethylarsine oxide) in different concentrations were added. The negative control consisted of untreated cells; the positive control was exposed to 1 mg/ml N-ethyl-nitrosourea. For exposure to the volatile species DMA(III) (dimethylarsinous acid) 1,000,000 cells/10 ml medium were seeded into 25 cm² cell culture flasks with vent caps.

After incubation for 30 min exposure media were removed and the cells were trypsinised as described above. The cells were resuspended in PBS and 5,000 cells were seeded into each agarose gel consisting of 0.79 % low melting point agarose in PBS. The gels were solidified on ice and the cells were lysed over night.

For electrophoresis the gels were washed with Ampuwa and incubated in 4 °C cold electrophoresis solution at pH 13 for 15 min. After electrophoresis for 30 min the gels were washed with Ampuwa and neutralised to pH 7.5. Finally the gels were washed with deionised water again and incubated in ethanol p.a. to remove the water residues. The gels were now dried over night at 4 °C.

Image analysis was performed with Comet Assay IV Software (Perceptive Instruments Ltd., Haverhill, UK) using a fluorescence microscope (Leica Microsystems GmbH, Wetzlar, Germany) and a digital camera (Leica Microsystems GmbH, Wetzlar, Germany). Therefore the cells were stained with SYBR GREEN (Sigma-Aldrich, Saint Louis, Missouri, USA) and 50 cells / gel were evaluated.

2.4 Colony formation assay

When a normal cell is transformed to a cancer cell it loses its ability to grow in monolayers. After cell transformation (a step towards malignancy) the cells grow in colonies. With help of the colony formation assay (Bredfeldt et al., 2006) the development of an anchorage independent growth after chronic exposure of cells to arsenic can be determined. The colony formation assay was prepared in a 24-well plate. First 500 µL of a base agar containing 0.6 % low melting point agarose in cell culture medium were added to each well, solidified at room temperature and sterilised under UV light over night.

UROtsa cells were seeded with a density of 10,000 cells / 500 µL into each well. Additional wells were prepared without cells containing only base and top agar for background detection. The cells were fed with 250 µL of fresh cell culture medium every 3 – 4 days.

Image analysis was performed after 2 weeks of incubation using an inverted microscope (Leica Microsystems GmbH, Wetzlar, Germany) combined with a Leica digital camera (Leica Microsystems GmbH, Wetzlar, Germany).

2.5 Cellular migration and invasion

Typical features of transformed and cancer cells are increased proliferation, migration and invasion. For the detection of invasion the xCELLigence DP system (Roche Applied Science, Mannheim, Germany) was conducted. Therefore CIM-Plates (Roche Applied Science, Mannheim, Germany) were coated with 50 µl of 0.02 % collagen (SERVA Electrophoresis GmbH, Heidelberg, Germany) on each side of the microporous membrane for 1 h. After removing the collagen residues the CIM-Plates were dried for approximately 1 h at room temperature under the laminar flow. In between UROtsa cells originated from the chronic exposure were trypsinised as described above and brought to a concentration of 1.5 Mio cells / ml. For the detection of migration uncoated CIM-Plates were conducted.

160 µl of the pre-warmed cell culture medium were added to each well of the lower chamber and 100 µl were added to each well of the upper chamber. The CIM-Plates were then placed into the xCELLigence devices and the background was measured. Now 100 µl of the prepared cell suspensions were added (duplicate wells) and the CIM-Plates were placed into the xCELLigence again. The measurement was performed for 24 h with intervals of 15 min.

2.6 Statistics

All experiments were performed in triplicate unless stated otherwise. The statistical evaluation for the Alkaline Comet Assay was performed using GraphPad Prism (GraphPad Software, San Diego, USA). The mean values of the detected Olive Tail Moments are presented in bar graphs with the standard error of mean. For statistical analysis the non-parametric Mann-Whitney-Test was applied, which approximates the Gaussian distribution for more than 20 random samples and compares each test group to the untreated control group. The results are given in significance levels p for the confidence interval of 95 %. Then one has $p > 0.05$: non-significant, $p \leq 0.05$: *, $p \leq 0.01$: **, $p \leq 0.001$: ***.

3. Results

3.1 Intracellular arsenic speciation and quantification

To study the intracellular arsenic biotransformation of MMA(III) we incubated UROtsa and HepG2 cells with 5 µM MMA(III) for 5 min up to 24 hours, followed by a newly developed sample preparation process (Hippler et al., 2011). Using HPLC-ICP/MS analysis we were able to detect more than 99.99% of the total arsenic in the non-soluble fraction of both cell lines and only 0.003% in the soluble fraction of UROtsa cells and 0.01% of HepG2 cells, respectively. While in the non-soluble fraction of UROtsa cells the arsenic content consisted only of a monomethylated species, in HepG2 cells a time dependent occurrence of a dimethylated arsenic species additionally to monomethylated arsenic was observed (Fig. 6.). The differentiation between trivalent and pentavalent arsenic metabolites was impossible due to their oxidative release from the cellular structures.

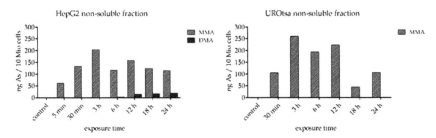

Fig. 6. Quantification of the metabolites in the non-soluble fraction after exposure of HepG2 and UROtsa cells to 5 μM MMA(III). The analysis was performed using HPLC-ICP/MS technique.

In the soluble fractions of both HepG2 and UROtsa cells only pentavalent arsenic species were detected (Fig 7.). In HepG2 cells a time dependent increase and decrease of MMA(V) was observed. Additionally we analysed the increase of DMA(V) by time. In contrast, in UROtsa cells only MMA(V) but no DMA(V) was detected. The occurrence of MMA(III) after 18 and 24 hours of exposure is believed to be the result of cytotoxic effects and can be correlated with membrane damage (data not shown).

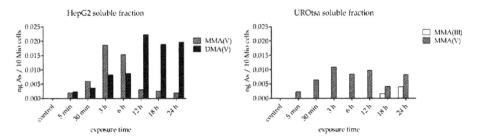

Fig. 7. Quantification of the metabolites in the soluble fraction after exposure of HepG2 and UROtsa cells to 5 μM MMA(III). The analysis was performed using HPLC-ICP/MS technique.

3.2 Alkaline Comet Assay

The Alkaline Comet Assay was conducted to examine the genotoxic effects of different arsenic metabolites. Testing the trivalent species we observed significant single and double strand breaks in UROtsa cells already after 30 min of exposure (Fig. 8.). Although the biotransformation initially was discussed to serve as a detoxification process, MMA(III) still is highly genotoxic and DMA(III) even exhibits the most genotoxic effects. In contrast, pentavalent arsenic species did not show any genotoxic effect except for As(V) at very high concentrations (Fig. 9).

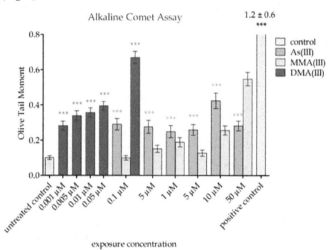

(mean ± SEM with p > 0.05: non-significant, p ≤ 0.05: *, p ≤ 0.01: **, p ≤ 0.001: ***)

Fig. 8. The Alkaline Comet Assay was conducted to assay single and double strand breaks of the DNA after 30 min of exposure to the trivalent arsenic species As(III), MMA(III) and DMA(III). The DNA damage is given in the Olive Tail Moment.

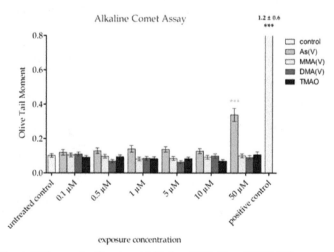

(mean ± SEM with p > 0.05: non-significant, p ≤ 0.05: *, p ≤ 0.01: **, p ≤ 0.001: ***)

Fig. 9. The Alkaline Comet Assay was conducted to assay single and double strand breaks of the DNA after 30 min of exposure to the pentavalent arsenic species As(V), MMA(V), DMA(V) and TMAO. The DNA damage is given in the Olive Tail Moment.

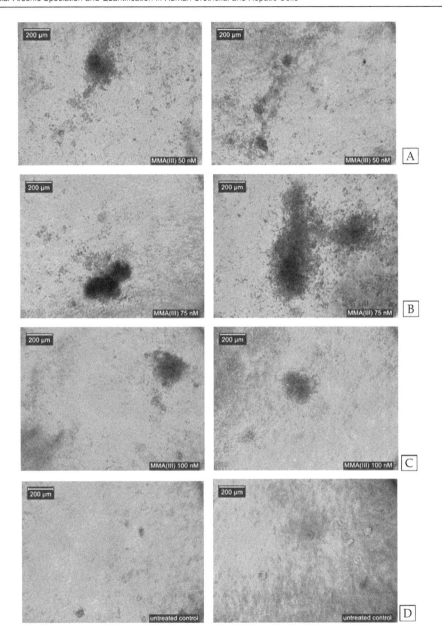

Fig. 10. The Colony formation assay was conducted for the analysis of an anchorage independent growth after chronic treatment of UROtsa cells with 50 nM (**A**), 75 nM (**B**), or 100 nM (**C**) MMA(III), respectively, for 93 weeks. The negative control (**D**) consisted of untreated UROtsa cells of the same passage. Given are two pictures of parallel treated samples.

3.3 Colony formation assay

To analyse the carcinogenic potential of one of the most important arsenic metabolites, MMA(III), UROtsa cells were cultured for 93 weeks and treated twice a week with fresh exposure medium containing 50 nM, 75 nM, and 100 nM MMA(III), respectively. Untreated UROtsa cells of the same passage served as negative control. The colony formation assay was determined to assay the loss of an anchorage dependent growth. As proven by the negative control, UROtsa cells are adherent cells and hence they cannot be cultured in soft agar (Bredfeldt et al., 2006). In contrast, after chronic exposure to MMA(III) UROtsa cells exhibit an anchorage independent growth and form notable colonies after two weeks of incubation in soft agar (Fig. 10.).

3.4 Cellular migration and invasion

To estimate the malignant potential of chronically exposed human urothelial cells to arsenic, their altered motility and invasiveness were examined. The xCELLigence system was conducted to assay the migration and invasion ability of UROtsa cells after 92 weeks of exposure to MMA(III). Hereby the cells moved through a microporous membrane and attached at the opposite side on the electrodes. For the analysis of the invasiveness the membranes and electrodes were coated with collagen, a typical extracellular matrix. The results show that after exposure to 75 nM and 100 nM MMA(III) for 92 weeks the motility of UROtsa cells was increased in comparison to the untreated control of the same passage. Only the exposure to 50 nM MMA(III) did not lead to an increase of migrated cells (Fig. 11.).

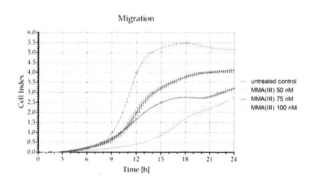

Fig. 11. The xCELLigence system was conducted for the analysis of the ability of migration after chronic treatment of UROtsa cells with 50 nM, 75 nM, or 100 nM MMA(III), respectively, for 92 weeks.

The examination of the invasion led to similar results. After coating the plate surface with collagen all samples exhibited an increased invasion property compared to the untreated control (Fig. 12.). In both migration and invasion assays the cells treated with 100 nM MMA(III) exhibited the strongest effects, leading to the assumption of an dose-dependent manner.

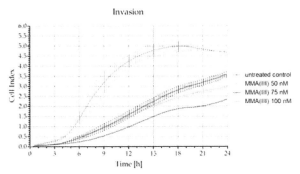

Fig. 12. The xCELLigence system was conducted for the analysis of the ability of invasion after chronic treatment of UROtsa cells with 50 nM, 75 nM, or 100 nM MMA(III), respectively, for 92 weeks. CIM-Plates were coated with collagen to simulate a biological matrix.

4. Discussion and conclusion

Arsenic is one of the most harmful toxins in drinking water worldwide and at many places on earth millions of people are at risk of arsenic induced diseases including cancer. In our study we have investigated the cellular uptake and biotransformation of arsenic species in non-methylating human urothelial (UROtsa) and methylating human hepatic cells (HepG2) using HPLC-ICP/MS technique. The induced genotoxic effects of several arsenic species in UROtsa cells were measured with the Alkaline Comet Assay and the malignant transformation after chronic arsenic treatment was assayed by using the Colony Formation Assay and the Migration and Invasion Assay.

The data presented here demonstrate that MMA(III) is rapidly taken up by human urothelial cells (UROtsa) and human hepatoma cells (HepG2). MMA(III) is known to be an important arsenic metabolite due to its high toxicity. Many studies report monomethylated and dimethylated arsenic species as the main metabolites in the urine (Aposhian et al., 2000; Fillol et al., 2010). Using an improved isolation method and HPLC-ICP/MS technique we were able to analyse not only the fast association of MMA(III) to large membrane structures, high-molecular-weight proteins, and other insoluble cell components, but also the presence of unbound pentavalent arsenic metabolites in the soluble fractions which only amount to 0.003% of the total intracellular arsenic in UROtsa cells and 0.01% in HepG2 cells, respectively. Furthermore we were able to differentiate between the various methylated metabolites and also their oxidation state in this complex cellular matrices.

The data demonstrate for both cell lines a fast cellular uptake of MMA(III) and the subsequent oxidation to MMA(V) already within 5 min of exposure and further increasing with time. Additionally, in HepG2 cells we observed a time dependent methylation to DMA(V). These findings appear to be in contrast to the reductive intracellular milieu (Du et al., 2009) due to glutathione concentrations up to millimolar ranges (Anderson, 1998). However, taking different cell compartments and specific metabolic effects of arsenic into account could provide a possible explanation. It is largely known from the literature that in contrast to their pentavalent analogues trivalent arsenicals bind to proteins (Styblo & Thomas, 1997; Yan et al., 2009). This leads to the assumption that MMA(III) rapidly binds to proteins after uptake, which is in compliance with the detection of more than 99.99 % of the total arsenic in the non-soluble fraction in both cell lines. We suggest that there is a fast subsequent degradation of at least part of the arsenic-conjugated or arsenic-inhibited proteins. Protein degradation is predominantly mediated by the proteasomes but can also take place in lysosomes, especially during turnover of membrane proteins (Clague & Urbé, 2010). An increased turnover of arsenic-bound proteins is in agreement with the evidence of the catabolism of arsenic-induced improperly folded or damaged proteins via the ubiquitin-dependent protein degradation pathway in zebrafish liver (Lam et al., 2006). Several studies report that protein ubiquitination not only targets protein degradation using the proteasome pathway but also the lysosomal pathway (Marques et al., 2004; Barriere et al.; 2007, Shenoy et al, 2008; Arancibia-Cárcamo et al, 2009). The lysosome is known to exhibit cellular oxidative activities (Chen, 2002) and during oxidative stress large amounts of hydrogen peroxide enter the lysosome, leading to the formation of hydroxyl radicals and lysosomal destabilisation (Terman et al., 2006). In addition, the lysosome is an important organelle in autophagy, helping the cells to remove toxic aggregation-prone proteins and even damaged organelles that are incompatible with the unfolding mechanism of the proteasome (Yang et al., 2008; Clague & Urbé, 2010; Mehrpour et al., 2010). The increase of protein catabolism, the elimination of excess or damaged organelles by autophagy, and the sequestering of toxicants is ubiquitous and believed to be a kind of "first-response reaction" to delay apoptosis (Kundu & Thompson, 2008; Yang et al., 2008). In the early stage of cell death autophagy is activated in HL60 cells soon after exposure to As$_2$O$_3$ to maintain cell survival under stress conditions (Yang et al., 2008).

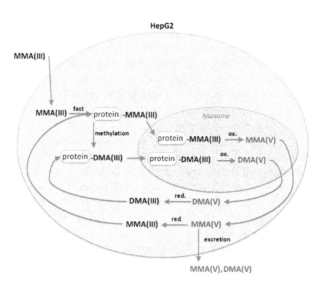

Fig. 13. Proposed arsenic cycle in HepG2 cells after exposure to MMA(III) (Hippler et al. 2011, modified)

Summarising all these data we conclude from our results that MMA(III) is immediately taken up and rapidly bound to proteins and other cellular structures, followed by, first, the generally accepted methylation to dimethylarsinic in HepG2 cells only, and second, the degradation of affected proteins and cellular structures in the lysosome in both HepG2 and UROtsa cells (Fig. 13. and 14.). During oxidative degradation in the lysosome arsenic is released as MMA(V) and DMA(V), which are either excreted from the cell or reduced by antioxidants in the cytosol. The reduced species MMA(III) and DMA(III) can then re-associate with proteins and cellular structures. In HepG2 cells most of the incorporated MMA(III) is methylated and oxidised to DMA(V) after passing this cycle; in UROtsa cells the cycle is limited to oxidation and reduction, and finally excretion, due to the fact that urothelial cells are non methylating (Hippler et al., 2011).

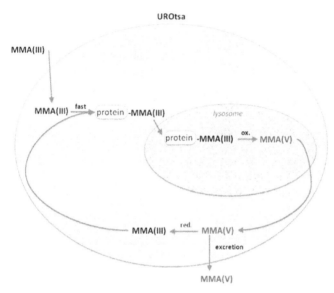

Fig. 14. Proposed arsenic cycle in UROtsa cells after exposure to MMA(III).

Especially the trivalent arsenicals are known to exhibit strong genotoxic effects (Dopp et al., 2010a). These effects can either be detected as DNA damage using the micronucleus test or the comet assay (Dopp et al., 2008), as oxidative damage by assaying the amount of 8-oxo-dG (8-Oxo-2'-deoxyguanosine) or in form of chromosomal aberrations (Dopp et al., 2004). In our study we determined the Alkaline Comet Assay to analyse single and double strand breaks of the DNA. We detected significant genotoxic effects of all tested trivalent arsenic compounds (As(III), MMA(III), and DMA(III)) and the pentavalent arsenate already after 30 min of exposure. These results are in compliance with the findings of previous studies using several mammalian cell types (Schwertdtle et al., 2003; Raisuddin & Jha, 2004; Dopp et al., 2005). This emphasises how urgently the knowledge of the tissue-dependent arsenic biotransformation (Fig. 13. and 14.) is needed, as the genotoxic effect of arsenic metabolites is not only dependent on its oxidative state but also on the state of methylation (Hirner & Rettenmeier, 2010; Dopp et al., 2010b). Wnek et al. (2009) reported that in UROtsa cells DNA damage caused by MMA(III) is not only a phenomenon of acute treatment but also an important effect in chronic, low-level exposure for 12 – 52 weeks.

The occurrence of single- and double-strand breaks is significantly decreased after the removal of MMA(III) for 2 weeks, but still significantly increased compared to the untreated control. The relative poly (ADP-ribose) polymerase (PARP) activity was significantly reduced during this chronic exposure and increased again after removal of MMA(III). Trivalent arsenic species are known to attach to zinc binding structures generally found in DNA repair enzymes and transcription factors, leading to alteration or inhibition of those proteins (Kitchin & Wallace, 2008). Together with the findings of Hu et al. (1998) it is likely that DNA repair is inhibited by both direct protein interaction and altered signal transduction or gene expression. Taken together, this leads to the fact that not only direct DNA damage plays a pivotal role in arsenic induced carcinogenesis. Inorganic arsenic and its metabolites are also known to be potent epigenetic modulators leading to (tissue specific) altered cellular functions, malignant transformation and tumorigenesis. Many studies report arsenic induced aberrant DNA methylation patterns (Sutherland & Costa, 2003; Smeester et al., 2011; Ren et al.; 2011), resulting in changes in the promoter activity that lead to altered gene expression (Jensen et al., 2009). Aberrant DNA methylation patterns might be the result of arsenic-induced altered global histone modification finally leading to, among others, the silencing of tumour suppressor genes (Zhou et al., 2008). Altered global DNA methylation levels have also been correlated with the arsenic metabolism as both systems use the same methyl donor SAM (S-adenosyl-methionine). Sam is known to transfer methyl groups to DNA methyltransferases on the one hand, and to AS3MT (arsenic (+3 oxidation state) methyltransferase) to the other hand (Ren et al., 2011). Jensen et al. (2009) correlated the occurrence of aberrant DNA methylation patterns after chronic low-dose exposure to MMA(III) with the development of a malignant phenotype of UROtsa cells (Table 2.).

Cell Line	Treatment	Exposure	Duration	Hyperproliferation	AIG	Tumors in mice
UROtsa	None	None	None	NA	No	No
URO-MSC12	MMA (III)	50 nM	12 weeks	Yes	No	No
URO-MSC24	MMA (III)	50 nM	24 weeks	Yes	Yes	No
URO-MSC36	MMA (III)	50 nM	36 weeks	Yes	Yes	ND
URO-MSC52	MMA (III)	50 nM	52 weeks	Yes	Yes	Yes
URO-MSC24 + 3mo	MMA (III)	50 nM	24 weeks	ND	Yes	ND
URO-MSC24 + 6mo	MMA (III)	50 nM	24 weeks	ND	Yes	ND
URO-MSC52 + 3mo	MMA (III)	50 nM	52 weeks	ND	Yes	Yes
URO-MSC52 + 6mo	MMA (III)	50 nM	52 weeks	ND	Yes	Yes
URO-ASSC	As (III)	1 μM	52 weeks	Yes	Yes	Yes
URO-CDSC	Cd (II)	1 μM	52 weeks	Yes	Yes	Yes

NA=not applicable; ND=not determined. (Jensen et al., 2009, modified)

Table 2. Cell line name, the treatment metal, concentration (exposure), and duration of treatment for each cell line are shown. In addition, the phenotypic properties of each cell line including increased growth rate relative to UROtsa (hyperproliferation), anchorage independent growth (AIG), and ability of each cell line to form tumours when injected subcutaneously into immunocompromised mice are described. The reference cites previous publications describing part or all of the information presented for a given cell line.

In our study we analysed the development of the malignant phenotype of UROtsa cells by assaying the ability of an anchorage independent growth as well as the ability of migration and invasion. Both characteristics are negative in untreated UROtsa cells, but occurred after chronic low-dose treatment to MMA(III) (50 nM, 75 nM, and 100 nM, respectively) for more than 90 weeks. The results of the soft agar assay do not provide evidence for a dose-dependent development of anchorage independent growth. In contrast, the data of the migration and invasion assays indicate that the motility of UROtsa cells is dose-dependently increased after chronic exposure to MMA(III). Both, the loss of anchorage independent growth and the increased motility / invasive potential, provide evidence for the formation of a malignant phenotype in UROtsa cells after chronic low-dose exposure to MMA(III). These *in vitro* results point to a possible model system to study the mechanisms of metastasis in arsenic-induced bladder cancer. Further studies have to be conducted analysing established molecular markers to support our presented data and proposals. For example, the analysis of cell-cell adhesion concerning the protein E-cadherin (encoded by the *CDH1* gene) and its regulation by the ZEB2 protein and *CDH1* promoter methylation would be of great interest for the investigation of the epithelial-mesenchymal transition (EMT), a basic mechanism required for the acquisition of an invasive and subsequently metastatic phenotype in epithelial tumours (Vandewalle et al., 2005). Furthermore, TWIST overexpression is known to increase migration and decrease the sensitivity to arsenic induced cell death in gastric cancer cells (Feng et al., 2009) and could serve as another interesting marker to study EMT and metastasis in arsenic-induced bladder cancer.

Fig. 15 summarises the molecular mechanisms of MMA(III)-induced toxicity and malignancy in UROtsa cells *in vitro* after chronic low-dose exposure. In this extended model we propose that after uptake and parallel to the fast conjugation to proteins and other cellular structures that is followed by lysosomal degradation and autophagy MMA(III) also induces DNA damage and epigenetic changes. This might lead to the observed alteration of signal transduction and cellular functions as well as the accumulation of (epi)genetic aberrations that are supposed to be the basis of transformation into a malignant phenotype.

Because this hypothetic model is based on *in vitro* research, there is an urgent need for further *in vivo* studies. While *in vitro* assays give important data for the investigation of molecular mechanisms, there is a lack of information concerning the defence of a whole organism against cancer including, e. g., the immune response.

In summary, we were able to present the tissue-dependent metabolism of MMA(III) in methylating HepG2 and non-methylating UROtsa cells. We analysed genotoxic effects of arsenic species in UROtsa cells and illustrated the dependence of genotoxicity on the methylation and oxidation state. This reveals how important the knowledge of the arsenic metabolism is, as each metabolite has its unique mechanisms of toxicity. MMA(III) is known as one of the most important metabolites due to its high toxicity. We analysed the malignant transformation of UROtsa cells after chronic low-dose exposure to MMA(III) and illustrated the loss of anchorage dependent growth and the development of increased migration and invasion properties. Both are serious phenotypical characteristics in the development of cancer. With our *in vitro* study we were able to give further evidence to arsenic-induced bladder cancer.

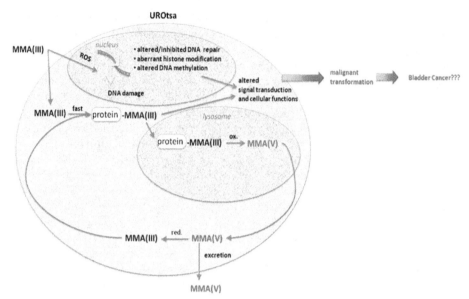

Fig. 15. Proposed molecular mechanisms of MMA(III) induced toxicity and malignancy in UROtsa cells after chronic low-dose exposure.

5. Acknowledgment

The authors would like to thank G. Zimmer, M. Gerhards and U. Zimmermann for their assistance of cell culturing. This work was kindly founded by the German research Foundation (DFG) Grant No: DO 332/8-1, JO 753/2-1 and HI 276/16-1.

6. References

Anderson, M. E. (1998). Glutathione: an overview of biosynthesis and modulation. *Chem Biol Interact*, Vol. 112, (April 1998), pp. 1-14, ISSN 0009-2797

Aposhian, H. V., Gurzau, E. S., Le, X. C., Gurzau, A., Healy, S. M., Lu, X. F., Ma, M. S., Yip, L., Zakharyan, R. A., Maiorino, R. M., Dart, R. C., Tircus, M. G., Gonzales-Ramirez, D., Morgan, D. L., Avram, D. & Aposhian, M. M. (2000). Occurrence of Monomethylarsonous acid in urine of humans exposed to inorganic arsenic. *Chem. Res. Toxicol.*, Vol. 13, No. 8, (August 2000), pp. 693-967, ISSN 0893-228X

Arancibia-Cárcamo I. L., Youen E. Y., Muir J., Lumb M. J., Michels G., Saliba R. S., Smart T. G., Yan Z., Kittler J. T. & Moss S. J. (2009). Ubiquitin-dependent lysosomal targeting of GABA(A) receptors regulates neuronal inhibition *PNAS*, Vol. 106, No. 41, (October 2009), pp. 17552-17557, ISSN 0027-8424

Barriere H., Nemes C., Du K. & Lukacs G. L. (2007). Plasticity of polyubiquitin recognition as lysosomal targeting signals by the endosomal sorting machinery. *MBoC*, Vol. 18, No. 10, (October 2007), pp. 3952-3965, ISSN 1059-1524

Bredfeldt, T. G., Jagadish, B., Eblin, K. E., Mash, E. A. & Gandolfi, A. J. (2006). Monomethylarsonous acid induces transformation of human bladder cells. *Toxicol. Appl. Pharmacol.*, Vol. 216, No. 1, (October 2006), pp. 69-79, ISSN 0041-008X

Chakraborti D., Sengupta M. K., Rahman M. M., Ahamed S., Chowdhury U. K., Hossain M. A., Mukherjee S. C., Pati S., Saha K. C., Dutta R. N. & Quamruzzaman Q. (2004). Groundwater arsenic contamination and its health effects in the Ganga-Meghna-Brahmaputra plain. *Journal of Environmental Monitoring*, Vol. 6, No. 6, (May 2004), pp. 74N-83N, ISSN 1464-0325

Chen C. L., Chiou H. Y., Hsu L. I., Hsueh Y. M., Wu M. M., Wang Y. H. & Chen C. J. (2010). Arsenic in Drinking Water and Risk of Urinary Tract Cancer: A Follow-up Study from Northeastern Taiwan. *Cancer Eepidemiology Biomarkers & Prevention*, Vol. 19, No. 1, (January 2010), pp. 101-110, ISSN 1055-9965

Chen C.-S. (2002). Phorbol ester induces elevated oxidative activity and alkalization in a subset of lysosomes. *BMC Cell Biology*, Vol. 3, (August 2002), pp. 21, doi:10.1186/1471-2121-3-21

Chiou H. Y., Hsueh Y. M., Liaw K. F., Horng S. F., Chiang M. H., Pu Y. S., Lin J. S. N., Huang C. H. & Chen C. J. (1995). Incidence of internal cancers and ingested Inorganic Arsenic - a 7- year follow-up-study in Taiwan. *Cancer Research*, Vol. 55, No. 6, (March 1995), pp. 1296-1300, ISSN 0008-5472

Clague M. J. & Urbé S. (2010). Ubiquitin: Same Molecule, Different Degradation Pathways. *Cell*, Vol. 143, No. 5, (November 2010), pp. 682-685, ISSN 0092-8674

Dopp E., Hartmann L. M., Florea A.-M., von Recklinghausen U., Pieper R., Shokouhi B., Rettenmeier A. W., Hirner A. V. & Obe G. (2004). Uptake of inorganic and organic derivates of arsenic associated with induced cytotoxic and genotoxic effects in Chinese hamster ovary (CHO) cells. *Toxicol Appl Pharmacol*, Vol. 201, No. 2, (December 2004), pp. 156-165, ISSN 0041-008X

Dopp E., Hartmann L. M., von Recklinghausen U., Florea A. M., Rabieh S., Zimmermann U., Shokouhi B., Yadav S., Hirner A. V. & Rettenmeier A. W. (2005). Forced Uptake of Trivalent and Pentavalent Methylated and Inorganic Arsenic and Its Cyto-/Genotoxicity in Fibroblasts and Hepatoma Cells. *Toxicol. Sciences*, Vol. 87, No. 1, (September 2005), pp. 46-56, ISSN 1096-6080

Dopp E. (2007) Neue Aspekte zur Arsen-induzierten Kanzerogenese. *ErgoMed*. Vol. 4, (n. d. 2007), pp. 100-1009

Dopp E., von Recklinghausen U., Hartmann L. M., Stueckradt I., Pollok I., Rabieh S., Hao L., Nussler A., Kartier C., Hirner A. V. & Retenmeier A. W. (2008). Subcellular Distributioan of Inorganic and Methylated Arsenic Compounds in Human Urothelial Cells and Human Hepatocytes. *Drug Metabolism and Disposition*, Vol. 36, No. 5, (May 2008), pp. 971-979, ISSN 0090-9556

Dopp E., von Recklinghausen U., Diaz-Bone R. A., Hirner A. V. & Rettenmeier A. W. (2010a). Cellular uptake, subcellular distribution and toxicity of arsenic compounds in methylating and non-methylating cells. *Environmental Research*, Vol. 110, No. 5, (July 2010), pp. 435-442, ISSN 0013-9351

Dopp E., Kligermann A. D. & Diaz-Bone R. A. (2010b). Organoarsenicals, Uptake, Metabolism, and Toxicity, In: *Metal Ions in Life Sciences*, Sigel A., Sigel H. & Sigel R.K.O. (Eds.), 231-265, RSC Publishing, ISSN 1559-0836, Cambridge, England

Du, Z.-X., Zhang, H.-Y., Meng, X., Guan, Y. & Wang, H.-Q. (2009). Role of oxidative stress and intracellular glutathione in the sensitivity to apoptosis induced by proteasome inhibitor in thyroid cancer cells. *BMC Cancer*, Vol. 9, No. 1, 56, DOI: 10.1186/1471-2407-9-56

Eblin, K. E., Hau, A. M., Jensen, T. J., Futscher, B.W. & Gandolfi, A. J. (2008). The role of arsenite and monomethylarsonous acid-induced signal transduction in human bladder cells: Acute studies. *Toxicology*, Vol. 250, No. 1, (August 2008), pp. 47-54, ISSN 0300-483X

Feng M.-Y., Wang K., Song H.-T., Yu H.W., Qin Y., Shi Q.-T. & Geng J.-S. (2009). Metastasis-induction and apoptosis-protection by TWIST in gastric cancer cells. *Clin Exp Metastasis*, Vol. 26, No. 8, (December 2008), pp. 1013-1023, ISSN 0262-0898

Fillol C., Dor F., Labat L., Boltz P., Le Bouard J., Mantey K., Mannschott C., Puskarczyk E., Viller F., Momas I. & Seta N. (2010). Urinary arsenic concentrations and speciation in residents living in an area with naturally contaminated soils. Science *of the Total Environment*, Vol. 408, No. 5, (February 2010), pp. 1190-1194, ISSN 0048-9697

Food Standards Agency of the UK, (2004). Seaweed warning. *Food Survey Information Sheet* (R938 - 28).

Francesconi K. A. (2010). Arsenic species in seafood: Origin and human health implications. *Pure and Applied Chemistry*, Vol. 82, No. 2, (February 2010), pp. 373-381, ISSN 0033-4545

Gorby M. S. & Albuquerque M. D., (1988). Arsenic Poisoning. *The Western Journal of Medicine*, Vol. 149, No. 3, (September 1988), pp. 308-315, ISSN 0093-0415

Hartwig A., Asmuss M., Ehleben I., Herzer U., Kostelac D., Pelzer A., Schwerdtle T. & Burkle A. (2002). Interference by toxic metal ions with DNA repair processes and cell cycle control: Molecular mechanisms. *Environmental Health Perspectives*, Vol. 110, Suppl. 5, (October 2002), pp. 797-799, ISSN 0091-6765

Hartwig A., Blessing H., Schwerdtle T. & Walter I. (2003), Modulation of DNA repair processes by arsenic and selenium compounds. *Toxicology*, Vol. 193, No. 1-2, (November 2003), pp. 161-169, ISSN 0300-483X

Hayakawa T., Kobayashi Y., Cui X. & Hirano S. (2005). A new metabolic pathway of arsenite: arsenic-glutathione complexes are substrates for human arsenic methyltransferase Cyt19. *Archives of Toxicology*, Vol. 79, No. 4, (April 2005), pp. 183-191, ISSN 0340-5761

Hippler J., Zdrenka R., Reichel R. A. D., Weber D. G., Rozynek P., Johnen G., Dopp E. & Hirner A. V. (2011). Intracellular, time resolved speciation and quantification of arsenic compound in human urothelial and hepatoma cells. *J. Anal. At. Spectrom.*, DOI:10.1039/C1JA10150A.

Hirner A. V. & Rettenmeier A. W. (2010). Methylated Metal(loid) Species in Humans, In: *Metal Ions in Life Sciences*, Sigel A., Sigel H. & Sigel R. K. O. (Eds.), pp. 465-512, RSC Publishing, ISSN 1559-0836, Cambridge, England

Hirner A. V. & Hippler J. (2011). Trace Metal(loids) (As, Cd, Cu, Hg, Pb, PGE, Sb, and Zn) and Their Species, In: *Treatise on water science,* Vol. 3, Wilderer P. (Ed.), pp. 31-57, Oxford: Academic Press, ISBN 0444531939

Hu, Y. Su, L. & Snow, E. T. (1998). Arsenic toxicity is enzyme specific and its affects on ligation are not caused by the direct inhibition of DNA repair enzymes. *Mutaion Research,* Vol. 408, No. 3, (September 1998), pp. 203-218, ISSN 0921-8777

Huang, C., Ke, Q., Costa, M. & Shi, x. (2004). Molecular Mechanisms of arsenic carcinogenesis. *Mol. Cell. Biochem.* Vol. 255, No. 1-2, (January 2004), pp. 57-66, ISSN 0300-8177

Jensen T. J., Novak P., Wnek S. M., Gandolfi A. J. & Futscher B. W. (2009). Arsenicals produce stable progressive changes in DNA methylation patterns that are linked to malignant transformation of immortalized urothelial cells. *Toxicol Appl Pharmacol,* Vol. 241, No. 2, (December 2009), pp. 221-229, ISSN 0041-008X

Kitchen, K. T. & Ahmad, S. (2003). Oxidative stress as a possible mode of action for arsenic carcinogenesis. *Toxicol. Lett.,* Vol. 137, No. 1-2, (January 2003), pp. 3-13, ISSN 0378-4274

Kitchen, K. T. & Wallace, K. (2008). The role of protein binding of trivalent arsenicals in arsenic carcinogenesis and toxicity. *J. Inorg. Biochem.,* Vol. 102, No. 3, (March 2008), pp. 532-539, ISSN 0162-0134

Kundu M. & Thompson C. B. (2008). Autophagy: Basic principles and relevance to disease. *Annu. Rev. Pathol. Mech. Dis.,* Vol. 3, (October 2008), pp. 427-455, ISSN 1553-4006

Lam S. H., Winata C. L., Tong Y., Korzh S., Lim W. S., Korzh V., Spitsbergen J., Mathavan S., Miller L. D., Liu E. T. & Gong Z. (2006). Transcriptome kinetics of arsenic-induced adaptive response in zebrafish liver. *Physiol. Genomics,* Vol. 27, No. 3, (November 2006), pp. 351-361, ISSN 1094-8341

Lozna, K. & Biernat, J. (2008). The occurrence of arsenc in the environment and food. *Rocz Panstw Zakl Hig,* Vol. 59, No. 1, (October 2008), pp. 19-31, ISSN 0035-7715

Marques C., Pereira P., Taylor A., Liang J. N., Reddy V. N., Szweda L. I. & Shang F.(2004). Ubiquitin-dependent lysosomal degradation of the HNE-modified proteins in lens epithelial cells. *The FASEB Journal,* Vol. 18, No. 10, (July 2004), pp. 1424-1426, ISSN 0892-6638

Meharg A. A., Ceacon C., Campbell R. C. J., Carey A. M., Williams P. N., Feldmann J. & Raab A. (2008). Inorganic arsenic levels in rice milk exceed EU and US drinking water standards. *Journal of Environmental Monitoring,* Vol. 10, No. 4, (March 2008), pp. 428-431, ISSN 1464-0325

Mehrpour M., Esclatine A., Beau I. & Codogno P. (2010). Overview of macroautophagy regulation in mammalian cells. *Cell Research,* Vol. 20, No. 7, (July 2010), pp. 748-762, ISSN 1001-0602

Nakajima Y., Endo Y., Inoue Y., Yamanaka K., Kato K., Wanibuchi H. & Endo G. (2006). Ingestion of Hijiki seaweed and risk of arsenic poisoning. *Applied Organometallic Chemistry,* Vol. 20, No. 9, (September 2006), pp. 557-564, ISSN 0268-2605

Naranmandura H., Suzuki N. & Suzuki K. T. (2006). Trivalent Arsenicals are bound to Proteins during reductive Methylation. *Chemical Research in Toxicology*, Vol. 19, No. 8, (August 2006), pp. 1010-1018, ISSN 0893-228X

Ng J. C., Wang J. & Shraim A. (2003). A global health problem caused by arsenic from natural sources. *Chemosphere*, Vol. 52, No. 9, (September 2003), pp. 1353-1359, ISSN 0045-6535

Planer-Friedrich B., Lehr C., Matschullat J., Merkel B. J., Nordstrom D. K. & Sandstrom M. W. (2006). Speciation of volatile arsenic at geothermal features in Yellowstone National Park. *Geochimica et Cosmochimica Acta*, Vol. 70, No. 10, (May 2006), pp. 2480-2491, ISSN 0016-7037

Planer-Friedrich B., London J., McCleskey R. B., Nordstrom D. K. & Wallschlaeger D. (2007). Thioarsenates in Geothermal Watersof Yellowstone National Park: Determination, Preservation, and Geochemical Importance. *Environmental Science & Technology*, Vol. 41, No. 15, (August 2007), pp. 5245-5251, ISSN 0013-936X

Raisuddin S. & Jha A. N. (2004). Relative Sensitivity of Fish and Mammalian Cells to Sodium Arsenate and Arsenite as Determined by Alkaline Single-Cell Gel Electrophoresis and Cytokinesis-Block Micronucleus Assay. *Environmental and Molecular Mutagenesis*, Vol. 44, No.1 , (June 2004), pp. 83-89, ISSN 0893-6692

Ren X., McHale C. M., Skibola C.F., Smith A. H., Smith M. T. & Zhang L. (2011). An Emerging Role for Epigenetic Dysregulation in Arsenic Toxicity and Carcinogenesis. *Environmental Health Perspectives*, Vol. 119, No. 1 (January 2011), pp. 11-19, ISSN 0091-6765

Rosen B. P., Ajees A. A. & McDermott T. R. (2011). Life and dead with arsenic, *Bioessays*, Vol. 33, No. 5, (May 2011), pp. 350-357, ISSN 0265-9247

Schwerdtle T., Walter I., Mackiw I. & Hartwig A. (2003). Induction of oxidative DNA damage by arsenite and its trivalent and pentavalent methylated metabolites in cultured human cells and isolated DNA. *Carcinogenesis*, Vol. 24, No. 5, (May 2003), pp. 967-974, ISSN 0143-3334

Shenoy S. K., Xiao K., Venkataramanan V., Snyder P. M., Freedmann N. J. & Weissmann A. M. (2008). Nedd4 mediates agonist-dependent ubiquitination, lysosomal targeting, and degradation of the beta(2)-adrenergic receptor. *J. Biol. Chem.*, Vol. 283, No. 32, (August 2008), pp. 22166-22176, ISSN 0021-9258

Signes-Pastor A. J., Deacon C., Jenkins R. O., Haris P. I., Carbonell-Barrachina A. A. & Meharg A. A. (2009). Arsenic speciation in Japanese rice drinks and condiments. *Journal of Environmental Monitoring*, Vol. 11, No. 11, (October 2009), pp. 1930-1934, ISSN 1464-0325

Smedley P. L. & Kinniburgh D. G. (2002). A review of the source, behaviour and distribution of arsenic in natural waters. *Applied Geochemistry*, Vol. 17, No. 5, (May 2002), pp. 517-568, ISSN 0883-2927

Smeester L. Rager J. E., Bailey K. A., Guan X., Smith N., Garcia-Vargas G., Del Razo L.-M., Drobná Z., Kelkar H., Stýblo M. & Fry R. C. (2011). Epigenetic Changes in Individuals with Arsenicosis. *Chem Res Toxicol*, Vol. 24, No. 2, (February 2011), pp. 165-167, ISSN 0893-228X

Smith A. H., Lingas E. O. & Rahman M. (2000). Contamination of drinking-water by arsenic in Bangladesh: a public health emergency. *Bulletin of the World Health Organization,* Vol. 78, No. 9, (n. d. 2000), pp. 1093-1103, ISSN 00429686

Styblo, M., Drobna, Z., Jaspers, I., Lin S. & Thomas, D. J. (2002). The role of biomethylation in toxicity and carcinogenicity of arsenic: a research update. *Environ. Health. Perspect.,* Vol. 110, Suppl. 5, (October 2002), pp. 767-771, ISSN 0091-6765

Styblo, M. & Thomas, D. J. (1997). Binding of arsenicals to proteins in an in vitro methylation system. *Toxicol Appl Pharmacol,* Vol. 147, No. 1, (November 1997), pp. 1-8, ISSN 0041-008X

Sun G. X., Williams P. N., Zhu Y. G., Deacon C., Carey A. M., Raab A., Feldmann J. & Meharg A. A. (2009). Survey of arsenic and its speciation in rice products such as breakfast cereals, rice crackers and Japanese rice condiments. *Environmental International,* Vol. 35, No. 3, (April 2009), pp. 473-475, ISSN 0160-4120

Sutherland J. E. & Costa M. (2003). Epigenetics and the Environment, In: *Ann. N.Y. Acad. Sci.,* Vol. 983, Verma M., Dunn B. K. & Umar A. (Ed.), pp. 151-160, NEW YORK ACAD SCIENCES, ISBN 1-57331-430-7

Terman A., Kurz T., Gustafsson B. & Brunk U. T. (2006). Lysosomal labilization. *IUBMB Life,* Vol. 58, No. 9, (September 2006), pp. 531-539, ISSN 1521-6543

Tseng C. H. (2007). Arsenic methylation, urinary arsenic metabolites and human diseases: Current perspective. *Journal of Environmental Science and Health, Part C Environmental Carcinogenesis and Ecotoxicology Reviews,* Vol. 25, No. 1, (2007), pp. 1-22, ISSN 1059-0501

Vandewalle C., Comijn J., De Craene B., Vermassen P., Bruyneel E., Andersen H., Tulchinsky E., Van Roy F. & Berx G. (2005). SIP1/ZEB2 induces EMT by repressing genes of different epithelial cell-cell junctions. *Nucleic Acids Research,* Vol. 33, No. 20, (November 2005), pp. 6566-6578, ISSN 0305-1048

Wei M., Wanibuchi H., Yamamoto S., Li W. & Fukushima S. (1999). Urinary bladder carcinogenicity of dimethylarsinic acid in male F344 rats. *Carcinogenesis,* Vol. 20, No. 9, (September 1999), pp. 1873–1876, ISSN 0143-3334

WHO (2001). *Arsenic compounds, Environmental health criteria 224, 2nd ed..* Geneva: World health organization

Wnek, S. M., Medeiros, M. K., Eblin, K. E. & Gandolfi A. J. (2009). Persistence of DNA damage following exposure of human bladder cells to chronic monomethylarsonous acid. *Toxicol. Appl. Pharmacol.,* Vol. 241, No. 2, (December 2009), pp. 202-209, ISSN 0041-008X

Wolfe-Simon F., Switzer Blum J., Kulp T. R., Gordon G. W., Hoeft S. E., Pett-Ridge J., Stolz J. F., Webb S. M., Weber P. K., Davies P. C. W., Anbar A. D. & Oremland R. S. (2010). A Bacterium That Can Grow by Using Arsenic Instead of Phosphorus. *Science,* Vol. 332, No. 6034, (June 2011) pp. 1163-1166, ISSN 0036-8075

Yan H. Wang N., Weinfeld M., Cullen W. R. &. Le X. C. (2009). Identification of Arsenic-Binding Proteins in Human Cells by Affinity Chromatography and Mass Spectrometry. *Anal. Chem.,* Vol. 81, No. 10, (May 2009), pp. 4144-4152, ISSN 0003-2700

Yang Y., Liang Z., Gao BJia., Y. & Qin Z. (2008). Dynamic effects of autophagy on arsenic trioxide-induced death of human leukemia cell line HL60 cells. *Acta Pharmacol Sin*, Vol. 29, No. 1, (January 2008), pp. 123-134, ISSN 1671-4083

Yoshida K., Inoue Y., Kuroda K., Chen H., Wanibuchi H., Fukushima S. & Endo G. (1998). Urinary excretion of arsenic metabolites after long-term oral administration of various arsenic compounds to rats. *J. Toxicol. Environ.Health*, Vol. 54, No. A, (June 1998), pp. 179-192, ISSN 0098-4108

Zhou X., Sun H., Ellen T. P., Chen H. & Costa M. (2008). Arsenite alters global histone H3 methylation. *Carcinogenesis*, Vol. 29, No. 9, (September 2008), pp. 1831-1836, ISSN 0143-3334

10

Animal Models for Basic and Preclinical Research in Bladder Cancer

Ana María Eiján[1,2], Catalina Lodillinsky[2] and Eduardo Omar Sandes[1]
[1]Research Area of the Institute of Oncology Angel H. Roffo, University of Buenos Aires,
[2]Consejo Nacional de Investigaciones Científicas y Técnicas (CONICET)
Argentina

1. Introduction

Bladder cancer is one of the most common cancers in the world. In 2006, there were about 61,240 diagnosed cases of bladder cancer and approximately 13,060 deaths attributable to this disease, being the prevalence estimated worldwide more than 1,000,000 patients (Jemal *et al.*, 2006; Lerner, 2005). Taking into account that its incidence seems to be increasing, bladder cancer is clearly a significant public health issue around the world. Thus, it is necessary to intensify research on this topic.

Urinary bladder cancer originates mainly from epithelial cells of the urothelium (Lopez-Beltran *et al.*, 2004; Montironi *et al.*, 2005). When initially diagnosed, most bladder cancers (about 70%) do not present muscle invasion, and are thus known as non-muscle invasive bladder cancer (pTa and pT1). In these cases, a simple transurethral resection is sufficient to remove the tumor. However, some patients experience recurrence or even tumor progression. The progression of the tumor involves invasion of tumor cells, which penetrate deeper layers of the bladder such as the detrusor muscle (pT2), perivesical tissue (pT3) and extravesical organs (pT4) (Figure 1). Since this progression threatens the patient's life, more aggressive therapies are necessary (Sobin *et al.*, 1997).

Intensive research in bladder cancer, as well as that in most tumors, is being carried out to elucidate the reason for the appearance of tumors, and to find out which factors are involved in their development and which are related to the tumor progression process. These investigations, which provide insights into the biology of the tumor, are essential for the implementation of new therapeutic and/or preventive modalities (Bhattacharya *et al.*, 2010; Zhang *et al.*, 2011).

Research on basic science is focused on the mechanisms that lead cells towards transformation and development of cancer, using simple experimental models where it is easier to interpret the results. Cell culture techniques are widely used to study different oncological processes. The cell culture is the growth of any cell type, usually tumor cells, in with nutrient-containing solutions. The cells grow attached to the plastic surface, forming a monolayer, usually in a two-dimensional way. This technique allows studying processes such as mutagenesis, invasion, migration, and production of proteolytic enzymes. Although cell culture is a very important tool, it has certain limitations. Many biological processes depend on the three-dimensional architecture. In addition, monolayer culture is usually restricted to a single or at most two cell types. In contrast, tumors are complex and consist of tumor cells and other cell types such as stroma and immune cells that interact to either promote or inhibit tumor growth. To overcome these limitations, it is necessary to use three-dimensional models, such as tissue or organ cultures (Varley *et al.*, 2011).

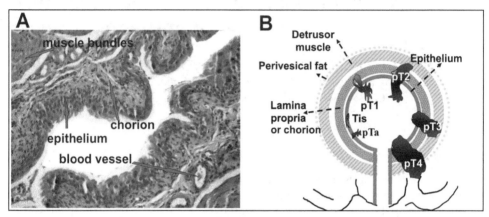

Fig. 1. A: Histology of a normal bladder from a C57BL/6J mouse (Hematoxylin- eosin). B: Scheme of the invasion status of bladder tumors. Non-muscle invasive tumors pTa when are confined to epithelium, and pT1 when penetrating into the chorion. Invasive tumors when penetrate deeper layers of the bladder such as the detrusor muscle (pT2), perivesical tissue (T3) and extravesical organs (pT4).

To corroborate in vitro results, the next step in the investigation is the assay in a living organism. Animal models are important tools which allow studying the mechanisms of carcinogenesis as well as carrying out preclinical studies of new therapeutic modalities. It is important to design a model as similar to human disease as possible, so that observations can be readily transferred to clinical studies.

2. General characteristics of animal models

Animal models constitute the essential link between cell-based experiments and the translation of novel agents into human patients with cancer. They are used to study the development and progression of diseases and to test new treatments before they are provided to humans. Therefore, models should be as close to human pathology as possible.
In evolutionary biological terms, large animals have more similarity to humans. However, the most widely used animal models are rodents, in particular mice and rats. Although imperfect in their translatability into clinical efficacy, these animals have the advantage that they reproduce easily in short time, are easy to maintain with low cost, and can be manipulated genetically, thus remaining a critical tool in bladder cancer research.
Models allow researchers to study different characteristics of the tumor biology such as tumor growth, latency, growth rate, invasion and metastasis. Studies of carcinogenic substances or prevention of carcinogenesis may be carried out in animal models. Also, analysis of the response to cytotoxicity and immunotherapy treatments can be performed (Bhattacharya *et al.*, 2010; Takeuchi *et al.*, 2011; Zhang *et al.*, 2011).

According to the site of tumor inoculation, models are classified as heterotopic or orthotopic (see points 2.1.4 and 2.1.5.). In addition, depending on the species in which the tumor cell lines are inoculated, models may be xenogeneic or syngeneic models (see below).

2.1 Mouse models in bladder cancer
2.1.1 Xenogeneic models

Animals with transplanted human cancers are called xenogeneic or xenograft models. Nude mice are commonly used to inoculate human tumor fragments or bladder cancer cells. These mice have a spontaneous mutation in chromosome 11 named *nude* (*nu*), which gives certain phenotypic and functional changes. Homozygous nude mice show absence of hair, the feature that gave the name to the mutation. However, a few years after the appearance of the mutation, it was found that nude mice do not have a functional thymus. As a consequence, these animals have a low number of mature T lymphocytes, which allows them to accept xenograft transplantation. This feature of nude mice has contributed to the development of research in cancer, making these animal models useful to study the in vivo growth of human tumors and human cancer cell lines in which the efficacy of therapeutic agents such as monoclonal antibodies, cytotoxic drugs and radiotherapy can be tested. Below are a few examples of the relevant experiments in bladder cancer therapy using xenograft models.

One of the main features of tumors is their capacity to grow uncontrollably, invading the surrounding tissue, inducing neoformation of blood (angiogenesis) and lymphatic vessels and spreading in the body, forming secondary tumors or metastasis. In most cases, the death of patients with bladder cancer is due to the generation of metastasis. Angiogenesis, which is intricately involved in growth and metastasis and is in fact a prerequisite for these processes (Fidler, 1990; Folkman, 1986), is regulated by a fine balance between stimulatory and inhibitory factors produced by the tumor and the surrounding stroma (Liotta *et al.*, 1991). Bladder tumors produce high levels of several stimulatory factors, being the vascular endothelial growth factor (VEGF) overexpressed in bladder cancer (Crew *et al.*, 1997; O'Brien *et al.*, 1995). The action of this factor is mediated by its membrane receptor (VEGFR). Both VEGF and VEGFR are considered as important therapeutic targets. Some papers have studied the effects of a neutralizing monoclonal antibody targeted at murine VEGFR by using a xenograft model. In combination with cytotoxic compounds, such as paclitaxel, this monoclonal antibody impairs tumor growth and angiogenesis and. thus prevents metastatic spread and prolongs mouse survival (Davis *et al.*, 2004; Inoue *et al.*, 2000).

Xenograft models have also been used in radiopharmaceutical studies (Pfost *et al.*, 2009). Pfost et al. coupled monoclonal antibodies that recognize epidermal growth factor receptors on bladder cancer cells with [213]Bi, a radioactive alpha particle emitter, and found that therapy with 0.37 MBq of radiation after tumor cell inoculation in the bladder of nude mice results in higher survival of mice when compared with conventional treatment with Mitomycin C. These authors were also able to show that Mitomycin C produces nephrotoxicity, whereas [213]Bi-anti-EGFR-mAb treatment showed no signs of nephrotoxicity. These results suggest that radioimmunotherapy using intravesically instilled [213]Bi-anti-EGFR-mAb is a promising option for the treatment of bladder cancer in patients.

Xenogeneic models have also been used for the detection of growth and metastasis spread by bioluminescence techniques (Hadaschik *et al.*, 2007). To monitor tumor growth and therapeutic efficacy, noninvasive imaging concepts are preferable. For that purpose, tumor cells are stably transfected with genes coding for fluorescent proteins (Tanaka et al., 2003) or enzymes catalyzing bioluminescence (Hadaschik et al., 2007), allowing for the continuous visualization of tumor development after intravesical instillation of tumor cells.

Although, as described above, xenograft models are important tools to study the behavior of human tumors in vivo, they also have an important limitation: they are immunodeficient. This makes this animal model not suitable to study interactions between the host immune system and the tumor. Furthermore, xenograft models are useless for research on the biological mechanisms related to carcinogenesis or on the possible compounds able to prevent carcinogenesis. In contrast, syngeneic animal models are more appropriate to approach these issues.

2.1.2 Syngeneic models

Syngeneic models include the appearance of spontaneous tumors, induction of tumors by chemical carcinogens, and inoculation of tumor cells in mice genetically identical to those in which tumors were developed. All of them are useful for studies in which the host-tumor interaction must be taken into account.

Immunotherapy

In patients, non-muscle invasive bladder cancers are usually managed with transurethral resection followed by the intravesical administration of Bacillus Calmette-Guerin (BCG). This immune therapy has been used without modification since 1976 (Morales et al., 1976). In addition to the direct anti-tumor effect (Sandes et al., 2007), it is widely recognized that intravesical BCG therapy is more potent in preventing tumor recurrence than any other intravesical chemotherapy (Sylvester, 2009). However, about 20% of patients either fail to respond initially or relapse within the first five years of treatment (Smaldone et al., 2009). The exact mechanisms of BCG action have not been completely elucidated yet. However, it is known that BCG generates a local immunological reaction with activation of immune cells as well as secretion of cytokines involving Th1 cell cytotoxicity (Riemensberger et al., 2002). To investigate the immune mechanisms by which BCG prevents bladder tumor recurrence and progression as well as the mechanisms of immune suppression to explain the lack of effectiveness of BCG observed in some patients, animal models with a competent immune system are needed. Syngeneic mouse bladder cancer models have thus been used for this purpose.

Animal models using subcutaneous or orthotopic inoculation of bladder cancer cell lines are being designed to study potential therapies to reverse these immune suppressive mechanisms. Mangsbo et al. have studied a syngeneic model by inoculating MB49 bladder cancer cell lines in the subcutis of C57BL/6J mice. This experimental model closely mimics human bladder cancer, because MB49 cells express negative regulatory proteins of the immune response (Inman et al., 2007; Nakanishi et al., 2007). Among others, the programmed death ligand 1 (PD-L1) and the cytotoxicity T lymphocyte antigen-4 (CTLA-4) render T regulatory cells (Tregs) that can oppose to BCG immunotherapy. Antibodies able to block PD-L1 and CTLA-4 administered intratumorally improves long-term survival and leads to increased levels of tumor-reactive T cells and decreased numbers of Tregs at the tumor site. Therefore, this experimental model has allowed an approach to the understanding of immune suppression during immune therapy with BCG and represents a new therapeutic option in the treatment of bladder cancer (Mangsbo et al., 2010).

It is known that BCG is neither free of mild or intermediate side effects such as fever and granulomatous prostatitis nor of severe side effects such as pneumonitis, hepatitis and BCG sepsis (DeHaven et al., 1992). To avoid such unfavorable events, it is necessary to develop a more active and less toxic immunotherapeutic agent. A mouse syngeneic model using subcutaneous inoculation of MBT2 bladder cancer cell lines has been used to evaluate the effectiveness of liposomes containing walls from BCG bacteria as immune therapy. With this experimental design, Joraku et al. have demonstrated inhibition of tumor growth with increased immunity. Thus, this non-live bacterial agent may contribute to providing a more active and less toxic tool as a substitute for live BCG in immunotherapy (Joraku et al., 2009). Besides the study of the immune mechanism, other studies involving the tumor-host interaction have used syngeneic models. For example, in our laboratory, we have evaluated the mechanism of action of BCG using animals inoculated subcutaneously with MB49 bladder cancer cells, and found that macrophages from tumor-bearing mice treated with BCG intratumorally were able to produce soluble factors including fibroblast growth factor-2 (FGF-2), which induces fibroblast proliferation. We also found that in vivo BCG therapy reduces tumor growth with a concomitant increase in collagen deposition and expression of alpha-smooth muscle actin and FGF-2. These results suggest that tissue repair mechanisms similar to healing are involved in BCG immunotherapy of bladder cancer (Lodillinsky et al., 2010).

Carcinogenesis and chemo-prevention

Bladder cancer is a candidate for chemo-prevention intervention for several reasons. In the first place, bladder cancer patients present successive recurrences that must be prevented. Also, in addition to genetic susceptibility, this cancer is closely related to exposure to environmental contaminants, including cigarette smoking, which implies the constant contact of carcinogenetic substances with the urothelium.

Animal models are widely used to select chemical synthesis products, purified natural products or even mixtures of natural products with potential to prevent tumor development, which can then be used in clinical trials. The idea is to use organ-specific animal models to determine which agents are likely to be helpful in preventing specific forms of cancer. These animal models can be obtained by chemical induction, spontaneous occurrence or use of transgenic animals.

To be useful, animal models must meet several characteristics. The model should be of clinical relevance, not only in terms of organ specificity but also in terms of the histology and the genetic abnormalities. Furthermore, premalignant lesions should be developed with genetic and histological features as similar as possible to those observed in the development of human cancer. In addition, the model must be consistent in generating tumors in a significant number of animals in a reasonable period. Finally, the model must be predictive in terms of clinical efficacy, i.e. that the positive or negative results obtained in the animal model should later correlate with positive and negative results in human trials (Steele et al., 2010).

One of most useful models is the induction of bladder cancer in mice and rats with hydroxybutyl(butyl)nitrosamine (OH-BBN). This carcinogen compound induces premalignant lesions that progress to transitional bladder tumors, and in little proportion of squamous tumors (Grubbs et al., 2000). Recent studies by Lu et al. have compared bladder tumors in rats and mice induced by OH-BBN with human bladder tumors, using a global gene expression approach cross-species analysis, and shown the similarity between this animal model and bladder cancer in humans. These genes are likely to have conserved functions contributing to bladder carcinogenesis. To strengthen this analysis, these authors studied the molecular pathway commonly activated in both human and rodent bladder cancer and found a number of pathways that affect the cell cycle, HIF-1 and MYC expression, and regulation of apoptosis in both rodent and human bladder cancer. Also, they compared expression changes at mRNA and protein levels in the rat model and identified several genes/proteins exhibiting concordant changes in human bladder tumors. They concluded that rodent models (in OH-BBN-treated B6D2F1 mice and Fischer-344 rats) of bladder cancer accurately represent the clinical situation to an extent that will allow successful miming of target genes, showing that these models are powerful tools for chemoprevention research (Lu et al., 2010). Using this experimental model, it has been demonstrated that NSAIDs (such as indomethacin, naproxen, NO-naproxen, and celecoxib), various EGFR inhibitors, and purified natural compounds (such as tea polyphenols and sulforaphane) have striking efficacy to prevent bladder tumor development (Ding et al., 2010; Grubbs et al., 2000; Lubet et al., 2005; Steele et al., 2009; Yao et al., 2004).

Two disadvantages inherent in these models are the long experimental times (usually periods between 8 to 12 months) and the occupational exposure of workers. To avoid the use of carcinogens, knockout or transgenic mouse models can be used. These models are used in chemoprevention trials as well as in studies on the relevance of each gene in tumor development.

2.1.3 Transgenic models

Activation of oncogenes or inactivation of tumor suppressors in the urothelium is considered critical for the development of urothelial cancer. Transgenic mice have proven to be powerful tools to unravel the mechanisms of carcinogenesis and to understand the molecular basis of the disease. Transgenic mice are a particular case of syngeneic models, which are genetically modified to study the importance of a particular gene in cancer development and progression. Knockout mice, which are genetically modified mice, can be used to study the effect on the deficiency of a particular gene.

Alterations in the suppressor genes RB1 and p53 as well as the activation of oncogenes such as Ha-ras are commonly found in human urothelial tumors. Transgenic mice with alterations in these genes have been designed. By way of example, we will next describe some of the models developed and the conclusions that have been reached.

Mouse embryos lacking the retinoblastoma (Rb) gene die 14 days into gestation and mice lacking the p53 gene succumb to thymic lymphomas at seven months of age. So, the role of these genes in the analysis of tumorigenesis was delayed until conditional transgenic mice were developed. These models achieve the loss of gene function only in a particular tissue. The specific urothelium knockout system was developed using the Cre/loxP strategy. Transgenic mouse lines in which a 3.6-kb mouse uroplakin II promoter is used to drive the expression of Cre recombinase (Cre) have been generated (Mo et al., 2005). The use of this model has allowed understanding the role of antitumor genes such as RB, p53 and PTEN in bladder carcinogenesis (Ahmad et al., 2011; Ayala de la Pena et al., 2011; He et al., 2009). Conditional inactivation of both RB1 alleles in the mouse urothelium instead of accelerate urothelial proliferation, profoundly activated the p53 pathway, leading to extensive apoptosis in urothelial cells. Thus, pRb loss triggers fail-safe mechanisms whereby urothelial cells can evade tumorigenesis. Additional loss of p53 in pRb-deficient urothelial cells can remove these p53-dependent tumor barriers, resulting in hyperplasia or umbrella cell nuclear atypia. Also, superficial papillary bladder tumors of low-grade (rare occurrence) but not invasive carcinomas have been detected. Furthermore, mice deficient in both pRb and p53 are highly susceptible to carcinogen exposure, developing invasive carcinomas that resemble human bladder cancer (He *et al.*, 2009). Another transgenic mouse with inactivation of the tumor suppressor p53 has been obtained by expression of SV40 large T antigen, directed to the urothelium with the specific promoter uroplakin-II. In the same way as in the transgenic mice described above, this construction has allowed demonstrating that the elimination of p53 alone is not sufficient for the generation of bladder tumor (Ayala de la Pena *et al.*, 2011). The function of proto-oncogene activation has been assessed by using Ha-ras trangenic mice (Zhang *et al.*, 2001).

Transgenic mice with compromised immune systems have also been developed. Mice knockout to IFN gamma (IFNγ -/-), interleukins 17, 12 and 23 (IL-17 -/-; IL-12-/- and IL-23 -/-), among others, are being used to understand how different components of the immune system either promote or inhibit the development of bladder tumors (Kortylewski et al., 2009; Langowski et al., 2006; Wang *et al.*, 2009).

In both syngeneic and xenogeneic models, tumors can grow in heterotopic or orthotopic sites. Below we describe the advantages and disadvantages of both modalities.

2.1.4 Heterotopic tumor growth

This site of inoculation refers to the growth of a tumor in a site different from its target organs, generally using subcutaneous inoculation. This approach is advantageous in cases where the orthotopic inoculation (see below) is complex such as in bladder, kidney, and bowels. Tumor inoculation is simple and can be carried out by an operator with minimum training. Furthermore, the tumor can be easily detected and the tumor evolution can be easily assessed by using palpation of the skin and measurement with a caliper, respectively. To assess tumor growth, at least two perpendicular diameters, the larger diameter (D) and the smaller diameter (d), must be measured. Some researchers also measure depth (Figure 2). However, the latter is difficult to determine and generally produces large errors. Tumor size can be calculated from these data, using various formulas such as geometric mean ($(Dxd)^{1/2}$ expressed in millimeters), arithmetic average ($Dxd/2$ expressed in mm²), or volume of the ellipsoid ($4/3 \pi Dxd^2$, expressed mm³). Not all tumors grow in the same way; some of them are more compact, whereas others develop necrosis. Therefore, to choose the most appropriate formula for each tumor, it is first necessary to validate the formula that best fits, when compared with tumor weight.

The main disadvantage of the heterotopic model is the fact that an anatomic site other than an orthotopic site can differentially develop tumor growth. The tumorigenesis and metastatic potential of tumors depend not only on the characteristics of the tumor cells, but also on the tumor environment and therefore on the site of injection. Human tumors can be formed by different cell subpopulations with varying ability to metastasize and susceptibility to treatment, depending on the site of inoculation (Fidler, 1986). It has been observed that subcutaneous inoculation of murine MB49 bladder cancer cell lines induces lung metastases, and that inoculation of these cells in the bladder does not (Lodillinsky *et al.*, 2009). Similar observations have been made for human tumors using 253J B-V cells (Black *et al.*, 2007). After 28 days of tumor growth either in the bladder or in the subcutis, Black et al. were able to determine that the tumor size was similar in both sites, but that only tumors growing orthotopically in the bladder developed metastasis to lymph nodes and lungs. The orthotopic tumors, as compared to the subcutaneous tumors, have an increased microvessel density, increase in growth factors expression and proteolytic enzyme activity. Therefore, models of orthotopic growth are more appropriate for studies related to metastasis dissemination or response to any treatment.

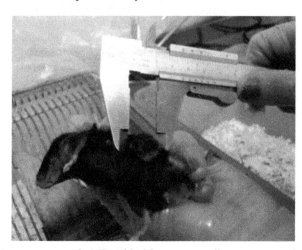

Fig. 2. Heterotopic tumor growth: MB49 bladder cancer cells growing in the subcutis of C57BL/6J mice.

There are some heterotopic models such as inoculation into the tail vein or the left ventricle of the heart which have been widely used to evaluate the process of extravasations and colonization in the lung or bone, respectively (Growcott, 2009; Wu *et al.*, 2010). Although very used, these models consider only a limited aspect of the metastatic process (Figure 3).

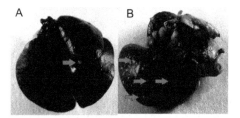

Fig. 3. Lung metastases: inoculation of MB49 (panel A) or MB49-I (panel B) bladder cancer cell lines into the tail vein induces lung metastasis. The lungs are colored in black by intratracheal inoculation of Indian ink. Metastases are seen in yellow by the stain and Bouin's fixative solution.

2.1.5 Orthotopic tumor growth

Growth in the target organ allows for better analysis of the interaction between the host and the tumor. When tumors are chemically induced, the carcinogen is chosen such that the tumor develops in the desired organ. Thus, tumor growth occurs in the orthotopic site. However, in the case that the tumor is generated by inoculation of a tumor fragment or tumor cell lines, the orthotopic inoculation is not always easy to perform. However, this difficulty must be overcome since the results obtained with heterotopic models are not always easy translated into clinical trials.

As previously mentioned, there are examples showing that different results are observed when the tumor is inoculated subcutaneously or orthotopically in the bladder. In studies of chemoprevention, inhibition of bladder cancer development by allyl isothiocyanate was detected for tumors growing orthotopically but not in the subcutis (Bhattacharya *et al.*, 2010). Furthermore, as described in the previous section, considerable variation has been detected between the two models in assays of immunotherapy, angiogenesis, invasion and metastatic spread, among others. Taking these limitations into account, to achieve a correct interpretation of results and a translatable preclinical model, it is necessary to inoculate the tumor in the bladder.

Inoculation into the bladder requires a qualified technician. Mice must first be anesthetized and subsequently, a 24-gauge Teflon i.v. catheter must be inserted through the urethra into the bladder using an inert lubricant to avoid discomfort in mice. For successful implantation of the bladder tumor cells, the urothelium must first be damaged. There are different techniques to induce such damage in the bladder. One of them involves the use of hydrochloric acid (0.1 ml 0.1 M HCl for 15 minutes) and subsequent neutralization with alkali and extensive washing with saline (Zhang *et al.*, 2011). Another technique involves instillation of a solution of silver nitrate (NO_3Ag) (Chade *et al.*, 2008). Both forms of injury allow the generation of tumors uniformly distributed in the bladder. The inoculation of MB49 tumor cells ($1x10^5$ to $5x10^5$) in syngeneic mice generates superficial tumors in about 7 to 15 days. Other techniques, using polylysine instillation, intramurally inoculation via laparotomy, or electro cauterization of the urothelium, are also used (Black *et al.*, 2010).

Cauterization of the bladder mimics transurethral resection of bladder tumor and therefore should facilitate adherence of instilled tumor cells to the bladder wall. The method was designed by Gunther et al. for the inoculation of MB49 cells in syngeneic mice (Gunther *et al.*, 1999). However, it is also used for inoculation of cells from human bladder tumors in nude mice (Pfost *et al.*, 2009). The technique involves the insertion of a guiding wire into the bladder of a mouse positioned dorsally on the ground plate of the cautery unit via the teflon catheter. When it is verified that the wire touches the bladder wall, the wire is attached to the cautery unit, and a monopolar coagulation mode is applied for 2 seconds at the lowest level (7 W). Then, via the same catheter, an appropriate number of tumor cells are inoculated and should remain in the bladder for at least 30 minutes (Figure 4A).

Another difficulty to be overcome is the determination of the evolution of bladder tumor growth. Unlike what happens in the case of a subcutaneous tumor growth, where its size can be easily determine at different times of evolution, the growth evolution in the bladder is more uncertain. However, hematuria is the hallmark of tumor presence (Figure 4B). Mice with $1x10^4$ or $1x10^5$ MB49 cell lines, inoculated by electrocautery, present hematuria about 15 or 9 days post-inoculation, respectively (Lodillinsky *et al.*, 2009). Inoculation of $5x10^3$ cells in the bladder previously treated with NO_3Ag generates hematuria in all mice about 7 days after tumor implantation (Chade *et al.*, 2008). Palpation of the bladder may give an idea of the extent of the tumor, but it is difficult to carry out because the bladder is retropubic. Also, in some cases, palpation could be given a wrong interpretation. When there is an obstruction of the urethra by blood clots, the bladder is greatly enlarged as a product of the accumulation of urine, and may thus lead to a wrong estimate of the extension of the tumor

(Figure 4C and D). Therefore, in these cases, the true evaluation of tumor size can be obtained at the end of the experiment, either by measuring the bladder with a caliper or by determining its weight (Figure 4E and F). Experiments of this type, also called end-point, have the disadvantage that they focus only on one measure of tumor size and not on its evolution throughout the experiment. This problem will soon be overcome by the design of non-invasive diagnostic equipment for small animals, similar to those used in medical practice in humans, such as ultrasound-doppler, infrared (IR) or bioluminescence imaging. By way of example, ultrasound-Doppler sagittal images have been used to evaluate angiogenesis in a mouse bladder cancer model (Sugano *et al.*, 2011). Also, bladder cancer cells that have been engineered to express certain proteins that emit fluorescence are being used in bioluminescence detection of tumor development (Black *et al.*, 2010).

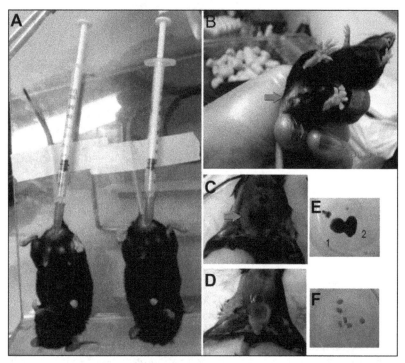

Fig. 4. Bladder tumor growth: A) orthotopic inoculation: after cauterization and inoculation of the appropriate number of tumor cells, mice should remain upside-down for at least 30 minutes so that cells can adhere to the bladder epithelium. B) Hematuria is the hallmark of tumor presence. C) Mouse with bladder tumor. D) Mouse with bladder containing urine but without tumor. E) Two bladders with tumor. F) Bladders from normal mice.

2.2 Mouse bladder cancer model for study of invasion and metastasis
2.2.1 Invasion and metastasis
The process of tumor invasion and metastasis is the most devastating stage of neoplastic disease and worsens prognosis of cancer patients. Adverse effects of systemic anti-tumor therapy and organ failure invaded with metastatic tissue are the leading causes of death in

these patients (Steeg *et al.*, 2006). It is currently accepted that tumors have a clonal origin, which means that they are derived from a single cell. The high proliferative capacity, coupled with the genetic instability of tumor cells, generates new mutations, and thus the generation of other cell populations conferring tumor heterogeneity. This is considered part of an evolutionary process of genetic and epigenetic changes that allow some of the primary tumor cells acquire an adaptive advantage to migrate and colonize new environments. However, new findings have shown the possibility of a parallel development of cells capable of early metastatic spread. This parallel progression model urges to review the current diagnostic and treatment (Klein *et al.* 2009).

The local invasion process that gives rise to metastatic spread is a multi-step event called metastatic cascade. This is a phenomenon with low efficiency, indicating that only a few of the cells that emerge from the primary tumor are able to generate metastases.

Initially, tumor cells release proteolytic enzymes, such as MMPs and cathepsins, which degrade the extracellular components of basement membrane, thereby creating gaps that allow the invasion of the underlying connective tissue. The tumor cells migrate through the extracellular matrix and some may penetrate the lymphatic and blood capillaries, a phenomenon knows as intravasation. Once in the bloodstream, cells that manage to survive must leave the vessel (extravasation) into different organs (Figure 5). When the microenvironment of the target organ is appropriate, colonizing tumor cells can form metastases.

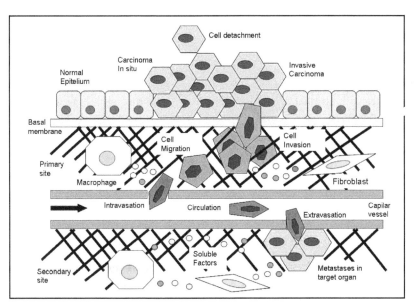

Fig. 5. During the metastatic cascade, tumor cells undergo genotypic and phenotypic changes that increase their capacity for invasion and migration. Some tumor cells are capable of degrading the basal membrane and migrating through connective tissue. Cells from connective tissue, such as macrophages and fibroblasts, through the release of growth factors, cytokines and proteolytic enzymes, can enhance the invasive behavior of tumor cells.

2.2.2 Metastogenes

The study of gene expression in primary tumor cells and metastatic cells has begun to lift the veil that prevented the understanding of the complex process of metastasis. These studies have identified a set of genes involved in the development of metastasis, called "metastogenic genes". Although there may be some overlap, these genes have been classified into three categories: a) initiation genes, b) progression genes and c) virulence genes (Nguyen et al., 2007).

Initiation genes are associated with the processes of invasion, angiogenesis and epithelial-mesenchymal transition (EMT). Since during invasion the migration of cells is an important step, genes encoding for GTPases involved in cytoskeleton remodeling such as RhoC have been included in this category. Among those involved in angiogenesis are those encoding the vascular endothelium growth factor, and matrix metalloproteinase 9 (MMP9). EMT allows changes that give advantages in terms of migration and invasion. Certain genes that encode for transcription factors associated with this transition such as TWIST1 are also included in this group.

Progression genes are linked to the negative regulation of the immune response, vascular remodeling and extravasations. Examples are the gene coding for cyclooxygenase 2 (COX-2), matrix metalloproteinase 1 (MMP-1) and angiopoietin-like 4 (ANGPTL4), among others.

Finally, virulence genes are those which give the tumor cell an adaptive advantage to survive within an organ-specific microenvironment (Chiang et al., 2008). Among them are intercellular signaling molecules such as cytokines and interleukins (CXCR4 and IL-11), molecules of the family of tumor necrosis factor (TNF) that are associated with bone metabolism (RANKL) and mediators of the angiogenic process such as the Endothelin-1.

Recent findings have identified the expression pattern characteristic of primary tumor gene, which is similar to a genetic signature that predicts the metastatic potential of the tumor (Bertucci et al., 2007, Van't Veer et al., 2002). This implies that the genetic profile expressed in metastases in specific organs is not always the same. Different groups of genes allow tumor cells to interact with stromal cells of the target organ. For example, the genes involved in breast cancer metastasis to bone are different from those involved in metastasis to the lung. This knowledge would allow the development of therapeutic strategies specific for each gene expression pattern or "signature " of a metastasis.

2.2.3 Epithelial-mesenchymal transition

During the invasion process, the tumor cells show a phenotypic change called epithelial-mesenchymal transition (EMT), which is characterized by a morphological change that is due to a genetic reprogramming process which normally occurs during embryonic development and tissue repair such as scarring (Peinado et al., 2007). This reprogramming involves the expression of a group of transcriptional repressors (Zeb-1 and 2, Twist, Snail and Slug) that recruit histone deacetylases, controlling the expression of genes associated with the epithelial phenotype. An example of this is the decreased expression of E-cadherin, which leads to a loss of homotypic adhesion. Certain cytokines of the family of transforming growth factor beta (TGFbeta) and bone morphogenetic protein (BMP) are responsible for increasing the expression of these repressors (McConkey et al., 2009).

Simultaneously with an underexpression of proteins of the epithelial phenotype, an overexpression of molecules associated with the mesenchymal phenotype has been detected. The expression of vimentin and loss of apical-basal polarization is a characteristic change of cells undergoing EMT (Peinado et al., 2007).

2.2.4 Proteolytic enzymes in bladder cancer invasion

Proteolytic activity is of fundamental importance for the development, growth and maintenance of homeostasis of all the tissues in any organism. In each particular tissue, the activity of proteolytic enzymes is regulated at different levels, both at gene expression, transcriptional regulation and by specific endogenous inhibitors (Durkan *et al.*, 2003; Kumar *et al.*, 2010). In addition, these enzymes can activate each other through a mechanism cascade that also regulates their activity. The genetic instability of tumor cells leads to alterations in the genes encoding proteolytic enzymes and/or their inhibitors, which lead to an increased proteolytic activity in the tumor. It is well documented that proteolytic enzymes are involved in the process of invasion and metastasis. Matrix metalloproteinases (MMPs),cathepsins (B, L) and urokinase-type plasminogen activator (uPA) are the three main groups of enzymes described in the process of tumor invasion.

MMPs, of which several isoforms are known, have a major role in matrix destruction and are involved in metastasis by mediating basement membrane destruction and angiogenesis (Kim *et al.*, 2004). Of all known isoforms, MMP-2 and MMP-9 are strongly associated with invasion in bladder cancer (Eissa *et al.*, 2007; Papathoma *et al.*, 2000).

Cathepsins have also been involved in cancer invasion. Cathepsin B (CB) is one of the most abundant lysosomal cysteine proteinase in mammalian tissue. It is synthesized as a glycosylated zymogen named pro-CB and subsequently converted to an active form of 33 kDa or 27-29 kDa. CB has an important role in the lysosomal degradation of proteins and is also involved in the degradation of the extracellular matrix in neoplastic and inflammatory diseases. Particularly, results from our laboratory have shown that the high expression of the active form of CB in transitional bladder tumors is associated with worse prognosis factors such as invasiveness and high histological grade (Eiján *et al.*, 2003).

The proteolytic activity of uPA is a system regulated by urokinase, its specific receptor uPAR and the specific plasminogen activator inhibitor 1 (PAI-1). This system plays a major role in tumorigenesis, tumor progression, tumor invasion and metastasis formation. It is generally assumed that the pro-malignant effect of the uPA-uPAR system is mediated by increased local proteolysis, thus favoring tumor invasion, as well as by the pro-angiogenic effect (Binder *et al.*, 2008). Consistent with this activity it has been shown, in a rat orthotopic model, that intravesical administration of PAI-1, which inhibits uPA activity in tumors, reduces the growth and progression of bladder cancer (Chen *et al.*, 2009).

2.2.5 Orthotopic mouse bladder cancer invasion model

Certain fundamental properties of metastatic cells such as migration and invasion can be studied in the laboratory using tumor cell cultures. Using various tools of genetic engineering, genes that encode molecules that emit fluorescence (green fluorescent protein), bioluminescent molecules (luciferase) or molecules with color (beta galactosidase) can be introduced into the cell. This technique is known as reporter gene and has allowed the analysis of molecular processes at the level of cell groups or isolated cells (Ghajar *et al.*, 2008; Menon *et al.*, 2009). In vitro experiments have also been useful to shed light on genes that might be involved in certain steps of the metastatic cascade. So, the use of genetic and pharmacological methods has shown that the expression of certain genes facilitate the assembly of new tumor blood vessels, tumor cells out of circulation and the passage of circulating tumor cells through the pulmonary capillaries to grow lung metastases (Gupta *et al.*, 2007; Valastyan *et al.*, 2009). However, in vitro models allow a simple analysis and do not always allow evaluating interactions with the tumor microenvironment. It is therefore important to develop animal models to analyze the factors associated with tumor progression (Bos *et al.*, 2010). To this end, we have added the advances in multiphoton intravital microscopy, which allows observing the in vivo behavior of tumor cells labeled with green fluorescent protein in the process of invasion and metastasis (Condeelis *et al.*, 2003).

There are only few useful animal models to study the processes of invasion and metastasis. Dinney et al. have designed an orthotopic murine model with different degrees of invasion. To this end, they seeded human 253J cells into the bladder wall of immunodeficient mice (nude) and then selected subpopulations of the parental line by in vivo reimplantation in the bladder. After five serial passages, tumors were more tumorigenic and showed metastatic capacity (Dinney *et al.*, 1995). These authors observed that these variants had a tumoral abnormal karyotype, increased expression of molecules such as epidermal growth factor receptor (EGFR), interleukin 8 (IL-8) and MMP-9, and also observed an increased anchorage-independent growth and increased capacity to migrate in Matrigel ® (trade name of a protein mixture secreted by mouse sarcoma cells Engelbreth-Holm-Swarm), commonly used in the study of invasive and migratory behavior of tumor cells in contact with extracellular matrix components.

This is a xenogeneic model in which it is possible to study the changes experienced by the tumor cells to acquire their invasive and metastatic phenotype. While this is an ingenious and very useful model, the fact that it is an immunodeficient mouse slightly restricts the applicability of the model.

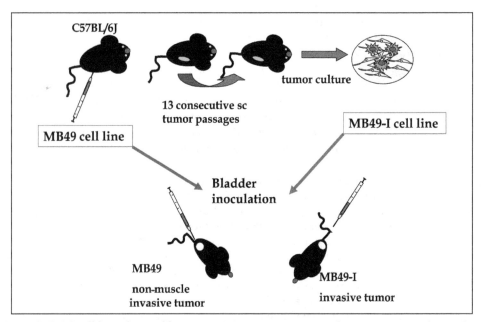

Fig. 6. MB49-I cell line obtained by successive in vivo passages of primary tumor obtained by inoculation of the MB49 bladder tumor cell line. The orthotopic inoculation in bladder of MB49 or MB49-I generates non-muscle invasive or muscle invasive tumors respectively.

In our laboratory, following the methodology of Dinney, but with subcutaneous inoculation, we developed a syngeneic murine model that reproduces the human pathology in terms of invasion status. A single cell suspension of the MB49 cell line was inoculated subcutaneously in the flank of syngeneic C57BL/6J mice. After 24 days, tumors were surgically removed and 2-mm tumor pieces were transplanted by trocar into the left flank of mice. This process was repeated 13 consecutive times. We found that the growth rate was increased in transplants #6 to #10 and then became stable. Therefore, primary culture from transplant #13 was carried out and the cell line originated was named MB49-I. The orthotopic inoculation of MB49 or MB49-I in the bladder generates non-muscle invasive or muscle invasive tumors respectively (Figure 6).

This new line has more aggressive characteristics. The MB49-I cell line has higher activity of the MMP-9, uPA and CB as well as increased in vitro invasion of Matrigel ®. Given the association of these enzymes with bladder cancer progression, our model has close similarities to human disease. The histopathological study in vivo showed results consistent with in vivo tests. Intravesical inoculation of MB49 cells was able to develop tumors without muscle invasion. By contrast, inoculation of the MB49-I cell line generated carcinoma with a disorganized structure and larger tumors with cellular atypia, muscle layer invasion and lung metastasis (Figure 7).

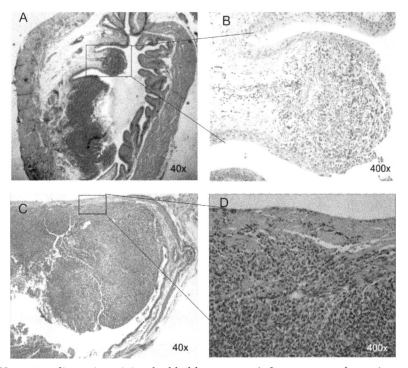

Fig. 7. Haematoxylin-eosin staining for bladder tumors. A: It can see two formations of a tumor of bladder MB49: one sessile and one pedunculated, which do not invade the muscle wall. B: MB49 the polypoid formation is magnified 400X. C: image of a tumor MB49-I, we observe a large tumor invading the muscular layer. D: MB49-I bladder tumor with higher magnification, where the tumor cells are intermingled with the muscle fibers.

Cellular plasticity is a fundamental process during tumor progression. It is now accepted that epithelial-mesenchymal transition is associated with tumor progression. A mark of this transition is the loss of cytokeratin and an increase in vimentin. MB49-I has not only morphological diversity, but also decreased cytokeratin and increased vimentin expression in vitro and in vivo.

Since both the xenogeneic and syngeneic models described here resemble human bladder cancer, they could be useful to study tumor progression, tissue remodeling, and invasive and metastatic processes, and to assay anti-invasive and metastatic agents.

3. Conclusions

Since animal models can reproduce the tumor-host interactions, performing studies using these models is a mandatory step to translate from basic research to the clinic. Taking into account that animal experiments are performed to obtain an improvement for human-health, but must generate a reduced impact on the animals, these experiments should be made according to international rules of bioethics. To accomplish the maximum welfare of the animal, every protocol, indicating the justification of each experiment and the methodology to be used, must be approved by the institutional ethics committee for the use of laboratory animals.

The ideal animal model should meet all the characteristics of the human pathology, such as growth parameters, histology, evolution and metastatic dissemination. However, in the practice, the ideal model does not always have a complete similarity. The researcher must thus decide which model best fits the question to be answered. Alternatively, the researcher can design his/her own model that most closely approaches the point of interest.

The generation of transgenic animals is one of the most developed branches in animal models. Technical refinements have allowed generating genetically modified mice either stable or conditional, making them a valuable tool.

Animal models that mimic human bladder cancer in terms of invasion have also been developed. The use of successive transplants of tumors derived from a cancer cell line can generate invasive bladder tumors. Both the syngeneic and xenogenic invasive models of tumor are useful in the study of tumor progression. Finally, it is important to note that for a better understanding of the tumor mechanism and the relationship with the host, the best models are those, like MB49-I, in which the tumor is inoculated in an orthotopic site.

4. Acknowledgments

This publication was supported by grants from the Consejo Nacional de Investigaciones Científicas y Técnicas (CONICET: www.conicet.gov.ar), and Universidad de Buenos Aires - UBACYT M017 (www.uba.ar). We thank M. Krasnapolsky and D. Belgorosky for their help in preparing the manuscript.

5. References

Ahmad, I.; Morton, J.P.; Singh, L.B.; Radulescu, S.M.; Ridgway, R.A.; Patel, S.; Woodgett, J.; Winton, D.J.; Taketo, M.M.; Wu, X.R.; Leung, H.Y. & Sansom, O.J. (2011). beta-Catenin activation synergizes with PTEN loss to cause bladder cancer formation. *Oncogene*, 30,2, (Jan 13, 2011), 178-89, 1476-5594 (Electronic) 0950-9232 (Linking).

Ayala De La Pena, F.; Kanasaki, K.; Kanasaki, M.; Tangirala, N.; Maeda, G. & Kalluri, R. (2011). Loss of p53 and acquisition of angiogenic microRNA profile is insufficient to facilitate progression of bladder urothelial carcinoma in situ to invasive carcinoma. *J Biol Chem*, (Mar 9, 2011), 1083-351X (Electronic) 0021-9258 (Linking).

Bertucci, F.; Cervera, N. & Birnbaum, D. (2007). A gene signature in breast cancer. *N Engl J Med*, 356,18, (May 3, 2007), 1887-8; author reply 1887-8, 1533-4406 (Electronic) 0028-4793 (Linking).

Bhattacharya, A.; Tang, L.; Li, Y.; Geng, F.; Paonessa, J.D.; Chen, S.C.; Wong, M.K. & Zhang, Y. (2010). Inhibition of bladder cancer development by allyl isothiocyanate. *Carcinogenesis*, 31,2, (Feb, 2010), 281-6, 1460 2180 (Electronic) 0143-3334 (Linking).

Binder, B.R. & Mihaly, J. (2008). The plasminogen activator inhibitor "paradox" in cancer. *Immunol Lett*, 118,2, (Jun 30, 2008), 116-24, 0165-2478 (Print) 0165-2478 (Linking).

Black, P.C. & Dinney, C.P. (2007). Bladder cancer angiogenesis and metastasis--translation from murine model to clinical trial. *Cancer Metastasis Rev*, 26,3-4, (Dec, 2007), 623-34, 0167-7659 (Print) 0167-7659 (Linking).

Black, P.C.; Shetty, A.; Brown, G.A.; Esparza-Coss, E.; Metwalli, A.R.; Agarwal, P.K.; Mcconkey, D.J.; Hazle, J.D. & Dinney, C.P. (2010). Validating bladder cancer xenograft bioluminescence with magnetic resonance imaging: the significance of hypoxia and necrosis. *BJU Int*, 106,11, (Dec, 2010), 1799-804, 1464-410X (Electronic) 1464-4096 (Linking).

Bos, P.D.; Nguyen, D.X. & Massague, J. (2010). Modeling metastasis in the mouse. *Curr Opin Pharmacol*, 10,5, (Oct, 2010), 571-7, 1471-4973 (Electronic) 1471-4892 (Linking).

Chade, D.C.; Andrade, P.M.; Borra, R.C.; Leite, K.R.; Andrade, E.; Villanova, F.E. & Srougi, M. (2008). Histopathological characterization of a syngeneic orthotopic murine bladder cancer model. *Int Braz J Urol*, 34,2, (Mar-Apr, 2008), 220-6; discussion 226-9, 1677-5538 (Print) 1677-5538 (Linking).

Chen, S.C.; Henry, D.O.; Hicks, D.G.; Reczek, P.R. & Wong, M.K. (2009). Intravesical administration of plasminogen activator inhibitor type-1 inhibits in vivo bladder tumor invasion and progression. *J Urol*, 181,1, (Jan, 2009), 336-42, 1527-3792 (Electronic) 0022-5347 (Linking).

Chiang, A.C. & Massague, J. (2008). Molecular basis of metastasis. *N Engl J Med*, 359,26, (Dec 25, 2008), 2814-23, 1533-4406 (Electronic) 0028-4793 (Linking).

Condeelis, J. & Segall, J.E. (2003). Intravital imaging of cell movement in tumours. *Nat Rev Cancer*, 3,12, (Dec, 2003), 921-30, 1474-175X (Print) 1474-175X (Linking).

Crew, J.P.; O'brien, T.; Bradburn, M.; Fuggle, S.; Bicknell, R.; Cranston, D. & Harris, A.L. (1997). Vascular endothelial growth factor is a predictor of relapse and stage progression in superficial bladder cancer. *Cancer Res*, 57,23, (Dec 1, 1997), 5281-5, 0008-5472 (Print) 0008-5472 (Linking).

Davis, D.W.; Inoue, K.; Dinney, C.P.; Hicklin, D.J.; Abbruzzese, J.L. & Mcconkey, D.J. (2004). Regional effects of an antivascular endothelial growth factor receptor monoclonal antibody on receptor phosphorylation and apoptosis in human 253J B-V bladder cancer xenografts. *Cancer Res*, 64,13, (Jul 1, 2004), 4601-10, 0008-5472 (Print) 0008-5472 (Linking).

DeHaven, J.I.; Traynellis, C.; Riggs, D.R.; Ting, E. & Lamm, D.L. (1992). Antibiotic and steroid therapy of massive systemic bacillus Calmette-Guerin toxicity. *J Urol*, 147,3, (Mar, 1992), 738-42, 0022-5347 (Print) 0022-5347 (Linking).

Ding, Y.; Paonessa, J.D.; Randall, K.L.; Argoti, D.; Chen, L.; Vouros, P. & Zhang, Y. (2010). Sulforaphane inhibits 4-aminobiphenyl-induced DNA damage in bladder cells and tissues. *Carcinogenesis*, 31,11, (Nov, 2010), 1999-2003, 1460-2180 (Electronic) 0143-3334 (Linking).

Dinney, C.P.; Fishbeck, R.; Singh, R.K.; Eve, B.; Pathak, S.; Brown, N.; Xie, B.; Fan, D.; Bucana, C.D.; Fidler, I.J. & Et Al. (1995). Isolation and characterization of metastatic variants from human transitional cell carcinoma passaged by orthotopic implantation in athymic nude mice. *J Urol*, 154,4, (Oct, 1995), 1532-8, 0022-5347 (Print) 0022-5347 (Linking).

Durkan, G.C.; Nutt, J.E.; Marsh, C.; Rajjayabun, P.H.; Robinson, M.C.; Neal, D.E.; Lunec, J. & Mellon, J.K. (2003). Alteration in urinary matrix metalloproteinase-9 to tissue inhibitor of metalloproteinase-1 ratio predicts recurrence in nonmuscle-invasive bladder cancer. *Clin Cancer Res*, 9,7, (Jul, 2003), 2576-82, 1078-0432 (Print) 1078-0432 (Linking).

Eijan, A.M.; Sandes, E.O.; Riveros, M.D.; Thompson, S.; Pasik, L.; Mallagrino, H.; Celeste, F. & Casabe, A.R. (2003). High expression of cathepsin B in transitional bladder carcinoma correlates with tumor invasion. *Cancer*, 98,2, (Jul 15, 2003), 262-8, 0008-543X (Print) 0008-543X (Linking).

Eissa, S.; Ali-Labib, R.; Swellam, M.; Bassiony, M.; Tash, F. & El-Zayat, T.M. (2007). Noninvasive diagnosis of bladder cancer by detection of matrix metalloproteinases (MMP-2 and MMP-9) and their inhibitor (TIMP-2) in urine. *Eur Urol*, 52,5, (Nov, 2007), 1388-96, 0302-2838 (Print) 0302-2838 (Linking).

Fidler, I.J. (1986). Rationale and methods for the use of nude mice to study the biology and therapy of human cancer metastasis. *Cancer Metastasis Rev*, 5,1, (1986), 29-49, 0167-7659 (Print) 0167-7659 (Linking).

Fidler, I.J. (1990). Critical factors in the biology of human cancer metastasis: twenty-eighth G.H.A. Clowes memorial award lecture. *Cancer Res*, 50,19, (Oct 1, 1990), 6130-8, 0008-5472 (Print) 0008-5472 (Linking).

Folkman, J. (1986). How is blood vessel growth regulated in normal and neoplastic tissue? G.H.A. Clowes memorial Award lecture. *Cancer Res*, 46,2, (Feb, 1986), 467-73, 0008-5472 (Print) 0008-5472 (Linking).

Ghajar, C.M. & Bissell, M.J. (2008). Extracellular matrix control of mammary gland morphogenesis and tumorigenesis: insights from imaging. *Histochem Cell Biol*, 130,6, (Dec, 2008), 1105-18, 0948-6143 (Print) 0948-6143 (Linking).

Growcott, J.W. (2009). Preclinical anticancer activity of the specific endothelin A receptor antagonist ZD4054. *Anticancer Drugs*, 20,2, (Feb, 2009), 83-8, 1473-5741 (Electronic) 0959-4973 (Linking).

Grubbs, C.J.; Lubet, R.A.; Koki, A.T.; Leahy, K.M.; Masferrer, J.L.; Steele, V.E.; Kelloff, G.J.; Hill, D.L. & Seibert, K. (2000). Celecoxib inhibits N-butyl-N-(4-hydroxybutyl)-nitrosamine-induced urinary bladder cancers in male B6D2F1 mice and female Fischer-344 rats. *Cancer Res*, 60,20, (Oct 15, 2000), 5599-602, 0008-5472 (Print) 0008-5472 (Linking).

Gunther, J.H.; Jurczok, A.; Wulf, T.; Brandau, S.; Deinert, I.; Jocham, D. & Bohle, A. (1999). Optimizing syngeneic orthotopic murine bladder cancer (MB49). *Cancer Res*, 59,12, (Jun 15, 1999), 2834-7, 0008-5472 (Print) 0008-5472 (Linking).

Gupta, G.P.; Nguyen, D.X.; Chiang, A.C.; Bos, P.D.; Kim, J.Y.; Nadal, C.; Gomis, R.R.; Manova-Todorova, K. & Massague, J. (2007). Mediators of vascular remodelling co-opted for sequential steps in lung metastasis. *Nature*, 446,7137, (Apr 12, 2007), 765-70, 1476-4687 (Electronic) 0028-0836 (Linking).

Hadaschik, B.A.; Black, P.C.; Sea, J.C.; Metwalli, A.R.; Fazli, L.; Dinney, C.P.; Gleave, M.E. & So, A.I. (2007). A validated mouse model for orthotopic bladder cancer using transurethral tumour inoculation and bioluminescence imaging. *BJU Int*, 100,6, (Dec, 2007), 1377-84, 1464-410X (Electronic) 1464-4096 (Linking).

He, F.; Mo, L.; Zheng, X.Y.; Hu, C.; Lepor, H.; Lee, E.Y.; Sun, T.T. & Wu, X.R. (2009). Deficiency of pRb family proteins and p53 in invasive urothelial tumorigenesis. *Cancer Res*, 69,24, (Dec 15, 2009), 9413-21, 1538-7445 (Electronic) 0008-5472 (Linking).

Inman, B.A.; Sebo, T.J.; Frigola, X.; Dong, H.; Bergstralh, E.J.; Frank, I.; Fradet, Y.; Lacombe, L. & Kwon, E.D. (2007). PD-L1 (B7-H1) expression by urothelial carcinoma of the bladder and BCG-induced granulomata: associations with localized stage progression. *Cancer*, 109,8, (Apr 15, 2007), 1499-505, 0008-543X (Print) 0008-543X (Linking).

Inoue, K.; Slaton, J.W.; Davis, D.W.; Hicklin, D.J.; Mcconkey, D.J.; Karashima, T.; Radinsky, R. & Dinney, C.P. (2000). Treatment of human metastatic transitional cell carcinoma of the bladder in a murine model with the anti-vascular endothelial growth factor receptor monoclonal antibody DC101 and paclitaxel. *Clin Cancer Res*, 6,7, (Jul, 2000), 2635-43, 1078-0432 (Print) 1078-0432 (Linking).

Jemal, A.; Siegel, R.; Ward, E.; Murray, T.; Xu, J.; Smigal, C. & Thun, M.J. (2006). Cancer statistics, 2006. *CA Cancer J Clin*, 56,2, (Mar-Apr, 2006), 106-30, 0007-9235 (Print) 0007-9235 (Linking).

Joraku, A.; Homhuan, A.; Kawai, K.; Yamamoto, T.; Miyazaki, J.; Kogure, K.; Yano, I.; Harashima, H. & Akaza, H. (2009). Immunoprotection against murine bladder carcinoma by octaarginine-modified liposomes incorporating cell wall of Mycobacterium bovis bacillus Calmette-Guerin. *BJU Int*, 103,5, (Mar, 2009), 686-93, 1464-410X (Electronic) 1464-4096 (Linking).

Kim, S.; Park, H.S.; Son, H.J. & Moon, W.S. (2004). [The role of angiostatin, vascular endothelial growth factor, matrix metalloproteinase 9 and 12 in the angiogenesis of hepatocellular carcinoma]. *Korean J Hepatol*, 10,1, (Mar, 2004), 62-72, 1738-222X (Print) 1738-222X (Linking).

Klein, C.A. (2009). Parallel progression of primary tumours and metastases. *Nat Rev Cancer*, 9,4, (Apr, 2009), 302-12, 1474-1768 (Electronic) 1474-175X (Linking).

Kortylewski, M.; Xin, H.; Kujawski, M.; Lee, H.; Liu, Y.; Harris, T.; Drake, C.; Pardoll, D. & Yu, H. (2009). Regulation of the IL-23 and IL-12 balance by Stat3 signaling in the tumor microenvironment. *Cancer Cell*, 15,2, (Feb 3, 2009), 114-23, 1878-3686 (Electronic) 1535-6108 (Linking).

Kumar, B.; Koul, S.; Petersen, J.; Khandrika, L.; Hwa, J.S.; Meacham, R.B.; Wilson, S. & Koul, H.K. (2010). p38 mitogen-activated protein kinase-driven MAPKAPK2 regulates invasion of bladder cancer by modulation of MMP-2 and MMP-9 activity. *Cancer Res*, 70,2, (Jan 15, 2010), 832-41, 1538-7445 (Electronic) 0008-5472 (Linking).

Langowski, J.L.; Zhang, X.; Wu, L.; Mattson, J.D.; Chen, T.; Smith, K.; Basham, B.; Mcclanahan, T.; Kastelein, R.A. & Oft, M. (2006). IL-23 promotes tumour incidence and growth. *Nature*, 442,7101, (Jul 27, 2006), 461-5, 1476-4687 (Electronic) 0028-0836 (Linking).

Lerner, S.P. (2005). Bladder cancer clinical trials. *Urol Oncol*, 23,4, (Jul-Aug, 2005), 275-9, 1078-1439 (Print) 1078-1439 (Linking).

Liotta, L.A.; Steeg, P.S. & Stetler-Stevenson, W.G. (1991). Cancer metastasis and angiogenesis: an imbalance of positive and negative regulation. *Cell*, 64,2, (Jan 25, 1991), 327-36, 0092-8674 (Print) 0092-8674 (Linking).

Lodillinsky, C.; Langle, Y.; Guionet, A.; Gongora, A.; Baldi, A.; Sandes, E.O.; Casabe, A. & Eijan, A.M. (2010). Bacillus Calmette Guerin induces fibroblast activation both directly and through macrophages in a mouse bladder cancer model. *PLoS One*, 5,10, 2010), e13571, 1932-6203 (Electronic) 1932-6203 (Linking).

Lodillinsky, C.; Rodriguez, V.; Vauthay, L.; Sandes, E.; Casabe, A. & Eijan, A.M. (2009). Novel invasive orthotopic bladder cancer model with high cathepsin B activity resembling human bladder cancer. *J Urol*, 182,2, (Aug, 2009), 749-55, 1527-3792 (Electronic) 0022-5347 (Linking).

Lopez-Beltran, A. & Montironi, R. (2004). Non-invasive urothelial neoplasms: according to the most recent WHO classification. *Eur Urol*, 46,2, (Aug, 2004), 170-6, 0302-2838 (Print) 0302-2838 (Linking).

Lu, Y.; Liu, P.; Wen, W.; Grubbs, C.J.; Townsend, R.R.; Malone, J.P.; Lubet, R.A. & You, M. (2010). Cross-species comparison of orthologous gene expression in human bladder cancer and carcinogen-induced rodent models. *Am J Transl Res*, 3,1, (2010), 8-27, 1943-8141 (Electronic)

Lubet, R.A.; Huebner, K.; Fong, L.Y.; Altieri, D.C.; Steele, V.E.; Kopelovich, L.; Kavanaugh, C.; Juliana, M.M.; Soong, S.J. & Grubbs, C.J. (2005). 4-Hydroxybutyl(butyl)nitrosamine-induced urinary bladder cancers in mice: characterization of FHIT and survivin expression and chemopreventive effects of indomethacin. *Carcinogenesis*, 26,3, (Mar, 2005), 571-8, 0143-3334 (Print) 0143-3334 (Linking).

Mangsbo, S.M.; Sandin, L.C.; Anger, K.; Korman, A.J.; Loskog, A. & Totterman, T.H. (2010). Enhanced tumor eradication by combining CTLA-4 or PD-1 blockade with CpG therapy. *J Immunother*, 33,3, (Apr, 2010), 225-35, 1537-4513 (Electronic) 1524-9557 (Linking).

McConkey, D.J.; Choi, W.; Marquis, L.; Martin, F.; Williams, M.B.; Shah, J.; Svatek, R.; Das, A.; Adam, L.; Kamat, A.; Siefker-Radtke, A. & Dinney, C. (2009). Role of epithelial-to-mesenchymal transition (EMT) in drug sensitivity and metastasis in bladder cancer. *Cancer Metastasis Rev*, 28,3-4, (Dec, 2009), 335-44, 1573-7233 (Electronic) 0167-7659 (Linking).

Menon, M.B.; Ronkina, N.; Schwermann, J.; Kotlyarov, A. & Gaestel, M. (2009). Fluorescence-based quantitative scratch wound healing assay demonstrating the role of MAPKAPK-2/3 in fibroblast migration. *Cell Motil Cytoskeleton*, 66,12, (Dec, 2009), 1041-7, 1097-0169 (Electronic) 0886-1544 (Linking).

Mo, L.; Cheng, J.; Lee, E.Y.; Sun, T.T. & Wu, X.R. (2005). Gene deletion in urothelium by specific expression of Cre recombinase. *Am J Physiol Renal Physiol*, 289,3, (Sep, 2005), F562-8, 1931-857X (Print)

Montironi, R. & Lopez-Beltran, A. (2005). The 2004 WHO classification of bladder tumors: a summary and commentary. *Int J Surg Pathol*, 13,2, (Apr, 2005), 143-53, 1066-8969 (Print) 1066-8969 (Linking).

Morales, A.; Eidinger, D. & Bruce, A.W. (1976). Intracavitary Bacillus Calmette-Guerin in the treatment of superficial bladder tumors. *J Urol*, 116,2, (Aug, 1976), 180-3, 0022-5347 (Print) 0022-5347 (Linking).

Nakanishi, J.; Wada, Y.; Matsumoto, K.; Azuma, M.; Kikuchi, K. & Ueda, S. (2007). Overexpression of B7-H1 (PD-L1) significantly associates with tumor grade and postoperative prognosis in human urothelial cancers. *Cancer Immunol Immunother*, 56,8, (Aug, 2007), 1173-82, 0340-7004 (Print) 0340-7004 (Linking).

Nguyen, D.X. & Massague, J. (2007). Genetic determinants of cancer metastasis. *Nat Rev Genet*, 8,5, (May, 2007), 341-52, 1471-0056 (Print) 1471-0056 (Linking).

O'Brien, T.; Cranston, D.; Fuggle, S.; Bicknell, R. & Harris, A.L. (1995). Different angiogenic pathways characterize superficial and invasive bladder cancer. *Cancer Res*, 55,3, (Feb 1, 1995), 510-3, 0008-5472 (Print) 0008-5472 (Linking).

Papathoma, A.S.; Petraki, C.; Grigorakis, A.; Papakonstantinou, H.; Karavana, V.; Stefanakis, S.; Sotsiou, F. & Pintzas, A. (2000). Prognostic significance of matrix metalloproteinases 2 and 9 in bladder cancer. *Anticancer Res*, 20,3B, (May-Jun, 2000), 2009-13, 0250-7005 (Print) 0250-7005 (Linking).

Peinado, H.; Olmeda, D. & Cano, A. (2007). Snail, Zeb and bHLH factors in tumour progression: an alliance against the epithelial phenotype? *Nat Rev Cancer*, 7,6, (Jun, 2007), 415-28, 1474-175X (Print) 1474-175X (Linking).

Pfost, B.; Seidl, C.; Autenrieth, M.; Saur, D.; Bruchertseifer, F.; Morgenstern, A.; Schwaiger, M. & Senekowitsch-Schmidtke, R. (2009). Intravesical alpha-radioimmunotherapy with ^{213}Bi-anti-EGFR-mAb defeats human bladder carcinoma in xenografted nude mice. *J Nucl Med*, 50,10, (Oct, 2009), 1700-8, 1535-5667 (Electronic) 0161-5505 (Linking).

Riemensberger, J.; Bohle, A. & Brandau, S. (2002). IFN-gamma and IL-12 but not IL-10 are required for local tumour surveillance in a syngeneic model of orthotopic bladder cancer. *Clin Exp Immunol*, 127,1, (Jan, 2002), 20-6, 0009-9104 (Print) 0009-9104 (Linking).

Sandes, E.; Lodillinsky, C.; Cwirenbaum, R.; Arguelles, C.; Casabe, A. & Eijan, A.M. (2007). Cathepsin B is involved in the apoptosis intrinsic pathway induced by Bacillus Calmette-Guerin in transitional cancer cell lines. *Int J Mol Med*, 20,6, (Dec, 2007), 823-8, 1107-3756 (Print) 1107-3756 (Linking).

Smaldone, M.C.; Gayed, B.A.; Tomaszewski, J.J. & Gingrich, J.R. (2009). Strategies to enhance the efficacy of intravescical therapy for non-muscle invasive bladder cancer. *Minerva Urol Nefrol*, 61,2, (Jun, 2009), 71-89, 0393-2249 (Print) 0393-2249 (Linking).

Sobin, L.H. & Fleming, I.D. (1997). TNM Classification of Malignant Tumors, fifth edition (1997). Union Internationale Contre le Cancer and the American Joint Committee on Cancer. *Cancer*, 80,9, (Nov 1, 1997), 1803-4, 0008-543X (Print) 0008-543X (Linking).

Steeg, P.S. (2006). Tumor metastasis: mechanistic insights and clinical challenges. *Nat Med*, 12,8, (Aug, 2006), 895-904, 1078-8956 (Print) 1078-8956 (Linking).

Steele, V.E. & Lubet, R.A. (2010). The use of animal models for cancer chemoprevention drug development. *Semin Oncol*, 37,4, (Aug, 2010), 327-38, 1532-8708 (Electronic) 0093-7754 (Linking).

Steele, V.E.; Rao, C.V.; Zhang, Y.; Patlolla, J.; Boring, D.; Kopelovich, L.; Juliana, M.M.; Grubbs, C.J. & Lubet, R.A. (2009). Chemopreventive efficacy of naproxen and nitric oxide-naproxen in rodent models of colon, urinary bladder, and mammary cancers. *Cancer Prev Res (Phila)*, 2,11, (Nov, 2009), 951-6, 1940-6215 (Electronic) 1940-6215 (Linking).

Sugano, G.; Bernard-Pierrot, I.; Lae, M.; Battail, C.; Allory, Y.; Stransky, N.; Krumeich, S.; Lepage, M.L.; Maille, P.; Donnadieu, M.H.; Abbou, C.C.; Benhamou, S.; Lebret, T.; Sastre-Garau, X.; Amigorena, S.; Radvanyi, F. & Thery, C. (2011). Milk fat globule--epidermal growth factor--factor VIII (MFGE8)/lactadherin promotes bladder tumor development. *Oncogene*, 30,6, (Feb 10, 2011), 642-53, 1476-5594 (Electronic) 0950-9232 (Linking).

Sylvester, R.J. (2009). Bacillus Calmette-Guerin versus mitomycin C for the treatment of intermediate-risk non-muscle-invasive bladder cancer: the debate continues. *Eur Urol*, 56,2, (Aug, 2009), 266-8; discussion 268-9, 1873-7560 (Electronic) 0302-2838 (Linking).

Takeuchi, A.; Dejima, T.; Yamada, H.; Shibata, K.; Nakamura, R.; Eto, M.; Nakatani, T.; Naito, S. & Yoshikai, Y. (2011). IL-17 production by gammadelta T cells is important for the antitumor effect of Mycobacterium bovis bacillus Calmette-Guerin treatment against bladder cancer. *Eur J Immunol*, 41,1, (Jan, 2011), 246-51, 1521-4141 (Electronic) 0014-2980 (Linking).

Tanaka, M.; Gee, J.R.; De La Cerda, J.; Rosser, C.J.; Zhou, J.H.; Benedict, W.F. & Grossman, H.B. (2003). Noninvasive detection of bladder cancer in an orthotopic murine model with green fluorescence protein cytology. *J Urol*, 170,3, (Sep, 2003), 975-8, 0022-5347 (Print) 0022-5347 (Linking).

Valastyan, S.; Reinhardt, F.; Benaich, N.; Calogrias, D.; Szasz, A.M.; Wang, Z.C.; Brock, J.E.; Richardson, A.L. & Weinberg, R.A. (2009). A pleiotropically acting microRNA, miR-31, inhibits breast cancer metastasis. *Cell*, 137,6, (Jun 12, 2009), 1032-46, 1097-4172 (Electronic) 0092-8674 (Linking).

Van 'T Veer, L.J.; Dai, H.; Van De Vijver, M.J.; He, Y.D.; Hart, A.A.; Mao, M.; Peterse, H.L.; Van Der Kooy, K.; Marton, M.J.; Witteveen, A.T.; Schreiber, G.J.; Kerkhoven, R.M.; Roberts, C.; Linsley, P.S.; Bernards, R. & Friend, S.H. (2002). Gene expression profiling predicts clinical outcome of breast cancer. *Nature*, 415,6871, (Jan 31, 2002), 530-6, 0028-0836 (Print) 0028-0836 (Linking).

Varley, C.L. & Southgate, J. (2011). Organotypic and 3D reconstructed cultures of the human bladder and urinary tract. *Methods Mol Biol*, 695, (2011), 197-211, 1940-6029 (Electronic) 1064-3745 (Linking).

Wang, L.; Yi, T.; Kortylewski, M.; Pardoll, D.M.; Zeng, D. & Yu, H. (2009). IL-17 can promote tumor growth through an IL-6-Stat3 signaling pathway. *J Exp Med*, 206,7, (Jul 6, 2009), 1457-64, 1540-9538 (Electronic) 0022-1007 (Linking).

Wu, Z.; Owens, C.; Chandra, N.; Popovic, K.; Conaway, M. & Theodorescu, D. (2010). RalBP1 is necessary for metastasis of human cancer cell lines. *Neoplasia*, 12,12, (Dec, 2010), 1003-12, 1476-5586 (Electronic) 1476-5586 (Linking).

Yao, R.; Lemon, W.J.; Wang, Y.; Grubbs, C.J.; Lubet, R.A. & You, M. (2004). Altered gene expression profile in mouse bladder cancers induced by hydroxybutyl (butyl) nitrosamine. *Neoplasia*, 6,5, (Sep-Oct, 2004), 569-77, 1522-8002 (Print) 1476-5586 (Linking).

Zhang, Z.; Xu, X.; Zhang, X.; Chen, X.; Chen, Q.; Dong, L.; Hu, Z.; Li, J. & Gao, J. (2011). The therapeutic potential of SA-sCD40L in the orthotopic model of superficial bladder cancer. *Acta Oncol*, (Jan 19, 2011), 1651-226X (Electronic) 0284-186X (Linking).

Zhang, Z.T.; Pak, J.; Huang, H.Y.; Shapiro, E.; Sun, T.T.; Pellicer, A. & Wu, X.R. (2001). Role of Ha-ras activation in superficial papillary pathway of urothelial tumor formation. *Oncogene*, 20,16, (Apr 12, 2001), 1973-80, 0950-9232 (Print) 0950-9232 (Linking).

Part 6

Chemoprevention

11

Chemoprevention and Novel Treatments of Non-Muscle Invasive Bladder Cancer

Adam Luchey, Morris Jessop, Claire Oliver, Dale Riggs,
Barbara Jackson, Stanley Kandzari and Stanley Zaslau
Division of Urology
West Virginia University
Morgantown, WV,
USA

1. Introduction

The Cancer Journal for Clinicians reports there will be 69,250 newly diagnosed cases of bladder cancer in 2011, with 52,020 being men and 17,230 being women with an increase by 50% of annual cases since 1985. Approximately 1 in 5 of those who develop bladder cancer will die due to the disease (relative mortality 20.8%, [Siegel et al., 2011, Golijanin et al., 2006]). Bladder cancer has become the second most prevalent cancer after cancer of the prostate in middle-aged to elderly male individuals. Many patients do not die from their disease, but typically have multiple recurrences (Pelucchi et al., 2006). This lends to a five-year cost to Medicare attributed to bladder cancer of over one billion dollars (Yabroff et al., 2008). Tobacco use and exposure to aromatic amines are well established etiologic contributors to bladder cancer and by eliminating or reducing contact with these substances has been shown to reduce such risk.

BCG (bacillus Calmette-Guerin) has become the standard of care in the treatment of carcinoma in situ as well as high grade T1 (invasion into the lamina propria) and when not appropriate, Mitomycin-C, has been proven to be an acceptable, albeit, less effective alternate. The goal of this chapter will be to describe novel agents that may show promise in the treatment of bladder cancer. This will include descriptions of the agents, their respective mechanism of action (e.g. molecular/biochemical pathways, cell cycle interaction, necrosis), clinical data, combinations of combinations of regimens and mode of delivery. and mode of delivery. A second goal of this chapter will be to consider whether any of these novel agents may have a role in the prevention of bladder cancer.

2. Chemoprevention

Kamat in his review of superficial bladder cancer stated that chemoprevention is needed for a multitude of reasons: high recurrence rates, increased morbidity from repeat resections, a tedious course of disease to see treatment outcomes, ability of agents to be concentrated in the urine, and the ability to monitor recurrence with cytology/cystoscopy (Kamat, 2003). Table 1 lists potential agents that may be considered for chemoprevention of bladder cancer.

POTENTIAL CHEMOPREVENTION AGENTS
• Vitamin A
• Vitamin E
• Vitamin C
• Selenium
• Cactus Pear
• Isoflavones
• Garlic
• Green Tea
• Difluoromethlyornithine (DFMO)
• Non-Steroidal Anti-Inflammatory Drugs
• Statins

Table 1. Potential Chemoprevention agents for Bladder Cancer

2.1 Vitamin A

Vitamin A is necessary for light absorption in the retina and is also known to have a role in epithelial growth. Additionally, vitamin A has been researched as a chemotherapeutic and chemopreventive agent for a variety of malignancies. Currently, it is utilized to treat acute promyelocytic leukemia (Zusi et al., 2002). The mechanism of vitamin A's inhibition of tumor growth is thought to work through modulation of gene expression in cell growth, differentiation, and apoptosis (Zanardi et al., 2006). Evidence suggests that it does this through a variety of molecular pathways including binding to nuclear retinoic acid receptors (RAR) and ligand activating transcription factors such as retinoid X receptors (RXR) (Simeone & Tari, 2004). Additionally, vitamin A's anti-tumor activity may involve, among others, interactions with growth factors and cytokines, neoplastic stem cell pathways such as WNT, cAMP pathways, mitogen activated protein kinases (MAPKs), PI3K/AKT, cyclin-dependent kinases (CDKs), protein kinase C, and epigenetic modulation of gene expression (Garattini et al., 2007). Other studies indicate that some synthetic retinoids may even reduce VEGF expression, which is an important angiogenic factor in bladder cancer growth (Hameed & el-Metwally, 2008).

Several studies have examined vitamin A and its derivatives for chemoprevention of bladder cancer. The first clinical trial was performed in 1978 (Gunby, 1978) and was followed by several other prospective and controlled trials. Results for these trials were mixed, with some showing significant preventative effects (Alfthan et al., 1983; Studer et al., 1995; Yoshida et al., 1986) and others showing less promising results (Decensi et al., 2000; Prout & Barton, 1992). Mild to severe toxicities were also noted in many of these studies and may potentially limit vitamin A's use as a chemopreventive agent (Hameed & el-Metwally, 2008). More recently, to enable lower doses of retinoic acids and decrease unwanted side effects, combinations of retinoic acid and inhibitors of the CYP26A enzyme (involved in degradation of vitamin A) have been explored with some success (Hameed & el-Metwally, 2008). Although a recent cohort study showed no significant association of several vitamins including retinoids with urothelial carcinoma risk (Hotaling et al., 2011), other past studies provide some compelling evidence for vitamin A's efficacy. Thus further research into vitamin A's use in preventing bladder cancer is warranted.

2.2 Vitamin E

Vitamin E is a lipid soluble anti-oxidant and is known to be important in a variety of biological processes. It is also thought to possibly lower the risk of many malignancies through free radical scavenging, inhibition of N-nitroso compound formation (Mirvish, 1995), immunological stimulation (Beisel et al., 1981), and potent induction of apoptosis (Kline et al., 2004; Sigounas et al., 1997).

The clinical evidence for vitamin E in bladder cancer prevention has mixed results. A large Cohort study with Vitamin E and C and risk of bladder cancer mortality showed a reduced risk of mortality with regular intake of vitamin E (Jacobs et al., 2002). A phase III clinical trial using megadoses of several vitamins including E, when compared to patients who just received the recommended daily allowance (RDA) of the same vitamins, had a 40% reduction in bladder tumor recurrence after the first 10 months of the study (Lamm et al., 1994). However, in this same study, patients also received BCG therapy, which is known to promote immune response to tumors and may have confounded the results (Coulter et al, 2006). Further support comes from a prospective study, which showed an inverse relationship between vitamin E supplement consumption and the risk of bladder malignancy in men (Michaud et al., 2000).

In contrast to studies supporting vitamin E, a recent cohort study suggested no association of vitamin E intake and risk of urothelial carcinoma (Roswall et al., 2009). In addition, a meta-analysis for vitamin E and C intake and prevention of cancer indicated overall poor evidence for vitamin E in reduction of bladder cancer recurrence (Coulter et al, 2006). Additionally, a recently published cohort study indicated that the use of a variety of vitamins and supplements including vitamin E had no significant association with urothelial carcinoma risk in age-adjusted or multi-variate models (Hotaling et al., 2011). It should be noted that several studies have indicated that high doses of vitamin E may actually increase the risk for bladder cancer (The New England Journal of Medicine [NEJM], 1994; Miller et al., 2005). Since the evidence for vitamin E as a chemopreventive agent is conflicting, further studies should be performed to assess its true value.

2.3 Vitamin C

Vitamin C is an important vitamin found abundantly in fruits and vegetables. Proven to be a powerful antioxidant and necessary for a variety of metabolic activities, vitamin C consumption has also been researched as a method to reduce the risk of bladder cancer. It is hypothesized that vitamin C's anti-tumor activity is derived from inhibition of p53-induced replicative senescence, by suppressing both reactive oxygen species production and p38 MAPK activity (Kim et al., 2008), and sparing vitamin E to jointly reduce reactive α-tocopheroxy radicals (Park et al., 2010). Malignant transformation may also be decreased by vitamin C through reduction of N-nitroso compounds, which are known to be carcinogenic (Wu et al., 2000).

Despite these mechanisms proposed, data to support vitamin C as a chemopreventive agent is conflicting. A cohort study using data from 1981-1989 showed a significant reduction in relative risk for bladder cancer in patients taking vitamin C (Shibata et al., 1992). A more recent prospective study found a strong inverse relationship between vitamin C intake and bladder cancer risk in ex-smokers and non-smokers, but did not show the same results with current smokers (Michaud et al., 2000). High doses of vitamin C in combination with megadoses of vitamins A, B6, E and zinc were also found to be beneficial, in combination with BCG therapy, in a phase III trial of Bladder cancer (Lamm et al., 1994). However, as mentioned earlier with Vitamin E, the results in this study may in part be confounded by BCG therapy (Coulter et al., 2006).

Other studies suggest less promising evidence. In a large cohort study of U.S. men and women, no associations were found between vitamin C use and bladder cancer death (Jacobs et al., 2002). This data is consistent with a cohort study by Hotaling et al. indicating the same relationship (Hotaling et al., 2011). A recent prospective study showed no significant effect of vitamin C, E or folate on prevention of urothelial carcinoma (Roswall et al., 2009) and there is evidence that doses of vitamin C beyond the RDA may contribute to oxalate stone formation (Taylor et al., 2004) and may even induce bladder carcinogenic activity (Mirvish, 1986). These studies indicating poor support for vitamin C's use, along with other studies supporting vitamin C as a bladder cancer chemopreventive agent, indicate that further investigation into vitamin C and bladder cancer prevention is required.

2.4 Selenium

An essential micronutrient that is primarily known for its function as a co-factor for reduction of antioxidant enzymes, selenium is also being researched for its potential in reducing the risk of several malignancies including bladder cancer (Silberstein & Parsons, 2010). A variety of mechanisms have been proposed for selenium's anti-tumor activity: free radical scavenging (Murawaki et al., 2008), modifying thiols, mimiching mimicking methionine methionine which leads to to higher methylating efficiency of RNA and thiols (Jackson & Combs, 2008), enhancement of p53 activity towards DNA repair or apoptosis (Smith et al., 2004) and anti-androgenic activity, which is especially relevant in prostate cancer (Husbeck et al., 2006; Gazi et al., 2007).

The clinical evidence for selenium's anti bladder cancer activity is somewhat controversial. A recent meta-analysis from seven epidemiological studies showed that the overall risk of bladder cancer was inversely associated with elevated levels of selenium in serum and toenail samples, with the greatest effect seen in women (Amaral et al., 2010). Additionally, Wallace et al. showed no association of selenium levels in toenail samples with bladder cancer, it did find a significant association with moderate smokers and p53 positive cancers, suggesting selenium may affect the risk of bladder malignancies with specific p53 immunophenotypes (Wallace et al., 2009). This was further demonstrated in a case control study performed in Belgium that showed an inverse association between serum selenium concentrations and bladder cancer risk (Kellen et al., 2006).

In contrast to studies supporting selenium, a recent cohort study mentioned earlier, showed no significant association with selenium and urothelial carcinoma risk in an age-adjusted or multi-variate models (Hotaling et al., 2011). Current literature reviewed, there is a lack of interventional studies examining selenium and bladder cancer risk (Silberstein & Parsons, 2010).

2.5 Cactus pear

Cactus fruit, or prickly pear, is a fruit generally used as a dietary supplement and has been widely researched for its anti-oxidant effects (Fernández-López et al., 2010; Tesoriere et al., 2004; Zou et al., 2005). These fruits have a variety of ingredients shown to have health benefits including phenolics, flavonoids, and betalains. Recently, cactus pear has also been studied for a possible application in cancer prevention. Although the mechanism is not completely understood, a recent study suggests it might be through increasing expression of annexin IV, a Ca2+ dependent membrane-binding protein important in apoptosis (Zou et al., 2005). Additionally, cactus pear extracts have been proposed to promote immune response and to decrease expression of VEGF (Liang et al., 2008), an important angiogenic factor in bladder and other malignancies (Zou et al., 2005).

Despite the proposed mechanisms, data supporting cactus pear for prevention of bladder cancer is limited, although some data exists to support use in other types of cancer. In a 2005 study, Arizona prickly cactus pear solution inhibited tumor growth in several different cancer cell cultures including ovarian and cervical (Zou et al., 2005). In another study, polysaccharides extracted from cactus pear fruit limited growth of S180 (sarcoma model) tumor cells in mice and induced features of apoptosis (Liang et al., 2008). In a 2010 study, cactus pear extracts induced reactive oxygen species production and apoptosis in ovarian cancer cells (Feugang et al., 2010). A specific species of cactus pear, Opuntia humifusa, was found to inhibit human glioblastoma cell lines (Hahm et al., 2010). Another study examining nine cactus pear species against prostate, colon, hepatic and mammary cancer cell lines showed some cytotoxic activity with certain species (Chavez-Santoscoy et al., 2009). However, normal fibroblast controls were also affected in this study with some of the pear species, thus the conclusions of this study are limited. More research, especially studies utilizing bladder cancer models, are necessary to determine the true potential of cactus pear as a chemopreventative agent for bladder cancer.

2.6 Isoflavones

Isoflavones are naturally occurring compounds found in soy and other products. They are primarily known for their phytoestrogen and anti-oxidant properties, although recent research has suggested they may also help in cancer prevention. Currently, isoflavones have shown at least some promise in preventing several types of cancers including but not limited to bladder, prostate (Yan & Spitznagel, 2005), breast (Bondesson & Gustafsson, 2010), lung (Hess & Igal, 2011), and liver (Ma et al., 2010).

Multiple mechanisms for this anti-tumor activity have been proposed. Several in vitro studies suggest that isoflavones may induce G2-M cycle arrest, apoptosis, and angiogenesis (Su et al., 2000; Zhou et al., 1998). Another study found that a possible mitochondrial mediated apoptosis pathway through regulation of AKT and MAPK pathways (Lin et al., 2010). Much of the research has focused on the specific isoflavone genistein, which has been shown to inhibit cancer through a variety of pathways. One study showed genistein inhibited EGF-R and EGF, of which the quantity and distribution are associated with urothelial abnormalities (Theodorescu et al., 1998). Another study on genistein showed that it might down regulate COX-2 (Hwang et al., 2009), which has been shown to play a role in tumorigenesis. A 2006 study indicated genistein down regulates nuclear factor kappa-B in bladder tumor tissue and reduces circulating insulin-like growth factor-1 levels, both important in tumor metastasis (Singh et al., 2006). Another more recent study showed that genistein modulates chromatin configuration and DNA methylation, thus activating tumor-suppressing genes (Zhang & Chen, 2011).

The clinical data for isoflavones as chemopreventive agents in bladder cancer has mixed results. In a 2000 study using seven human cancer cell lines, the isoflavone genistein significantly decreased bladder cancer cell growth and two other isoflavones directly induced apoptosis (Su et al., 2000). Another study examining the effect of soy phytochemicals on poorly differentiated and highly metastatic human bladder cancer cell lines in vitro showed significant inhibition by cell cycle arrest in G2-M phases in addition to significant apoptosis (Singh et al., 2006). This same study also showed significant inhibition of clinically relevant orthotopic bladder tumor models by induction of tumor cell apoptosis and reduction of tumor angiogenesis. A study examining the effects of 13-Methyltetradecanoic acid (13-MTD), a soy fermentation product, on human bladder cancer cells found that 13-MTD induced apoptosis (Lin et al., 2010). In contrast to evidence supporting use, epidemiological studies have suggested an increased risk for bladder cancer with consumption of soy (Brinkman & Zeegers, 2008). Since the evidence is contradictory, more research needs to be performed into the potential of soy and soy products to act as chemopreventive agents.

2.7 Garlic

Garlic is considered both a food and supplement with medicinal properties. Extensive research has been performed into the health benefits of garlic and more recently garlic has been examined for cancer prevention. Studies suggest it may induce or prevent suppression of the immune response (Miroddi et al., 2011), induce cytokine production (Lamm & Riggs, 2000), scavenge free radicals (Butt et al., 2009), and bind thiol compounds important in crucial regulatory functions (Cerella et al., 2011). Numerous other mechanisms have also been proposed for specific components of garlic supported by in vitro studies (Shukla & Kaira, 2007).

Although many studies provide evidence of the anti-tumor activity of garlic on other types of cancer (Shukla & Kaira, 2007), research into garlic's anti-tumorigenic properties for prevention of bladder cancer is relatively sparse. A 1986 study using urothelial cancer lines in transplanted into the hind legs of mice, found a therapeutic effect of garlic when intraperitoneally injected (Lau et al., 1986). Another later study found a significant anti-tumor efficacy of garlic when given orally and subcutaneously in mice with injected urothelial carcinoma (Riggs et al., 1997).

Although some studies support the use of garlic, others fail to support garlic or garlic derivatives for chemoprevention of bladder cancer. In a 1993 study, diallyl sulfide, a primary component of garlic, failed to prevent the formation of urinary bladder papillomas in a rat model (Hadjiolov et al., 1993). A recently published cohort study indicated that the use of a variety of vitamins and supplements, including garlic, had no significant association with risk of urothelial carcinoma when adjusted for age and in multi-variate models (Hotaling et al., 2011). Due to these mixed results and lack of clinical studies, further research is needed into garlic and its potential as a chemopreventive agent for bladder cancer.

2.8 Green tea

Green tea is a widely consumed supplement worldwide with a variety of ingredients that have been researched for their health benefits. One application may be for cancer chemoprevention. Green tea has shown inhibitory activity on a variety of tumors in animal models including skin, lung, oral cavity, esophagus, stomach, intestine, colon, liver, pancreas, mammary gland, prostate, and bladder cancers (Lubet et al., 2007; Yang et al., 2011). Several mechanisms have been proposed. For example, one ingredient, polyphenols, has been shown to have antioxidant properties and may prevent cancer through neutralization of free radicals (Forester & Lambert, 2011). Polyphenols also block ornithine decarboxylase (Messing et al., 1987), which is a key enzyme in polyamine synthesis and plays a major role in cell division and proliferation (Pegg, 2006). Another ingredient, catechins, may exhibit anti-tumor activity through inhibition of nitrosamine formations and decreased chromosomal damage (Kamori et al., 1993). Additional research on green tea suggests other possible mechanisms for a variety of its ingredients including caspase mediation (Oz & Ebersole, 2010), inhibition of angiogenesis (Tsao et al., 2009), and others.

Evidence for green tea in prevention of bladder cancer is variable. In rat models, green tea reduced bladder tumor incidence in several studies (Lubet et al., 2007; Sato, 1999; Sato & Matsushima, 2003). Additionally, great tea mixture modulated actin remodeling (through Rho activity) in an in vitro human bladder cancer model of non-transformed urothelial cell lines as well as reducing tumor growth (Lu et al., 2005). Since malignant cells require actin remodeling in a variety of malignant behaviors (altering morphology, loss of cohesion, invasiveness), this study may point out an additional mechanism for green tea's potential to inhibit bladder cancer (Lu et al., 2005). However, a recent review of the literature suggests caution promoting green tea as a chemopreventative agent for bladder cancer due to conflicting evidence (Boehm et al., 2009), citing two studies that either showed no association (Chyou et al., 1993) or an increased risk of developing bladder cancer (Wakai et al., 2004).

2.9 Difluoromethylornithine (DFMO)

Although originally tested for prevention of bladder and renal cancers (Dunzendorfer, 1981), Difluoromethylornithine (DFMO) is a drug primarily used for the treatment of hirsutism and trypanosomiasis (African sleeping sickness). Recently, there has been renewed interest in using DFMO to prevent a variety of malignancies, including bladder cancer. Although DFMO's mechanism of cancer prevention is not completely understood, it is well established as an irreversible inhibitor of ornithine decarboxylase, which plays a role in cell division and proliferation (Kelloff et al., 1994). A recent study showed that DFMO, when combined with sulindac (an NSAID), significantly reduced the risk of recurring colorectal polyps (Meyskens et al., 2008). Another controlled phase III clinical trial showed that DFMO might reduce the recurrence of basal cell carcinoma (Balley et al., 2010). In addition, DFMO is currently being researched in prevention of esophageal cancer (Sinicrope et al., 2011) and breast cancer (Izbicka et al., 2010). However, past studies assessing DFMO's possible efficacy in reducing recurring bladder cancer have mixed results. Initial studies using DFMO to suppress malignant urothelial cells from human cell lines (Messing et al., 1988) as well as suppressing BBN-induced urothelial carcinoma in mice (Boon et al., 1990) demonstrated selective inhibition of malignant cells. However, a recent controlled phase III clinical trial showed no difference in bladder tumor recurrence rates between placebo and DFMO treated patients (Messing et al., 2006). Due to the variable results, further research into DFMO as a chemopreventive agent in bladder cancer is recommended.

2.10 Non-steroidal anti-inflammatory drugs

NSAIDs, well known for their anti-inflammatory abilities, have also been recently proposed as chemopreventative agents. Studies suggest that cyclooxygenase enzymes may have a key role in carcinogenesis, thus inhibitors have the potential for cancer prevention (Axelsson et al., 2010; Flossmann et al., 2007; Khan & Lee, 2011). Recent studies suggest an important role of COX-2 inhibitors in bladder cancer therapy. Several studies support increased COX-2 expression in bladder tumor stage and/or grade (Wadhwa et al., 2005; Yildirim et al., 2010; Yu et al., 2008). The primary mechanisms in which NSAIDs are thought to inhibit bladder cancer are through stimulation of apoptosis and reduction of angiogenesis (Thun et al., 2002). Another recent study suggested that COX-2 dependent and independent activation of downstream signals, such as CK2α-Akt/uPA, may play a critical role in urothelial carcinoma cell survival and is neutralized by selective COX-2 inhibitors (Shimada et al., 2011).

Clinical data has mixed results for support of NSAID use in bladder and other cancer chemoprevention. A recent pooled analysis of three prospective cohort studies indicated a reduced risk in bladder cancer, particularly in non-smokers, with increased use of non-aspirin NSAIDs, but found no associated decrease in risk of bladder cancer with aspirin use (Daughtery et al., 2011). An in vivo bladder cancer model recently showed some efficacy of naproxen (Lubet et al., 2010). In a bladder tumor mouse model, rofecoxib, a selective COX-2 inhibitor, provided a significant reduction in incidence of neoplastic bladder lesions (D'Arca et al., 2010). Another study that examined multiple randomized trials using daily aspirin versus no aspirin on risk of gastrointestinal and other types of cancer death revealed increased survival, although bladder cancer was not specifically included in the analysis (Rothwell et al., 2011). Further research is needed into the possibility that NSAID's may prevent bladder cancer.

2.11 Statins

Statins are a class of drugs used to lower cholesterol levels through inhibition of 3-hydroxy-3-methylglutaryl coenzyme A (HMG-CoA) reductase. However, there is some evidence suggesting that statins may have other properties in addition to their effect on lowering cholesterol. It is hypothesized that statins may inhibit tumor growth by neutralization of protein prenylation of GTPases, affecting downstream isoprenoids (Demierre et al., 2005), which in turn affect immune response, apoptosis, and cell maturation (Issat et al., 2011).

Currently statins are being researched for their efficacy in preventing a variety of cancers, including bladder malignancies. In a study examining atorvastatin and human bladder cancer cell lines, a significant anti-proliferative effect was observed when compared to controls (Kamat & Nelkin, 2005). In another study using mouse cells transfected with H-ras oncogene from human bladder carcinoma, researchers observed a significant in vivo inhibition of ras-oncogene transformed cells (Sebti et al., 1991). Other studies also point out additional reasons to use statins, since use may also improve local control in patients undergoing concurrent therapy for muscle invasive bladder cancer (Tsai et al., 2006).

However, not all studies support statin efficacy in preventing bladder and other types of cancers. A recent cohort study looking at statins and the occurrence of 10 types of cancer including bladder, showed no significant association with statin use (Jacobs et al., 2011). Using a female rat model, another recent study showed no significant difference in mammary carcinogenesis with simvastatin use (Kubatka et al., 2011). Additionally, a phase II clinical trial using atorvastatin with sulindac (NSAID) and probiotic dietary fiber failed to provide convincing evidence of decreased recurrence of colorectal carcinoma (Limburg et al., 2011). Adding to the controversy, some data suggest that concurrent statin therapy with BCG may reduce clinical efficacy of the BCG therapy (Hoffmann et al., 2006), although this has not been consistent in all studies (Burglund et al., 2008) and not all literature supports discontinuation of the statin (Kamat & Wu, 2007). These results, in contrast with previous studies supporting anti-tumor growth, warrant further investigation into statin use in bladder cancer chemoprevention.

• Vitamin A	Alters cell growth, differentiation, and apoptosis through growth factors, cytokines, and neoplastic stem cell pathways
• Vitamin E	A free radical scavenger, inhibits N-nitroso compound formation as well as inducing apoptosis (some reports state may be a carcinogen)
• Vitamin C	Anti-oxidant, inhibits p-53 and p38 MAPK pathways
• Selemium	Works through methlyation of RNA, anti-androgen, and promotes DNA repair
• Cactus Pear	Increases expression of Annexin IV, decreases VEGF, and promotes immune response
• Isoflavones	Induction of G2-M cell cycle arrest, apoptosis, and angiogenesis
• Garlic	Free radical scavenger, increases cytokines production, a thiol binder along with preventing suppression of the immune response
• Green Tea	Caspase mediator, angiogensis inhibitor, and decreases chromosomal damage
• DFMO	Inhibits malignant urothelial cells through mostly unknown mechanisms, possibly inhibition of ornithine decarboxylase
• NSAIDS	Stimulates apoptosis and inhibits angiogenesis
• Statins	A neutralizer of protein prenylation of GTPases

Table 2. Key features of potential chemopreventative agents for bladder cancer.

3. Inheritance/biomarkers of bladder cancer

In a review article of the epidemiology of bladder cancer by Peluchhi et al., the risk of bladder cancer is increased by 50-100% in first-degree relatives in those that have the disease. Similar to cardiac disease, the risk for first-degree relatives is increased if the patient is diagnosed earlier than the age of 60 (Peluchhi et al., 2006; Goldgar et al., 1994). Current literature suggests a possible X-linked inheritance due to the increased incidence in siblings that are brothers (Pina & Hemminki, 2001).

It is well known of the increased risk that cigarette/tobacco consumption has on bladder cancer, Okkels and associates demonstrated the increased risk through the accumulation of slow acetylators with the Arylamine N-acetyltransferase 2 (NAT 2) genotype (Okkels et al., 1997). The relationship between NAT 1 and NAT 2 leads to the formation of DNA-binding metabolites for aromatic amines (carcinogens) in the bladder (Badawi et al., 1995).

Tobacco smoke also contains 4-aminobiphenyl (4-ABP), an aromatic amine, and for individuals with the NAT 2 phenotype, there is a stronger association, again with the slower acetylators (Yu et al., 1994).
Patients with inherited deletions of the gene, GSTN1, which encodes glutathione S-transferase M1, is associated with bladder cancer. This is in part due to the role of the gene, detoxification of carcinogens, being absent (Brockmoler et al., 1994). Although the aforementioned markers have shown an association with bladder cancer, the question that has still yet to be answered, is to what degree do GSTN1, NAT 1 and NAT 2, among others have on a patient and their risk of bladder cancer, especially with the exposure to carcinogens such as tobacco smoke and aromatic amines.

4. Gene therapy/ γδ T-CELLS

The immunotherapy action of BCG works through binding and availability to major histocompatibility complex (MHC) class I expression on cancer cells (Kitamura et al., 2006). In a murine model, Yuasa et al. investigated, using γδ T-cells (subset of human peripheral T cells), to augment immunotherapy in MHC-diminished superficial bladder cancer, which has been shown to be more aggressive then MHC-conservative bladder cancer. They demonstrated, by examining 123 patients undergoing either TUR or radical cystectomy, that not only was MHC class I expression diminished in lymph node and invasive bladder cancer, but they also experienced a shorter disease free and overall survival.
In their murine model (BALB/c SCID mice), using Luc-labeled bladder cancer cells and ex-vivo γδ T-cells from peripheral blood from healthy patients, mice were treated with γδ T-cells alone or in combination with zoledronic acid. Bladders were examined histologically with hematoxylin-eosin staining and immunohistochemically by with ani-human CD3. Using zoledronic acid to alter the cytotoix effect, γδ T-cells showed dose-dependent cytotoxicty (Kitamura et al., 2009). This shows potential for using γδ T-cells to augment other intravesical treatments to accentuate their benefits.

5. Novel treatments

5.1 Silibinin
Silibinin, a flavonoid phytochemical found in milk thistle, has been shown in vitro, with TCC-SUP (high-grade invasive) and T-24 (high grade), to cause cell cycle arrest along with apoptosis. An induction of G_1 arrest along with cell growth inhibition was determined by various methods including: flow cytometry, cell growth assays (24, 48, and 72 hours of treatments), cell cultures, immunoprecipitation and immunoblottin. Cyclin-dependent kinase activity when uncontrolled, will lead to continuous cell progression. Cyclins are also a determining factor in G_1/S and G_2/M transition (Singh et al., 2002). Both cyclins and cyclin-dependent kinases are reduced with Silibinin as determined by antibodies against CDK2 or CDK4 and kinase assays. Cell death through apoptosis, which was only seen with high-grade invasive cancer, was determined by Annexin V and Propidium Iodide. For the previous experiments, doses of Silibinin varied from 50 to 200 micromolars (Tyagi et al., 2004). Later, the same investigators, with bladder transitional-cell papilloma RT4 cells, induced apoptosis with Slibinin through p53-caspace activation (Tyagi et al., 2006). Through further understanding of the biochemical/cell cycle pathways of bladder cancer, the effects of Silibinin will be better understood.

5.2 Keyhole Limpet Hemocyanin (KLH)

KLH is a copper-containing, extracellular, respiratory protein that was first investigated by Curtis et al., to have immunostimulatory properties (Curtis et al., 1970). Its potential role in the treatment of bladder cancer may be in a cytolytic reduction of tumor growth through a humoral response and an increase in natural killer cells. There have been reports when treating non-muscle invasive bladder cancer to have recurrence rates as low as 31% with less side effects (sepsis, cystitis) than BCG (Harris & Markl, 1999; Nseyo & Lamm, 1997).

Jurincic-Winkler et al. treated thirteen patients with CIS with intravesical KLH (20 mg) on a weekly schedule for 6 weeks, then monthly for one year, and bimonthly for a total of 3 years. Overall, only two patients were free of disease at 66 and 82 months of follow up with the majority requiring BCG or cystectomy (Jurincic-Winkler et al., 2000).

When reviewed, KLH could also be beneficial for carbohydrate-based immunuotherapy in the appropriate adenocarcinoma when there are mucin-like epitopes as well as a potential treatment for melanomas (Harris & Markl, 1999). Overall, the evidence is lacking for KLH to be a major treatment for non-muscle invasive bladder cancer.

5.3 Apaziquone

Apaziquone, also referred commonly as EO9, is an indolequinone compound. Through an activation mechanism with NAD(P)H: Quinone oxidoreductase-1 (NQO1), Apaziquone, in an aerobic environment, has been shown to impact DNA-damaging species (Phillips et al., 2004). Increase in cell kill is also achieved through alklyating byproducts through redox cycling leading to single-strand breaks and DNA cross-linking (Comer & Murphy, 2003). In vivo, it has demonstrated activity against colon, non-small cell lung, renal, melanoma and central nervous system tumor models (Hendricks et al., 1993). With early promising results, it has failed to show favorable phase II outcomes with Phillips et al. citing its rapid pharmacokinetic elimination and poor penetration in avascular tissues (Phillips et al., 1998). In humans, Apaziquone's half-life is less than 10 minutes, via extra-hepatic metabolism by red blood cells, with its metabolites, EO5a, having decreased cytotoxicity (Schelens et al., 1994; Vainchtein et al., 2007).

Current research is aimed at finding adjunct compounds to improve its pharmokinetic properties. A quinone-based bioreductive drug, 2,3-bis(aziridinyl)-5-hydroxy-1,4-naphthoquinone, through its selectivity for NQO1-rich cells under hypoxic conditions, has shown such potential (Phillips et al., 2004).

5.4 Mycobacterium phlei

This agent, has shown anti-tumor activity, is a cell wall extract, composed of carbohydrates, peptides, and lipids that is commonly found on the outer capsule of Mycobacterium phlei, a gram-positive microorganism that is located in soil, plants, and drinking water (Chin et al., 1996; & Mallick et al., 1985). Commonly prepared as a mineral oil emulsion, it has demonstrated inhibitory effects on bladder cancer cell lines through inhibition of cellular proliferation via apoptosis, as well as by an increase in the production of interleukin-12 though stimulation of cancer-infiltrating monocytes and macrophages. Bladder cancer cell lines, in a study by Filion et al., that have been tested include: HT-1197 along with HT-1376 (which are derived from anaplastic transitional cell carcinomas of the bladder from humans, both grade IV and grade III respectively). Cytokine analysis and cellular apoptosis were detected using ELISA and cell death was determined by dimethylthiazoldiphenyltetrazolium bromide

(MTT), (Filion et al., 1999) . When tested in a murine model, mycobacterium phlei induced similar effects that are seen with BCG, namely a CD4+ T cell infiltrate when compared to control. Although the antitumor effect wasn't as significant as that seen with BCG, treatment was better tolerated overall (Chin et al., 1996).

5.5 Docetaxel
Docetaxel, a member of the taxane family, works through microtubule depolymerization inhibition and is commonly used in treatment of prostate and breast cancer, among others. Barlow et al., originally showed a 56% response rate in 18 patients who initially failed BCG therapy and refused to undergo cystectomy. The treatment regimen consisted of 6 weekly bladder instillations on a dose-escalation protocol (McKiernan et al., 2006) They continued their protocol, with the addition of 15 patients, for a median follow up of 29 months and had a 1 and 2 year recurrence-free survival rates of 45 and 32%. Adverse reactions to docetaxel included: dysuria, hematuria, facial flushing, frequency, rash, urinary tract infection, and premature voiding during instillation of the medication. Overall, they concluded that the data is very promising and offers an alternative treatment to those that have failed BCG and do not undergo cystectomy, however, large, multi-institutional, prospective trials are needed to concur effectiveness (Barolw et al., 2009).

Gefitinib, a selective epidermal growth factor receptor tyrosine kinase inhibitor, was studied by Kassouf et al., to determine its effect, in vitro, on enhancing the role of docetaxel on bladder cancer. Four bladder cancer cell lines were studied: 253J B-V, UM-UC-3, KU-7, and UM-UC-13. Through the use of flow cytometry and propidium iodide to determine cell cycle Analysis, along with Western Blot to establish EGFR downstream signaling, it was shown that when combined, gefitinib enhanced both the antiproliferative and apoptotic properties of docetaxel, but only when administered after the docetaxel (Kassouf et al., 2006).

5.6 Hyperthermia
A novel approach of combining local microwave hyperthermia along with Mitomcyin C after undergoing transurethral resection was reported by Colombo et al., with 83 patients who were followed for 24 months. They take into account the detrimental effect that heat has on malignant cells (which are more sensitive to thermal changes in the environment than that of normal cells) such as inhibition of DNA synthesis, RNA, cellular protein, and DNA duplication in the cell cycle. In their study, 83 patients were randomly assigned (after undergoing transurethral resection of primary or recurrent noninvasive bladder cancer) to either receiving Mitomycin C alone or in conjunction with local microwave-induced hyperthermia. Hyperthermia was administered using the Synergo SB-TS:101-1, which consists of a 915 MHz intravesical microwave applicator, to reach a temperature of 42°C ± 2°C and maintained for 40 minutes.

The patients were all followed with urine cytology as well as cystoscopy every 3 months for 2 years, with biopsies taken if suspicious lesions were noted. Abdominal and pelvic ultrasound was also obtained on a bi-annual basis. Overall, 75 patients completed the protocol and those receiving the hyperthermia experienced more severe side effects: cystitis, suprapubic pain, and thermal reaction. Only six patients (17.1%) had recurrence with the combination therapy as compared to 23 patients (57.5%) receiving only Mitomycin C (P value = 0.0002). There was one patient with disease progression in the chemotherapy only treatment group. Overall, the idea of combining intravesical chemotherapy along with hyperthermia is an attractive option for enhancing the effectiveness of chemotherapeutic agents especially for those that are not surgical candidates for radical cystectomy (Colombo et al., 2003).

A more recent study was carried out by Nativ et al., to examine those patients that experience recurrence of papillary non-muscle invasive bladder cancer after undergoing BCG treatment. They looked at 111 patients and followed them for 2 years with urine cytology and cystoscopy every 3 months. All patients were treated with hyperthermia, 42°C $\pm$ 2°C, for two cycles of 30 minute instillations of 20mg of Mitomycin C, for 6 weekly treatments followed by 6 maintenance sessions at 4 to 6 week intervals.

Adverse reactions were similar as compared to the earlier study with pain and bladder spasms being the most common (transient to mild at worse). Recurrence-free rates at one and two years were 85% and 56% respectively. There were 3 patients (3%) that progressed to muscle invasive bladder cancer during the follow up. Interestingly, those patients that received fewer than 10 maintenance treatments, had a tumor recurrence rate of 61% compared to 39% that completed the two year regimen (p value = 0.01) (Nativ et al., 2009). The combination of hyperthermia with intravesical treatment is very promising and should be considered very strongly for future trials in those patients that are considered BCG failures.

5.7 Inositol Hexaphosphate

Inositol Hexaphosphate (IP-6) is a naturally occurring polyphosphorylated carbohydrate that is found in foods that are high in fiber such as cereals, legumes, and grains (Fox & Eberl, 2002). It has already been shown to possess anti-tumor effects in numerous cancer cell lines: colon, hepatocellular, breast, lung, prostate, pancreas and melanoma among others while not being cytotoxic or cytostatic against normal cells (Shamsuddin et al., 1997). Zaslau et al., displayed its mechanism of action against bladder cancer cell lines (HTB9 [grade II], T24 [grade III], TCCSUP [grade IV]) via modulation of the cell cycle and induction of cellular apoptosis as well as necrosis (Zaslau et al., 2009).

Already demonstrating reduction in cellular proliferation, they tested IP-6's clinical efficacy with a 2-hour exposure time. All three cell lines (HTB9, T24, and TCCSUP) were plated and cultured with 2.5 and 4.5 mM of IP-6 for 2 hours and then had their supernatant incubated for an additional 24 and 48 hours. Cell viability was assessed though MTT colorimetric assay and cell cycle analysis though flow cytometry. All three cell lines, at all times tested, noted a significant reduction in cellular growth when treated with IP-6 with only a 2 hour incubation. Interestingly, when looking at cell cycle inhibition, IP-6 produced different results with the varying degrees of bladder cancer cell lines, which can be related to the different tumor grades replicating at different rates corresponding to diverse responses to the IP-6 treatments. There was an increase in cells in the $G_0/G1$ phase, reduction in G2/M, while no change in the S phase with the TCCSUP cell line. The T24 cell line was determined to be accelerating and not dividing through observances of cell reduction with 4.5 mM IP-6 in the $G_0/G1$ phase and no change in both the S and G2/M phases. Lastly, with the HTB9 cell line, as with the T24 cell line, no change was noted in G2/M, however, there was an induction in the arrest at $G_0/G1$ while a decrease in S phase (Zaslau et al., 2009).

IP-6 was later tested, with the same bladder cancer cell lines, using Annexin V-Fluorescein Isothiocyanate (FITC) and Propidium Iodine along with flow cytometry to determine method of cell kill. Using the same concentrations, 2.5 and 4.5 mM, at 2 hour incubations, HTB9 was effected by necrotic mechanisms, and T24 and TCCSUP went through an induction of apoptosis (Zaslau et al., 2010). The authors, with promising results thus far, state the Phase II clinical trials are needed to evaluate the safety and clinical utility of IP-6 for the intravesical use in bladder cancer.

5.8 HTI-286
HTI-286 is a synthetic analogue of the marine sponge product hemiasterlin. In a similar fashion to the taxanes, HTI-286 works through inhibition of tubulin polymerization with strong cytotoxic potential. In an in vitro study, HTI-286 was compared to MMC when tested in human bladder cancer cell lines RT4, MGH-U3, KU-7, as well as UM-UC3. In this study, it showed comparable cytotoxicity, inhibition of cell growth, and induction of apoptosis in all cell lines tested. An in vivo study using 8-week old nude mice demonstrated delayed cancer growth in a dose dependent manner (Hadaschik et al., 2008).

5.9 Suramin
Suramin, a polysulphonated naphthylurea, has anticancer functions that are comprised of growth factor antagonism and cellular DNA synthesis suppression (Walther et al., 1994; La Rocca et al., 1990).
Serious side effects including neurologic, renal, and metabolic Have been caused by systemic administration of suramin (La Rocca et al, 1990; Figg et al, 1994; Bowden et al, 1996) secondary to the compound having a 40-day plasma half-life in humans (Hawking, 1978). Suramin possesses several structural advantages for use intravesically in bladder cancer: its' high molecular mass (1429 Da) and negative ionic charge hamper systemic absorption (Ord et al, 2005); and its tendency to bind to protein favors growth factor antagonism in urine, which contains low protein levels (Ord et al, 2005). In particular, suramin inhibits the binding of epidermal growth factor (EGF) to its receptor, which are prevalent in high numbers in bladder cancer (Walther et al, 1996).
A phase I clinical trial found that intravesical treatment with suramin for cases of recurrent superficial bladder cancer was safe up to a 153mg/ml dose (Uchio et al, 2003). However, suramin's effects on bladder tumors has not yet been evaluated. Noted complications included bladder spasms and vesicoureteral reflux in a small percentage of the individual treatments, all of which completely abated within 48 hours (Uchio et al, 2003). Even at the highest dosages, plasma concentrations of suramin were minimal and further trials are warranted to decipher its usefulness.

5.10 Gemcitabine
Gemcitabine, as reported by Karak and Flechon, is a deoxycytidine analogue, a pyrimidine antimetabolite that is similar to cytarabine that works through inhibition of DNA synthesis (Karak & Flechon, 2007). Its effect on bladder cancer's cell cycle is via a blockage of cells progressing through the G1/S phase and a cytotoxic effect in S-phase (Guchelaar et al., 1996). It has already been approved through the Food and Drug Administration as a first line treatment for solid tumors of the pancreas as well as for inoperable, metastatic non-

small cell lung and breast cancer (Karak & Flechon, 2007). Gemcitabine has been known to cause is myelosuppression (Aapro et al., 1998).

Gemcitabine has also been used as single agent for those patients that were considered BCG failures. In a phase II trial Dalbagni et al. examined 30 patients that were refractory to BCG treatment. Treatment was given twice weekly for 3 weeks and surveillance was conducted at 8 weeks and then every 3 months for one year. Although there was a complete response in 50% of patient at 3 months, this was reduced to only 10% at one year (Dalbagni et al., 2006).

5.11 Mitomycin-C & Gemcitabine

Gemcitabine, as described by Breyer et al., is 2′,2′-difluoro-2′-deoxycytidine, that has shown broad spectrum anti-tumor activity. In their study, 10 patients that were either BCG refractory or BCG intolerant were treated with Gemcitabine (1000mg in 50cc sterile water) then MMC (40mg in 20cc sterile water) once a week for 6 weeks as their induction treatment. This was then followed by maintenance treatment (same dosage) once a month for 12 months. Median follow up for the patients (with median age of 67 years) was 26.5 months. Six out of ten patients were recurrence free at 14 months, with 4 patients having biopsy proven recurrence at a median of 6 months. Overall, the treatment was well tolerated with no major complications. Of note, 9 out of 10 patients had either high grade bladder cancer or carcinoma in situ before beginning treatment and had a median of five recurrences (Breyer et al, 2010). The same authors cited another study by Maymi and O'Donnell that compared Gemcitabine versus Gemicitabine in combination with MMC in 39 patients that have failed multiple, previous intravesical treatments. Alone, the median disease free survival was 6.5 months compared to 20 months for the combination of Gemicitabine and MMC (Maymi et al.). In a comparison study, Malmstrom et al. found only 4 out of 21 patients disease free that were treated with MMC for noninvasive bladder cancer at 3 years (Malmostrom et al., 1999). The literature that has been reviewed supports the use of MMC In combination with other intravesical agents to increase its effectiveness.

5.12 Mitomycin-C and BCG

The two leading intravescial treatments for non-muscle invasive bladder cancer are Mitomycin-C and BCG. There have been many studies that have looked to find an additive effect with the combination of the two agents (chemoimmunotherapy), but in whole, have not produced significant results. Witjes and colleagues examined 90 patients that underwent 4 weekly instillations of 40 mg of MMC followed by 6 weekly instillations of BCG (group 1) and compared them to 92 patients that just underwent 10 weekly instillations of MMC (group 2). Surprisingly, there was no significant difference seen between the two groups in regards to bacterial cystitis, chemical cystitis, and other local side effects. Eleven patients had fever (>38.5C) in group 1 compared to only 3 patients in group 2. Median follow up was 32 months. There were 35/90 patients with recurrence and 5/90 patients with progression in group 1 and 42/92 and 4/92 respectively, in group 2 (Witjes et al., 1998).

A prospective, randomized comparison of BCG alone with that of BCG and electromotive MMC was carried out by Di Stasi and colleagues. After being diagnosed with pT1 bladder cancer, 212 patients were randomly assigned to induction of either 81 mg of BCG for 2 hours once a week for 6 weeks or 81 mg of BCG over 2 hours once a week for 2 weeks, then 40 mg of electromotive MMC (intravesical electric current 20 mA for 30 min) once a week for three weeks. Exclusion criteria included previous treatment with either BCG or electromotive

MMC, any intravesical agent in the last 6 months, upper tract disease, and previous radiotherapy to the pelvis or chemotherapy among others. Maintenance for the BCG alone group consisted of 81 mg BCG once a month for 10 months compared to the group being treated with BCG and electromotive MMC which received the combination once a month for 2 months, then 81 mg of BCG once a month for three months. Of critical importance is that the authors defined the primary endpoint being disease-free survival with secondary endpoints being time to progression, overall survival and disease specific survival. Median follow-up was an impressive 88 months.

The patients that received the combination had a higher disease-free survival at 69 months compared to the patients that received only BCG, which was 21 months. Follow-up consisted of abdominal ultrasound, cystourethroscopy, and urine cytology every 3 months for the first three years and then every 6 months thereafter. If a patient was originally diagnosed with carcinoma in situ, the follow-up also included random bladder biopsies at 3 and 6 months. The combination group also has a lower rate of progression at 9.3% compared to 21.9% of BCG alone group, with 10 and 23 patients progressing to muscle-invasive bladder cancer respectively. Also, the BCG and electromotive MMC group only had 6 reported deaths due to bladder cancer compared to 23 in the BCG alone group. Adverse effects were similar between the two groups with each having 3 patients withdrawing from the trial. According to the authors, the benefit of the combination may be attributed to BCG-induced inflammation increasing the bladder mucosa permeability to the effects of the MMC, allowing it to reach the target tissue (Di Stasi et al., 2007).

• γδ T-cells	Enhances immunotherapy by increasing MHC class I expression
• Silibinin	Induced G1 cell cycle arrest and reduces cyclin and cyclin-dependent kinases which decreases cell progression
• KLH	Possible mechanism of action could include an increase in humoral response in an association with an increase of natural killer cells
• Apaziquone	Needs to be combined with another agent or treatment modality to better its pharmokinetics to lengthen its half-life and therapeutic effect
• Mycobacterium Phlei	Increases production of IL-12, induces apoptosis, as well as promoting a CD4+ T cell response
• Docetaxel	Inhibits microtubule depolymerization
• Hyperthermia	Environmental/thermal changes which malignant cells are more sensitive to and causes inhibition of DNA and RNA synthesis among other cellular pathways
• IP-6	Modulates cell cycle and induces cellular apoptosis and necrosis
• HTI-286	Similar mechanism of action as the taxanes (Docetaxel)

• Suramin	Growth factor antagonist and suppresses DNA synthesis
• Gemcitabine	Inhibits DNA synthesis and through a cystotoxic effect, inhibits malignant cells in G1/S and S-phase
• MMC and Gemcitabine	Overall, a well tolerated combination with beneficial results when compared to each agent alone.
• MMC and BCG	BCG may increase bladder mucosa permeability through an inflammatory response allowing MMC to reach its target at a more optimal level

Table 3. Mechanism of action of Novel Treatments for Bladder Cancer

6. Conclusion

Further advancement in the treatment of non-muscle invasive bladder cancer will come in the understanding of the disease's molecular/biochemical pathways and the effect on these pathways that chemopreventive and intravesical agents have on them. Certainly there are some areas that are more promising than others, especially with the combination of agents as well as the addition of hyperthermia to treatment regimens that are already producing significant positive results. As a review of the many agents discussed, table 2 provides the key features of potential chemopreventative agents for bladder cancer. Table 3 reviews the mechanism of action of Novel Treatments for Bladder Cancer. As always, it is not just the initial resection, or even the induction treatment that reduces recurrence and progression, but the role of maintenance therapy that is crucial for the patient to remain disease free. Again, with the new discoveries of cell signaling, cell cycle/death/apoptosis, interleukin, humoral and cell mediated responses, there will be more specific target treatments with the hopes of minimal side effects.

7. References

Aapro, M., Marin, C. & Hatty, S. (1998). Review Paper: Gemcitabine – a Safety Review. *Anti Cancer Drugs,* Vol.9, No.3, (March 1998), pp. 191-201, ISSN 1473-5741.

Alfthan, O., Tarkkanen, J., Gröhn, P., et al. (1983). Tigason (Etretinate) in Prevention of Recurrence of Superficial Bladder Tumors. A Double-blind Clinical Trial. *European Urology,* Vol.9, No.1, pp. 6-9, ISSN 0302-2838.

Amaral, A., Cantor, K., Silverman, D. & Malats, N. (2010). Selenium and Bladder Cancer Risk: A Meta-analysis. *Cancer Epidemiology, Biomarkers, and Prevention,* Vol.19, No.9, (September 2010), pp. 2407-2415, ISSN 1538-7755.

Axelsson, H., Lönnroth, C., Andersson, M. & Lundholm, K. (2010). Mechanisms Behind COX-1 and COX-2 Inhibition of Tumor Growth In Vivo. *International Journal of Oncology,* Vol.37, No.5, (November 2010), pp. 1143-1152, ISSN 1791-2423.

Badawi, A., Hirvonen, A., Bell, D., Lang, N. & Kadlubar, F. Role of Aromatic Amine Acetlytrasnferase, NAT1 and NAT2, in carcinogen-DNA Adduct Formation in the Human Urinary Bladder. *Cancer Res,* Vol.55, No.22, (November 1995), pp. 5230-5237, ISSN 1538-7445.

Balley, H., Kim, K., Verma, A., et al. (2010). A Randomized, Double-blind, Placebo-controlled Phase 3 Skin Cancer Prevention Study of {Alpha}-difluoromethylornithine in Subjects with Previous History of Skin Cancer. *Cancer Prevention Research,* Vol.3, No.1, (January 2010), pp. 35-47, ISSN 1940-6215.

Barlow, L., McKiernan, C. & Benson M. (2009). The Novel Use of Intravesical Docetaxel for the Treatment of Non-Muscle Invasive Bladder Cancer Refractory to BCG Therapy: a Single Institution Experience. *World J Urol,* Vol.27, No.3, (June 2009), pp. 331-335, ISSN 1433-8726.

Beisel, W., Edelman, R., Nauss, K. & Suskind, R. (1981). Single-nutrient Effects on Immunologic Functions. Report of a Workshop Sponsored by the Department of Food and Nutrition and its Nutrition Advisory Group of the American Medical Association. *The Journal of the American Medical Association,* Vol.245, No.1, (January 1981), pp. 53-58, ISSN 1538-3598.

Boehm, K., Borrelli, F., Ernst, E., et al. (2009). Green Tea (Camellia sinensis) for the Prevention of Cancer. *Cochrane Database of Systematic Reviews,* Issue.3: CD005004, (July 2009), ISSN 1469-493X.

Bondesson, M. & Gustafsson, J. (2010). Does Consuming Isoflavones Reduce or Increase Breast Cancer Risk? *Genome Medicine,* Vol.2, No.12, (December 2010), pp. 90, ISSN 1756-904X.

Boon, C., Kelloff, G. & Malone, W. (1990). Identification of Candidate Cancer Chemopreventive Agents and Their Evaluation in Animal Models and Human Clinical Trials: A Review. *Cancer Research,* Vol.50, No.1, (January 1990), pp. 2-9, ISSN 1538-7445.

Bowden, C., Figg, W., Dawson, N., et al. (1996). A Phase I/II Study of Continuous Infusion Suramin in Patients with Hormone-Refractory Prostate Cancer: Toxicity and Response. *Cancer Chemother Pharmacol,* Vol.39, No.1-2, (1996), pp. 1-8, ISSN 1432-0843.

Breyer, B., Whitson, J., Carroll, P. & Konety, B. (2010). Sequential Intravesical Gemcitabine and Mitomycin C Chemotherapy Regimen in Patients with Non-Muscle Invasive Bladder Cancer. *Urologic Oncology,* Vol.28, No.5, (September-October 2010), pp. 510-514, ISSN 1873-2496.

Brinkman, M. & Zeegers, M. (2008). Nutrition, Total Fluid and Bladder Cancer. *Scandinavian Journal of Urology and Nephrology. Supplementum,* Vol.218, (September 2008), pp. 25-36, ISSN 1651-2537.

Brockmoller, J., Kerb, R., Drakoulis, N., Staffeldt, B. & Roots, I. Glutathione S-Transferase M1 and its Variants A and B as Host Factors of Bladder Cancer Susceptibility: a Case-Control Study. *Cancer Res,* Vol.54, No.15, (August 1994), pp. 4103-4111, ISSN 1538-7445.

Burglund, R., Savage, C., Vora, K., Kurta, J. & Cronin, A. (2008). An Analysis of the Effect of Statin Use on the Efficacy of Bacillus Calmette-guerin Treatment for Transitional Cell Carcinoma of the Bladder. *The Journal of Urology,* Vol.180, No.4, (October 2008), pp. 1297-1300, ISSN 1527-3792.

Butt, M., Sultan, M., Butt, M. & Iqbal, J. Garlic: Nature's Protection Against Physiological Threats. *Critical Reviews in Food Science and Nutrition*, Vol.49, No.6, (June 2009), pp. 538-551, ISSN 1549-7852.

Cerella, C., Dicato, M., Jacob, C. & Diederich, M. (2011). Chemical Properties and Mechanisms Determining the Anti-cancer Action of Garlic-derived Organic Sulfur Compounds. *Anti-cancer Agents in Medicinal Chemistry*, Vol.11, No.3, (March 2011), pp. 267-271, ISSN 1875-5992.

Chavez-Santoscoy, R., Gutierrez-Uribe, J. & Serna-Saldívar, S. (2009). Phenolic Composition, Antioxidant Capacity and in Vitro Cancer Cell Cytotoxicity of Nine Prickly Pear (Opuntia Spp.) Juices. *Plant Foods for Human Nutrition*, Vol.64, No.2, (June 2009), pp. 146-152, ISSN 1573-9104.

Chin, J., Kadhim, S., Batislam, E. et al. (1996). Mycobacterium Cell Wall: an Alternative to Intravesical Bacillus Calmette Guerin (BCG) Therapy in Orthotopic Murine Bladder Ccancer. *J Urol*, Vol.156, No.3, (September 1996), pp. 1189-93, ISSN 1527-3792.

Chyou, P., Nomura, A. & Stemmermann, G. (1993). A Prospective Study of Diet, Smoking, and Lower Urinary Tract Cancer. *Annals of Epidemiology*, Vol.3, No.3, (May 1993), pp. 211-216, ISSN 1873-2585.

Columbo, R., Da Pozzo, L., Salonia, A. et al. (2003). Multicentric Study Comparing Intravesical Chemotherapy Alone and with Local Microwave Hyperthermia for Prophylaxis of Recurrence of Superficial Transitional Cell Carcinoma. *Journal of Clinical Oncology*, Vol.21, No.23, (December 2003), pp. 4270-4276, ISSN 1572-7755.

Comer, E. & Murphy, W. (2003). The Bromoquinone Annulation Reaction: a Formal Total Synthesis of EO9. *ARKIVOC*, Vol.7, (June 2003), pp. 286-296, ISSN 1551-7012.

Coulter, I., Hardy, M., Morton, S., et al. (2006). Antioxidants Vitamin C and Vitamin E for the Prevention and Treatment of Cancer. *Journal of General Internal Medicine*, Vol.21, No.7, (July 2006), pp. 735-744, ISSN 1525-1497.

Curtis, J., Hersh, E., Harris, J., et al. (1970). The Human Primary Immune Response to Keyhole Limpet Hemocyanin: Interrelationships of Delayed Hypersensitivity, Antibody Response and In Vitro Blast Transformation. *Clin. Exp.*, Vol.56, No.130, (April 1970), pp. 473-491, ISSN 1365-2249.

Dalbagni, G., Russo, P., Bochner, B., et al. (2006). Phase II Trial of Intravesical Gemcitabine in Bacilli Calmette-Guerin-Refractory Transitional Cell Carcinoma of the Bladder. *J Clin Oncol*, Vol.24, No.18, (June 2006), pp. 2729-2734, ISSN 1527-7755.

D'Arca, D., LeNoir, J., Wildemore, B., et al. (2010). Prevention of Urinary Bladder Cancer in the FHIT Knock-out Mouse with Rofecoxib, a Cox-2 Inhibitor. *Urologic Oncology*, Vol.28, No.2, (March-April 2010), pp. 189-194, ISSN 1873-2496.

Daughtery, S., Pfeiffer, R., Sigurdson, A., et al. (2011). Nonsteroidal Antiinflammatory Drugs and Bladder Cancer: A Pooled Analysis. *American Journal of Epidemiology*, Vol.173, No.7, (April 2011), pp. 721-730, ISSN 1476-6256.

Decensi, A., Torrisi, R., Bruno, S., et al. (2000). Randomized Trial of Fenretinide in Superficial Bladder Cancer Using DNA Flow Cytometry as an Intermediate End Point. *Cancer Epidemiology, Biomarkers & Prevention*, Vol.9, No.10, (October 2000), pp. 1071-1078, ISSN 1055-7755

Demierre, M., Higgins, P., Gruber, S., Hawk, E & Lippman, S. (2005). Statins and Cancer Prevention. *Nature Reviews. Cancer*, Vol.5, No.12, (December 2005), pp. 930-942, ISSN 1474-1768.

Di Stasi, S., Giannantoni, A., Giurioli, A. et al. (2006). Sequential BCG and Electromotive Mitomycin Versus BCG Alone for High-Risk Superficial Bladder Cancer: a Randomized Controlled Trial. *Lancet Oncol*, Vol.7, No.1, (January 2006), pp. 43-51, ISSN 1474-5488.

Dunzendorfer, U. (1981). The Effect of Alpha-difluoromethyl-ornithine on Tumor Growth, Acute Phase Reactants, Beta-2-microglobulin and Hydroxyproline in Kidney and Bladder Carcinomas. *Urologia Internationalis*, Vol.36, No.2, pp. 128-136, ISSN 1423-0399.

Fernández-López, J., Almela, L., Obón, J. & Castellar, R. (2010). Determination of Antioxidant Constituents in Cactus Pear Fruits. *Plant Foods for Human Nutrition*, Vol.65, No.3, (September 2010), pp. 253-259, ISSN 1573-9104.

Feugang, J., Ye, F., Zhang, D., et al. (2010). Cactus Pear Extracts Induce Reactive Oxygen Species Production and Apoptosis in Ovarian Cancer Cells. *Nutrition and Cancer*, Vol.62, No.5, pp. 692-699, ISSN 1532-7914.

Figg, W., Cooper, M., Thibault, A., Headlee, D., et al. (1994). Acute Renal Toxicity Associated with Suramin in the Treatment of Prostate Cancer. *Cancer*, Vol.74, No.5, (September 1994), pp. 1612-1614, ISSN 1097-0142.

Filion, M., Lepicier, P., Morales, A. & Phillips, N. Mycobacterium Phlei Cell Wall Complex Directly Induces Apoptosis in Human Bladder Cancer Cells. *British Journal of Cancer*, Vol.79, No.2, (January 1999), pp. 229-235, ISSN 1532-1827.

Flossmann, E., Rothwell, P., British Doctors Aspirin Trial and the UK-TIA Aspirin Trial. (2007). Effect of Aspirin on Long-term Risk of Colorectal Cancer: Consistent Evidence from Randomized and Observational Studies. *Lancet*, Vol.369, No.9573, (May 2007), pp. 1603-1613, ISSN 1474-547X.

Forester, S. & Lambert, J. (2011). The Role of Antioxidant Versus Pro-oxidant Effects of Green Tea Polyphenols in Cancer Prevention. *Molecular Nutrition & Food Research*, Vol.55, No.6, (June 2011), pp. 844-854, ISSN 1613-4133.

Fox, C. & Eberl, M. (2002). Phytic Acid (IP6), Novel Broad Spectrum Anti-Neoplastic Agent: a Systematic Review. *Complement Ther Med*, Vol.10, No. 4, (December 2002), pp. 229-234, ISSN 1873-6963.

Garattini, E., Gianni, M. & Terao, M. (2007). Retinoids as Differentiating Agents in Oncology: a Network of Interactions with Intracellular Pathways as the Basis for Rational Therapeutic Combinations. *Current Pharmaceutical Design*, Vol.13, No.13, pp. 1375-1400, ISSN 1381-6128.

Gazi, M., Gong, A., Donkena, K. & Young, C. (2006). Sodium Selenite Inhibits Interleukin-6-mediated Androgen Receptor Activation in Prostate Cancer Cells Via Upregulation of c-Jun. *Clinical Chimica Acta*, Vol. 380, No.1-2, (May 2007), pp. 145-150, ISSN 1873-3492.

Goldgar, D., Easton, D., Cannon-Albright, L. & Skolnick, M. (1994). Systematic Population-Based Assessment of Cancer Risk in First-Degree Relatives of Cancer Probands. *J Natl Cancer Inst*, Vol.86, No.21, (November 1994), pp. 1600-1608, ISSN 1460-2105.

Golijanin, D., Kiakiashvili, D,. Madeb, R., et al. (2006). Chemoprevention of Bladder Cancer. *World J Urol*, Vol. 24, No. 5, (November 2006), pp. 445-472, ISSN 1433-8726.

Guchelaar, H., Richel, D. & Van Knapen, A. (1996). Clinical Toxicological and Pharmacological Aspects of Gemcitabine. *Cancer Treat. Rev*, Vol.22, No.1, (January 1996), pp. 15-31, ISSN 1532-1967.

Gunby, P. (1978). Retinoid Chemoprevention Trial Begins Against Bladder Cancer. *The Journal of the American Medical Association*, Vol.240, No.7, (August 1978), pp. 609-610 & 614, ISSN 0098-7484.

Hadaschik, B., Adomat, H., Fazli, L. et al. (2008). Intravesical Chemotherapy of High-Grade Bladder Cancer with HTI-286, a Synthetic Analogue of the Marin Sponge Product Hemiasterlin. *Clin Cancer Res*, Vol.14, No.5, (March 2008), pp. 1510-1518, ISSN 1078-0432.

Hadjiolov, D., Fernando, R., Schmeiser, H., et al. (1993). Effect of Diallyl Sulfide on Aristolochic Acid-induced Forestomach Carcinogenesis in Rats. *Carcinogenesis*, Vol.14, No.3, (March 1993), pp. 407-410, ISSN 1460-2180.

Hahm, S., Park, J. & Son, Y. (2010). Opuntia humifusa Partitioned Extracts Inhibit the Growth of U87MG Human Glioblastoma Cells. *Plant Foods for Human Nutrition*, Vol.65, No.3, (September 2010), pp. 247-252, ISSN 1573-9104.

Hameed, D. & el-Metwally T. (2008). The Effectiveness of Retinoic Acid Treatment in Bladder Cancer: Impact on Recurrence, Survival and TGFalpha and VEGF as End-point Biomarkers. *Cancer Biology & Therapy*, Vol.7, No.1, (January 2008), pp. 92-100, ISSN 1538-4047.

Harris, J. & Markl, J. (1999). Keyhole Limpet Hemocyanin (KLH): a Biomedical Review. *Micron*, Vol.30, No.6, (December 1999), pp. 597-623, ISSN 1878-4291.

Hawking, F. (1978) Suramin: with Special Reference to Onchocerciasis. *Adv Pharmacol Chemother*, Vol.15, (1978), pp. 289-322, ISSN 0065-3144.

Hendriks, H., Pizao, P., Berger, D., et al. (1993). EO9: a Novel Bioreductive Alkylating Indoloquinone with Preferential Solid Tumour Activity and Lack of Bone Marrow Toxicity in Preclinical Models. *Eur J Cancer*, Vol.29, No.6, (1993), pp. 897-906, ISSN 0014-2964.

Hess, D. & Igal, R. (2011). Genistein Downregulates De Novo Lipid Synthesis and Impairs Cell Proliferation in Human Lung Cancer Cells. *Experimental Biology and Medicine*, Vol.236, No.6, (June 2011), pp. 707-713, ISSN 1535-3699.

Hoffmann, P., Roumeguère, T., Schulman, C. & van Velthoven, R. (2006). Use of Statins and Outcome of BCG Treatment for Bladder Cancer. *The New England Journal of Medicine*, Vol.355, No.25, (December 2006), pp. 2705-2707, ISSN 1533-4406.

Hotaling, J., Wright, J., Pocobelli, G., et al. (2011). Long-term Use of Supplemental Vitamins and Minerals Does Not Reduce the Risk of Urothelial Cell Carcinoma of the Bladder in the Vitamins And Lifestyle Study. *Journal of Urology*, Vol.185, No.4, (February 2011), ISSN 1527-3792.

Husbeck, B., Bhattacharyya, R., Feldman, D. & Knox, S. (2006). Inhibition of Androgen Receptor Signaling by Selenite and Methylseleninic Acid in Prostate Cancer Cells: Two Distinct Mechanisms of Action. *Molecular Cancer Therapeutics*, Vol.5, No.8, (August 2006), pp. 2078-2085, ISSN 1538-8514.

Hwang, J., Lee, Y., Shin, J. & Park, O. (2009). Anti-inflammatory and Anticarcinogenic Effect of Genistein Alone or in Combination with Capsaicin in TPA-treated Rat Mammary Glands or Mammary Cancer Cell Line. *Annals of the New York Academy of Sciences*, Vol.1171, (August 2009), pp. 415-420, ISSN 1749-6632.

Issat, T., Nowis, D., Bil, J., et al. (2011). Antitumor Effects of the Combination of Cholesterol Reducing Drugs. *Oncology Reports*, Vol.26, No.1, (July 2011), pp. 169-176, ISSN 1791-2431.

Izbicka, E., Streeper, R., Yeh, I., et al. (2010). Effects of Alpha-difluoromethylornithine on Markers of Proliferation, Invasion, and Apoptosis in Breast Cancer. *Anticancer Research*, Vol.30, No.6, (June 2010), pp. 2263-2269, ISSN 1791-7530.

Jackson, M. & Combs, G. Jr. (2008). Selenium and Anticarcinogenesis: Underlying Mechanisms. *Current Opinion in Clinical Nutrition and Metabolic Care*, Vol.11, No.6, (November 2008), pp. 718-726, ISSN 1535-3885.

Jacobs, E., Henion, A., Briggs, P., et al. (2002). Vitamin C and Vitamin E Supplement Use and Bladder Cancer Mortality in a Large Cohort of US Men and Women. *American Journal of Epidemiology*, Vol.156, No.1, (December 2002), pp. 1002-1010, ISSN 1476-6256.

Jacobs, E., Newton, C., Thun, M. & Gapstur, S. (2011). Long-term Use of Cholesterol-lowering Drugs and Cancer Incidence in a Large United States Cohort. *Cancer Research*, Vol.71, No.5, (March 2011), pp. 1763-1771, ISSN 1538-7445.

Jurincic-Winkler, C., Metz, K., Beuth, J. & Klippel, K. (2000). Keyhole Limpet Hemocyanin for Carcinoma in Situ of the Bladder: a Long-Term Follow-Up Study. *Eur Urol*, Vol.57, No.3, (2000), pp. 45-49, ISSN 1873-7860.

Kamat, A. (2003). Chemoprevention of Superficial Bladder Cancer. *Expert Rev. Anticancer Ther*, Vol. 6, No.6, pp. 799-808, ISSN 1744-8328.

Kamat, A. & Nelkin, G. (2005). Atorvastatin: A Potential Chemopreventive Agent in Bladder Cancer. *Urology*, Vol.66, No.6, (December 2005), pp.1209-1212, ISSN 1527-9995.

Kamat, A. & Wu, X. (2007). Statins and the Effect of BCG on Bladder Cancer. *The New England Journal of Medicine*, Vol.356, No.12, (March 2007), pp. 1276-1277, ISSN 1533-4406.

Kamori, A., Yatsunami, J., Okabe, S., Abe, S., Hara, K., Suganuma, M., Kim, S. & Fujiki, H. (1993). Anticarcinogenic Activity of Green Tea Polyphenols. *Japanese Journal of Clinical Oncology*, Vol.23, No.3, (June 1993), pp. 186-190, ISSN 1465-3621.

Karak, F. & Flechon, A. (2007). Gemcitabine in Bladder Cancer. *Expert Opin. Pharmacothe*, Vol.8, No.18, (December 2007), pp. 3251-3256, ISSN 1744-7666.

Kassouf, W., Luongo, T., Brown, G., Adam, L. & Dinney, C. (2006). Schedule dependent efficacy of Gefitinib and Docetaxel for bladder cancer. *J Urol*, Vol.176, No.2, (August 2006), pp. 787-792, 1527-3792.

Kellen, E., Zeegers, M. & Buntinx, F. (2006). Selenium is Inversely Associated with Bladder Cancer Risk: A Report from the Belgian Case-control Study on Bladder Cancer. *International Journal of Urology*, Vol.13, No.9, (September 2006), pp. 1180-1184, ISSN 1442-2042.

Kelloff, G., Crowell, J., Boone, C., et al. (1994). Strategy and Planning for Chemopreventive Drug Development: Clinical Development Plans. Chemoprevention Branch and

Agent Development Committee. National Cancer Institute. *Journal of Cellular Biochemistry. Supplement*, Vol.20, pp. 55-62, ISSN 0733-1959.

Khan, M. & Lee, Y. (2011). Cyclooxygenase Inhibitors: Scope of Their Use and Development in Cancer Chemotherapy. *Medicinal Research Reviews*, Vol.31, No.2, (March 2011), pp. 161-201, ISSN 1098-1128.

Kim, J., Jin, D., Lee, SD., et al. (2008). Vitamin C Inhibits p53-induced Replicative Senescence Through Suppression of ROS Production and p38 MAPK Activity. *International Journal of Molecular Medicine*, Vol.22, No.5, (November 2008), pp. 651-655, ISSN 1791-244X.

Kitamura, H., Torigoe, T., Honma, I., et al. (2006). Effect of Human Leukocytes Antigen Class I Expression of Tumor Cells on Outcome of Intravesical Instillation of Bacillus Calmette-Guerin Immunotherapy for Bladder Cancer. *Clin Cancer Res.*, Vol.12, No.15, (August 2006), pp. 4461-4464, ISSN 1078-0432.

Kline, K., Yu, W. & Sanders, B. (2004). Vitamin E and Breast Cancer. *The Journal of Nutrition.* Vol.134, No.12 Supplement, (December 2004), pp. 3458S-3462S, ISSN 1541-6100.

Kubatka, P., Zihlavnikóva, K., Kajo, K., et al. (2011). Antineoplastic Effects of Simvastatin in Experimental Breast Cancer. *Klinická Onkologie*, Vol.24, No.1, pp. 41-45, ISSN 1802-5307.

Lamm, D., Riggs, D., Shriver, J., et al. (1994). Megadose Vitamins in Bladder Cancer: A Double-blind Clinical Trial. *The Journal of Urology*, Vol.151, No.1, (January 1994), pp. 21-26, ISSN 1527-3792.

Lamm, D. & Riggs, D. (2000). The Potential Application of Allium Sativum (Garlic) for the Treatment of Bladder Cancer. *The Urologic Clinics of North America*, Vol.27, No.1, (February 2000), pp. 157-162, ISSN 1558-318X.

La Rocca, R., Stein, C., Danesi, R. et al. (1990). Suramin in Adrenal Cancer: Modulation of Steroid Hormone Production, Cytotoxicity In Vitro, and Clinical Antitumor Effect. *J Cin Endoctrinol Metab*, Vol. 71, No.2, (August 1990), pp. 497-504, ISSN 1945-7197.

Lau, B., Woolley, J., Marsh, C., et al. (1986). Superiority of Intralesional Immunotherapy with Corynebacterium parvum and Allium sativum in Control of Murine Transitional Cell Carcinoma. *The Journal of Urology*, Vol.136, No.3, (September 1986), pp. 701-705, ISSN 1527-3792.

Liang, B., Liu, H. & Cao, J. (2008). Antitumor Effect of Polysaccharides from Cactus Pear Fruit in S180-bearing Mice. *Chinese Journal of Cancer*, Vol.27, No.6, (June 2008), pp. 580-584, ISSN 1000-467X.

Limburg, P., Mahoney, M., Ziegler, K., et al. (2011). Randomized Phase II Trial of Sulindac, Atorvastatin, and Prebiotic Dietary Fiber for Colorectal Cancer Chemoprevention. *Cancer Prevention Research*, Vol.4, No.2, (February 2011), pp. 259-269, ISSN 1940-6215.

Lin, T., Yin, X., Cai, Q., et al. (2010). 13-Methyltetradecanoic Acid Induces Mitochondrial-mediated Apoptosis in Human Bladder Cancer Cells. *Urologic Oncology*, Epub ahead of print, (September 2010), ISSN 1873-2496.

Lu, Q., Jin, Y., Pantuck, A., et al. (2005). Green Tea Extract Modulates Actin Remodeling Via Rho Activity in an In Vitro Multistep Carcinogenic Model. *Clinical Cancer Research*, Vol.11, No.4, (February 2005), pp. 1675-1683, ISSN 1078-0432.

Lubet, R., Yang, C., Lee, M., et al. (2007). Preventative Effects of Polyphenon E on Urinary Bladder and Mammary Cancers in Rats and Correlations with Serum and Urine Levels of Tea Polyphenols. *Molecular Cancer Therapeutics*, Vol.6, No.7, (July 2007), pp. 2022-2028, ISSN 1538-8514.

Lubet, R., Steele, V., Julianna, M. & Grubbs, C. (2010). Screening Agents for Preventive Efficacy in a Bladder Cancer Model: Study Design, End Points, and Gefitinib and Naproxen Efficacy. *The Journal of Urology*, Vol.183, No.4, (April 2010), pp. 1598-1603, ISSN 1527-3792.

Ma, Y., Wang, J., Liu, L., et al. (2011). Genistein Potentiates the Effect of Arsenic Trioxide Against Human Hepatocellular Carcinoma: Role of Akt and Nuclear Factor κB. *Cancer Letters*, Vol.301, No.1, (February 2010), pp. 75-94, ISSN 1872-7980.

Mallick, B., Kishore, S., Das, S. & Garg A. (1995). Non-Specific Immunostimulation Against Viruses. *Comp Immunol Microbiol Infect Dis*, Vol.8, No.1, (1985), pp. 55-63, ISSN 1878-1667.

Malmostrom, P., Wijkstrom, H., Lundholm, C. et al. (1999). Five-Year Follow-Up of a Randomized Prospective Study Comparing Mitomycin C and Bacillus Calmette-Guerin in Patients with Superficial Bladder Carcinoma. *J Urol*, Vol.161, No.4, (1999), pp. 1124-1127, ISSN 1527-3792.

McKiernan, J., Masson, P., Murphy, A. et al. (2006). Phase I Trial of Intravesical Docetaxel in the Management of Superficial Bladder Cancer Refractory to Standard Intravesical Therapy. *J Clin Oncol*, Vol.19, No.1, (July 2006), pp. 3075-3080, ISSN 1527-7755.

Messing, E., Hanson, P., Ulrich, P. & Erturk, E. (1987). Epidermal Growth Factor-interactions with Normal and Malignant Urothelium: In Vivo and In Situ Studies. *The Journal of Urology*, Vol.138, No.5, (November 1987), pp. 1329-1335, ISSN 1527-3792.

Messing, E., Hanson, P. & Reznikoff, C. (1988). Normal and Malignant Human Urothelium: In Vitro Response to Blockade of Polyamine Synthesis and Interconversion. *Cancer Research*, Vol.48, No.2, (January 1988), pp. 357-361, ISSN 1538-7445.

Messing, E., Kim, K., Sharkey, F., et al. (2006). Randomized Prospective Phase III Trial of Difluoromethylornithine Vs. Placebo in Preventing Recurrence of Completely Resected Low Risk Superficial Bladder Cancer. *The Journal of Urology*, Vol.176, No.2, (August 2006), pp. 500-504, ISSN 1527-3792.

Meyskens, F., McLaren, C., Pelot, D., et al. (2008). Difluoromethylornithine Plus Sulindac for the Prevention of Sporadic Colorectal Adenomas: A Randomized Placebo-controlled, Double-blind Trial. *Cancer Prevention Research*, Vol.1, No.1, (June 2008), pp. 32-38, ISSN 1940-6215.

Michaud, D., Spiegelman, D., Clinton, S., et al. (2000). Prospective Study of Dietary Supplements, Macronutrients, Micronutrients, and Risk of Bladder Cancer in US Men. *American Journal of Epidemiology*, Vol.152, No.12, (December 2000), pp. 1145-1153, ISSN 1476-6256.

Miller, E., Pastor-Barriuso, R., Dalal, D., et al. (2005). Meta-analysis: High-dosage Vitamin E Supplementation May Increase All-cause Mortality. *Annals of Internal Medicine*, Vol.142, No.1, (January 2005), pp. 37-46, ISSN 1539-3704.

Miroddi, M., Calapai, F. & Calapai, G. (2011). Potential Beneficial Effects of Garlic in Oncohematology. *Mini Reviews in Medicinal Chemistry*, Vol.11, No.6, (June 2011), pp. 461-472, ISSN 1875-5607.

Mirvish, S. (1986). Effects of Vitamins C and E on N-nitroso Compound Formation, Carcinogenesis, and Cancer. *Cancer*, Vol.58 (8 Supplement), (October 1986), pp. 1842-1850, ISSN 1097-0142.

Mirvish, S. (1995). Role of N-nitroso Compounds (NOC) and N-nitrosation in Etiology of Gastric, Esophageal, Nasopharyngeal and Bladder Cancer and Contribution to Cancer of Known Exposures to NOC. *Cancer Letters*, Vol.93, No.1, (June 1995), pp. 17-48, ISSN 1872-7980.

Murawaki, Y., Tsuchiya, H., Kanbe, et al. (2008). Aberrant Expression of Selenoproteins in the Progression of Colorectal Cancer. *Cancer Letters*, Vol.259, No.2, (February 2008), pp. 218-230, ISSN 1872-7980.

Maymi, J., N, Saltsgaver. & O'Donnell, M. Intravesical sequential gemcitabine-mitomycin chemotherapy as salvage treatment for patient with refractory superficial bladder cancer. *J Urol*, Vol.175, No.4, Abstract 840.

Nativ, O., Witjes, J., Hendricksen, K. et al. (2009). Combined Thermo-Chemotherapy for Recurrent Bladder Cancer After Bacillus Calmette-Guerin. *J Urol*, Vol.182, No.4, (October 2009), pp. 1313-1317, ISSN 1527-3792.

Nseyo, U. & Lamm, D. (1997). Immunotherapy of Bladder Cancer. *Semin. Surg Oncology*, Vol.13, No.5, (September-October 1997), pp. 342-349, ISSN 1098-2388.

Okkels, K., Sigsgaard, T., Wolf, H. & Autrup, H. (1997). Arylamine N-Acetyltransferase 1 (NAT1) and 2 (NAT 2) Polymorphisms in Susceptibility to Bladder Cancer: the Influence of Smoking. *Cancer Epidemiol Biomarkers Prev*, Vol.6, No.4, (April 1997), pp. 225-231, ISSN 1538-7757.

Oz, H. & Ebersole, J. (2010). Grean Tea Polyphenols Mediated Apoptosis in Intestinal Epithelial Cells by a FADD-Dependent Pathway. *Journal of Cancer Therapy*, Vol.1, No.3, (September 2010), pp. 105-113, ISSN 2151-1942.

Park, Y., Spiegelman, D., Hunter, D., et al. (2010). Intakes of Vitamins A, C, and E and Use of Multiple Vitamin Supplements and Risk of Colon Cancer: A Pooled Analysis of Prospective Cohort Studies. *Cancer Causes & Control*, Vol.21, No.11, (November 2010), pp. 1745-1757, ISSN 1573-7225.

Pelucchi, C., Bosetti, C., Negrie, E., et al. (2006). Mechanisms of Disease: the Epidemiology of Bladder Cancer. *Nat Clin Pract Urol*, Vol. 3, No. 6, (June 2006), pp. 327-340, ISSN 1743-4289.

Pegg. A. (2006). Regulation of Ornithine Decarboxylase. *The Journal of Biological Chemistry*, Vol.281, No.21, (May 2006), pp. 14529-14532, ISSN 1083-351X.

Pelucchi, C., Bosetti, C., Negri, E., Malvezzi, M. & La Vecchia, C. (2006). Mechanisms of Disease: the Epidemiology of Bladder Cancer. *Nat Clin Pract Urol*, Vol.3, No.6, (June 2006), pp. 327-340, ISSN 1743-4289.

Phillips, R., Loadman, P. & Cronin, B. (1998). Evaluation of a Novel In Vitro Assay for Assessing Drug Penetration into Avascular Regions of Tumours. *Br J Cancer*, Vol.77, No.12, (June 1998), pp. 2112-9, ISSN 1532-1827.

Phillips, R., Jaffar, M., Maitland, D., et al. (2004). Pharmacological and Biological Evaluation of a Series of Substituted 1,4-Naphthoquinone Bioreductive Drugs. *Biochemical Pharmacology*, Vol.68, No.11, (December 2004), pp. 2107-2116, ISSN 1873-2968.

Pina, K. & Hemminki, K. (2001). Familial Bladder Cancer in the National Sweedish Family Cancer Database. *J Urol*, Vol.166, No.6, (December 2001), pp. 2129-2133, ISSN 1527-3792.

Prout, G. & Barton, B. (1992). 13-cis-retinoic Acid in Chemoprevention of Superficial Bladder Cancer. The National Bladder Cancer Group. *Journal of Cellular Biochemistry, Supplement*, Vol.16I, pp. 148-152, ISSN 0733-1959.

Riggs, D., DeHaven, J. & Lamm, D. (1997). Allium sativum (Garlic) Treatment for Murine Transitional Cell Carcinoma. *Cancer*, Vol.79, No.10, (May 1997), pp. 1987-1994, ISSN 1097-0142.

Roswall, N., Olsen, A., Christensen, J., et al. (2009). Micronutrient Intake and Risk of Urothelial Carcinoma in a Prospective Danish Cohort. *European Urology*, Vol.56, No.5, (November 2009), pp. 764-770, ISSN 1873-7560.

Rothwell, P., Fowkes, F., Belch, J., et al. (2011). Effect of Daily Aspirin on Long-term Risk of Death Due to Cancer: Analysis of Individual Patient Data from Randomized Trials. *Lancet*, Vol.377, No.9759, (January 2011), pp. 31-41, ISSN 1474-547X.

Sato, D. (1999). Inhibition of Urinary Bladder Tumors Induced by N-butyl-N-(4-hydroxybutyl)-nitrosamine in Rats by Green Tea. *International Journal of Urology*, Vol.6, No.2, (February 1999), pp. 93-99, ISSN 1442-2042.

Sato, D. & Matsushima, M. (2003). Preventative Effects of Urinary Bladder Tumors Induced by N-butyl-N-(4-hydroxybutyl)-nitrosamine in Rat by Green Tea Leaves. *International Journal of Urology*, Vol.10, No.3, (March 2003), pp. 160-166, ISSN 1442-2042.

Sebti, S., Tkalcevic, G. & Jani, J. (1991). Lovastatin, a Cholesterol Biosynthesis Inhibitor, Inhibits the Growth of Human H-ras Oncogene Transformed Cells in Nude Mice. *Cancer Communications*, Vol.3, No.5, (May 1991), pp. 141-147, ISSN 0955-3541.

Shamsuddin, A., Vucenik, I. & Cole, K. (1997). IP6: A novel Anti-Cancer Agent. *Life Sci*, Vol.61, No.4, (1997), pp. 343-354, ISSN 1879-0631.

Shibata, A., Paganini-Hill, A., Ross, R. & Henderson, B. (1992). Intake of Vegetables, Fruits, Beta-carotene, Vitamin C and Vitamin Supplements and Cancer Incidence Among the Elderly: A Prospective Study. *British Journal of Cancer*, Vol.66, No.4, (October 1992), pp. 673-679, ISSN 1532-1827.

Shimada, K., Anai, S., Marco, D., Fujimoto, K. & Konishi, N. (2011). Cyclooxygenase 2-dependent and Independent Activation of Akt Through Casein Kinase 2α Contributes to Human Bladder Cancer Cell Survival. *BMC Urology*, Vol.11, (May 2011), pp. 8, ISSN 1471-2490.

Shukla, Y. & Kaira, N. (2007). Cancer Chemoprevention with Garlic and its Constituents. *Cancer Letters*, Vol.247, No.2, (March 2007), pp. 167-181, ISSN 1872-7980.

Siegel, R., Ward, E., Brawley, O., & Jemal, A. (2011). Cancer statistics, 2011: The impact of eliminating socioeconomic and racial disparities on premature cancer deaths. *CA Cancer J Clin*, Vol. 61, No. 4, (July/August 2011), pp. 212-236, ISSN 1542-4863.

Sigounas, G., Anagnostou, A. & Steiner, M. (1997). Dl-alpha-tocopherol Induces Apoptosis in Erythroleukemia, Prostate, and Breast Cancer Cells. *Nutrition and Cancer,* Vol.28, No.1, pp. 30-35, ISSN 1532-7914.

Silberstein, J. & Parsons, J. (2010). Evidence-based Principles of Bladder Cancer and Diet. *Urology,* Vol.75, No.2, (February 2010), pp. 340-346, ISSN 1527-9995.

Simeone, A. & Tari A. (2004). How Retinoids Regulate Breast Cancer Cell Proliferation and Apoptosis. *Cellular and Molecular Life Sciences,* Vol.61, No.12, (June 2004), pp. 1475-1484, ISSN 1420-9071.

Singh, A., Franke, A., Blackburn, G. & Zhou, J. (2006). Soy Phytochemicals Prevent Orthotopic Growth and Metastasis of Bladder Cancer in Mice by Alterations of Cancer Cell Proliferation and Apoptosis and Tumor Angiogenesis. *Cancer Research,* Vol.66, No.3, (February 2006), pp. 1851-1858, ISSN 1538-7445.

Singh, R., Dhanalakshmi, S. & Agarwal, R. (2002). Phytochemicals as Cell Cycle Modulators-A Less Toxic Approach in Halting Human Cancers. *Cell Cycle,* Vol.1, No.3, (May-June 2002), pp. 156-61, ISSN 1551-4005.

Sinicrope, F., Broaddus, R., Joshi, N., et al. (2011). Evaluation of Difluoromethylornithine for the Chemoprevention of Barrett's Esophagus and Mucosal Dysplasia. *Cancer Prevention Research,* Vol.4, No.6, (June 2011), pp. 829-839, ISSN 1940-6215.

Smith, M., Lancia, J., Mercer, T. & Ip, C. (2004). Selenium Compounds Regulate p53 by Common and Distinctive Mechanisms. *Anticancer Research,* Vol.24, No.3a, (May-June 2004), pp. 1401-1408, ISSN 1791-7530

Studer, U., Jenzer, S., Biedermann, C., et al. (1995). Adjuvant Treatment with a Vitamin A Analogue (Etretinate) After Transurethral Resection of Superficial Bladder Tumors. Final Analysis of a Prospective, Randomized Multicenter Trial in Switzerland. *European Urology,* Vol.28, No.4, pp. 284-290, ISSN 0302-2838.

Su, S., Yeh, T., Lei, H. & Chow, N. (2000). The Potential of Soybean Foods as a Chemoprevention Approach for Human Urinary Tract Cancer. *Clinical Cancer Research,* Vol.6, No.1, (January 2000), pp. 230-236, ISSN 1078-0432.

Taylor, E., Stampfer M. & Curhan, G. (2004). Dietary Factors and the Risk of Incident Kidney Stones in Men: New Insights After 14 Years of Follow-up. *Journal of the American Society of Nephrology,* Vol.15, No.12, (December 2004), pp. 3225-3232, ISSN 1533-3450.

Tesoriere, L., Butera, D., Pintaudi, A., Allegra, M. & Livrea, M. (2004). Supplementation with Cactus Pear (Opuntia ficus-indica) Fruit Decreases Oxidative Stress in Healthy Humans: A Comparative Study with Vitamin C. *The American Journal of Clinical Nutrition,* Vol.80, No.2, (August 2004), pp. 391-395, ISSN 1938-3207.

The New England Journal of Medicine. (1994). The Effect of Vitamin E and Beta Carotene on the Incidence of Lung Cancer and Other Cancers in Male Smokers. The Alpha-Tocopherol, Beta Carotene Cancer Prevention Study Group. *The New England Journal of Medicine,* Vol.330, No.15, (April 1994), pp. 1029-1035, ISSN 1533-4406.

Theodorescu, D., Laderoute, K., Calaoagan, J. & Guilding, K. (1998). Inhibition of Human Bladder Cancer Cell Motility by Genistein is Dependent on Epidermal Growth Factor Receptor but Not p21ras Gene Expression. *International Journal of Cancer,* Vol.78, No.6, (December 1998), pp. 775-782, ISSN 1097-0215.

Thun. M., Henley, S. & Patrono, C. (2002). Nonsteroidal Anti-inflammatory Drugs as Anticancer Agents: Mechanistic, Pharmacologic, and Clinical Issues. *Journal of the National Cancer Institute*, Vol.94, No.4, (February 2002), pp. 252-266, ISSN 1460-2105.

Tsai, H., Katz, M., Coen, J., et al. (2006). Association of Statin Use with Improved Local Control in Patients Treated with Selective Bladder Preservation for Muscle-invasive Bladder Cancer. *Urology*, Vol.68, No.6, (December 2006), pp. 1188-1192, ISSN 1527-9995.

Tyagi, A., Agarwal, C., Harrison, G., et al. (2004). Silibinin Causes Cell Cycle Arrest and Apoptosis in Human Bladder Transitional Cell Carcinoma Cells by Regulating CDKI-CDK-Cyclin Cascade, and Caspase 3 and PARP Cleavages. *Carcinogenesis*, Vol.1, No.9, (September 2004), pp. 1711-20, ISSN 1460-2180.

Tyagi, A., Singh, R., Agarwal, C. & Agarwal, R. (2006). Silibinin Activates p53-caspase 2 Pathway and Causes Caspase-Mediated Cleavage of Cip1/p21 in Apoptosis Induction in Bladder Transitional-Cell Papilloma RT4 cells: Evidence for a Regulatory Loop Between p53 and Caspace 2. *Carcinogenesis*, Vol.27, No.11, (November 2006), pp. 2269-2280, ISSN 1460-2180.

Tsao, A., Liu, D., Martin, J., et al. (2009). Phase II Randomized, Placebo-controlled Trial of Green Tea Extract in Patients with High-risk Oral Premalignant Lesions. *Cancer Prevention Research*, Vol.2, No.11, (November 2009), pp. 931-941, ISSN 1940-6215.

Wadhwa, P., Goswami, A., Joshi, K. & Sharma, S. (2005). Cyclooxygenase-2 Expression Increases with the Stage and Grade in Transitional Cell Carcinoma of the Urinary Bladder. *International Urology and Nephrology*, Vol.37, No.1, pp. 47-53, ISSN 1573-2584.

Wakai, K., Hirose, K., Takezaki, T., et al. (2004). Foods and Beverages in Relation to Urothelial Cancer: Case-control Study in Japan. *International Journal of Urology*, Vol.11, No.1, (January 2004), pp. 11-19, ISSN 1442-2042.

Wallace, K., Kelsey, K., Schned, A., Morris, J., Andrew, A. & Karagas, M. (2009). Selenium and Risk of Bladder Cancer: A Population-based Case-control Study. *Cancer Prevention Research*, Vol.2, No.1, (January 2009), pp. 70-73, ISSN 1940-6215.

Walther, M., Trahan, E., Cooper, M., Venzon, D. & Linehan, W. (1994) Suramin Inhibits Proliferation and DNA Synthesis in Ttransitional Carcinoma Cell Lines. *J Uro*, Vol.152, No.5, (November 1994), pp. 1599-1602, ISSN 1527-3792.

Witjes, J., Caris, C., Mungan, N., Debruyne, M. & Witjes, W. (1998). Results of a Randomized Phase III Trial of Sequential Intravesical Therapy with Mitomycin C and Bacillus Calmette-Guerin Verus Mitomcyin C Alone in Patients with Superficial Bladder Cancer. *J Urol*, Vol.160, No.5, (November 1998), pp. 1668-1672, ISSN 1527-3792.

Wu, H., Lu, H., Hung, C. & Chung, J. (2000). Inhibition of Vitamin C of DNA Adduct Formation and Arylamine N-acetyltransferase Activity in Human Bladder Tumor Cells. *Urology Research*, Vol.28, No.4, (August 2000), pp. 235-240, ISSN 1434-0879.

Yabroff, K., Lamont, E., Mariotto. A., et al. (2008). Cost of Care for Elderly Cancer Patients in the United States. *J Natl Cancer Inst*, Vol.100, No.9, (May 2008), pp. 630-641. ISSN 1460-2105.

Yan, L. & Spitznagel, E. (2005). Meta-analysis of Soy Food and Risk of Prostate Cancer in Men. *International Journal of Cancer*, Vol.117, No.4, (November 2005), pp. 667-669, ISSN 1097-0215.

Yang, C., Wang, H., Li, G., et al. (2011). Cancer Prevention by Tea: Evidence from Laboratory Studies. *Pharmacological Research*, Vol.64, No.2, (August 2011), pp. 113-122, ISSN 1096-1186.

Yildirim, U., Erdem, H., Kayikci, A., Sahin, A., Uzunlar, A. & Albayrak, A. (2010). Cyclooxygenase-2 and Survivin in Superficial Urothelial Carcinoma of the Bladder and Correlation with Intratumoural Microvessel Density. *The Journal of International Medical Research*, Vol.38, No.5, (September-October 2010), pp. 1689-1699, ISSN 1473-2300.

Yoshida, O., Miyakawa, M., Watanabe, H., et al. (1986). Prophylactic Effect of Etretinate on the Recurrence of Superficial Bladder Tumors – Results of a Randomized Control Study. *Acta Urologica Japonica*, Vol.32, No.9, (September 1986), pp. 1349-1358, ISSN 0018-1994.

Yu, L., Chen, X., Shi, P., et al. (2008). Expression of Cyclooxygenase-2 in Bladder Transitional Cell Carcinoma and the Significance Thereof. *Zhonghua Yi Xue Za Zhi*, Vol.88, No.38, (October 2008), pp. 2683-2684, ISSN 0376-2491.

Yu, M., Skipper, P., Taghizadeh, K. et al. (1994). Acetylator Phenotype, Aminobiphenyl-Hemoglobin Adduct Levels, and Bladder Cancer Risk in White, Black, and Asian Men in Los Angeles, California. *J Natl Cancer Inst*, Vol.86, No.9, (May 1994), pp. 712-716, ISSN 1460-2105.

Yuasa, T., Sato, K., Ashihara, E., et al. (2009). Intravesical administration of gammadelta T cells Successfully Prevents the Growth of Bladder Cancer in the Murine Model. *Cancer Immunol Immunother*, Vol.58, No.4, (April 2009), pp/ 493-502, ISSN 1432-0851.

Zanardi, S., Serrano, D., Argusti, A., Barile, M., & Decensi, A. (2006). Clinical Trials with Retinoids for Breast Cancer Chemoprevention. *Endocrine Related Cancer*, Vol.13, No.1, (March 2006), pp. 51-68, ISSN 1351-0088.

Zaslau, S., Riggs, D., Jackson, B., Talug, C., & Kandzari, S. (2009). Inositol Hexaphosphate (IP6): Modulation of Cell Cycle and Proliferation of Bladder Cancer In Vivo. *Curr Urol*, Vol.3, No.3, (2009), pp. 136-140, ISSN 0025-3371.

Zaslau, S., Riggs, D., Jackson, B., Luchey, A. & Kandzari, S. (2010). In vitro inositol Hexaphosphate Treatment for Bladder Cancer: Evaluation of Short Versus Continual Exposure Time. Presented at the 2010 Annual Mid-Atlantic Meeting, September 23-26, Farmington, PA.

Zhang, Y. & Chen, H. (2011). Genistein, an Epigenome Modifier During Cancer Prevention. *Epigenetics*, Vol.6, No.7, (July 2011), ISSN 1559-2308.

Zhou, J., Mukherjee, P., Gugger, E., et al. (1998). Inhibition of Murine Bladder Tumorigenesis by Soy Isoflavones Via Alterations in the Cell Cycle, Apoptosis, and Angiogenesis. *Cancer Research*, Vol.58, No.22, (November 1998), pp. 5231-5238, ISSN 1538-7445.

Zou, D., Brewer, M., Garcia, F., et al. (2005). Cactus Pear: A Natural Product in Cancer Chemoprevention. *Nutrition Journal*, Vol.8, No.4, (September 2005), pp. 25, ISSN 1475-2891.

Zusi, F., Lorenzi, M., & Vivat-Hannah, V. (2002). Selective Retinoids and Rexinoids in Cancer Therapy and Chemoprevention. *Drug Discovery Today*, Vol.7, No.23, (December, 2002), pp. 1165-1174, ISSN 1359-6446.

Permissions

The contributors of this book come from diverse backgrounds, making this book a truly international effort. This book will bring forth new frontiers with its revolutionizing research information and detailed analysis of the nascent developments around the world.

We would like to thank Dr. Abdullah Erdem Canda, for lending his expertise to make the book truly unique. He has played a crucial role in the development of this book. Without his invaluable contribution this book wouldn't have been possible. He has made vital efforts to compile up to date information on the varied aspects of this subject to make this book a valuable addition to the collection of many professionals and students.

This book was conceptualized with the vision of imparting up-to-date information and advanced data in this field. To ensure the same, a matchless editorial board was set up. Every individual on the board went through rigorous rounds of assessment to prove their worth. After which they invested a large part of their time researching and compiling the most relevant data for our readers. Conferences and sessions were held from time to time between the editorial board and the contributing authors to present the data in the most comprehensible form. The editorial team has worked tirelessly to provide valuable and valid information to help people across the globe.

Every chapter published in this book has been scrutinized by our experts. Their significance has been extensively debated. The topics covered herein carry significant findings which will fuel the growth of the discipline. They may even be implemented as practical applications or may be referred to as a beginning point for another development. Chapters in this book were first published by InTech; hereby published with permission under the Creative Commons Attribution License or equivalent.

The editorial board has been involved in producing this book since its inception. They have spent rigorous hours researching and exploring the diverse topics which have resulted in the successful publishing of this book. They have passed on their knowledge of decades through this book. To expedite this challenging task, the publisher supported the team at every step. A small team of assistant editors was also appointed to further simplify the editing procedure and attain best results for the readers.

Our editorial team has been hand-picked from every corner of the world. Their multi-ethnicity adds dynamic inputs to the discussions which result in innovative outcomes. These outcomes are then further discussed with the researchers and contributors who give their valuable feedback and opinion regarding the same. The feedback is then collaborated with the researches and they are edited in a comprehensive manner to aid the understanding of the subject.

Apart from the editorial board, the designing team has also invested a significant amount of their time in understanding the subject and creating the most relevant covers. They scrutinized every image to scout for the most suitable representation of the subject and create an appropriate cover for the book.

The publishing team has been involved in this book since its early stages. They were actively engaged in every process, be it collecting the data, connecting with the contributors or procuring relevant information. The team has been an ardent support to the editorial, designing and production team. Their endless efforts to recruit the best for this project, has resulted in the accomplishment of this book. They are a veteran in the field of academics and their pool of knowledge is as vast as their experience in printing. Their expertise and guidance has proved useful at every step. Their uncompromising quality standards have made this book an exceptional effort. Their encouragement from time to time has been an inspiration for everyone.

The publisher and the editorial board hope that this book will prove to be a valuable piece of knowledge for researchers, students, practitioners and scholars across the globe.

List of Contributors

Sergio Arancibia, Fabián Salazar and María Inés Becker
Fundación Ciencia y Tecnología para el Desarrollo (FUCITED), Chile

María Inés Becker
Biosonda Corporation, Chile

Unyime O. Nseyo
North Florida-South Georgia Veterans Health System, Gainesville, Florida, USA

Katherine A. Corbyons
University of Florida, Gainesville, Florida, USA

Hari Siva Gurunadha Rao Tunuguntla
Robert Wood Johnson Medical School, New Brunswick, New Jersey, USA

Takehiro Sejima, Shuichi Morizane, Akihisa Yao, Tadahiro Isoyama and Atsushi Takenaka
Division of Urology, Department of Surgery, Tottori University Faculty of Medicine, Japan

Beate Köberle and Andrea Piee-Staffa
Institute of Toxicology, University of Mainz Medical Center, Mainz, Germany

Abdullah Erdem Canda, Ali Fuat Atmaca and Mevlana Derya Balbay
Ankara Atatürk Training and Research Hospital, 1st Urology Clinic, Ankara, Turkey

Martin C. Schumacher
Dept. of Urology, Karolinska University Hospital, Stockholm, Sweden
Hirslanden Klinik Aarau, Switzerland

S. Siracusano, S. Ciciliato, F. Visalli, N. Lampropoulou and L. Toffoli
Department of Urology – Trieste University, Italy

Imad Matouk
Department of Biological Chemistry, Institute of Life Sciences, The Hebrew University of Jerusalem, Jerusalem, Israel
Department of Biology, Science and Technology, Alquds Abu-Dis University, Jerusalem, Israel

Naveh Evantal, Doron Amit, Patricia Ohana, Vladimir Sorin, Tatiana Birman, Eitan Gershtain and Abraham Hochberg
Department of Biological Chemistry, Institute of Life Sciences, The Hebrew University of Jerusalem, Jerusalem, Israel

Ofer Gofrit
Department of Urology, Hadassah Hebrew University Medical Center, Jerusalem, Israel

Ricarda Zdrenka, Joerg Hippler, Georg Johnen, Alfred V. Hirner and Elke Dopp
University of Duisburg-Essen, Ruhr-University Bochum, University Hospital Essen, Germany

Ana María Eiján, Catalina Lodillinsky and Eduardo Omar Sandes
Research Area of the Institute of Oncology Angel H. Roffo, University of Buenos Aires, Argentina

Ana María Eiján and Catalina Lodillinsky
Consejo Nacional de Investigaciones Científicas y Técnicas (CONICET), Argentina

Adam Luchey, Morris Jessop, Claire Oliver, Dale Riggs, Barbara Jackson, Stanley Kandzari and Stanley Zaslau
Division of Urology, West Virginia University, Morgantown, WV, USA

Printed in the USA
CPSIA information can be obtained
at www.ICGtesting.com
JSHW011435221024
72173JS00004B/813